WHAT TO EXPECT®

EATING WELL WHEN YOU'RE EXPECTING

by HEIDI MURKOFF

with SHARON MAZEL

WORKMAN PUBLISHING • NEW YORK

To the three people in the world
I most love eating well with
(and just plain most love):
Erik, Emma, and Wyatt

And to Arlene, always and forever

▼ ▼ ▼

Library of Congress Cataloging-in-Publication Data
Murkoff , Heidi
What to Expect® Eating Well When You're Expecting, with Sharon Mazel.
p. cm.
Includes index.
ISBN 978-0-7611-3326-1 (alk. paper)
1. Pregnancy—Nutritional aspects. 2. Mothers—Nutrition. 3. Recipes.
I. Mazel, Sharon. II. Title.

RG559.E43 2004
6182'42—dc22   2004052950

Recipe consultant: Rena Coyle

Book design: Lisa Hollander
Cover illustration: Tim O'Brien
Cover photography: Gamma One Conversions, Inc.
Cover quilt: Margaret Cusack
Book illustration; Judy Francis

Workman books are available at special discounts when purchased in bulk for premiums and
sales promotions as well as for fund raising or educational use. Special editions or book excerpts
can be created to specification. For details, contact the Special Sales Director at the address below
or send an e-mail to specialmarkets@workman.com.

Workman Publishing Company, Inc.
225 Varick Street
New York, NY 10014-4381
www.workman.com
Printed in the U.S.A.
First printing: April 2005
20 19 18 17 16 15 14 13 12 11

Thanks Again!

I've often said that writing books is a little like making babies (and I speak from experience in both departments, though at this point in my life, my books comfortably outnumber my babies...and trust me, will continue to). You conceive (in my experience, making babies generally outrates making books here), you're pregnant, you expend a lot of energy, lose a lot of sleep, and finally . . . you deliver (hopefully, on time).

And you can't do either one on your own. Fortunately, I've never had to try. From day (and book) one, I've had the support of more amazing people than I can count and, certainly, more people than I can list. Which always makes writing these acknowledgments particularly challenging, but especially important. So thanks a million to:

My husband and partner (in every sense of the word, including the really good ones), Erik, for always being there for me (even in places I'm pretty sure he doesn't want to be). And this book around, for being an ever-willing (if not ever-eager, especially where ginger was concerned) recipe taster—even when it meant swilling mocktails when he'd rather be sipping cocktails, or going yet another round with those blueberry pancakes. And to those full-grown babies of ours, Emma and Wyatt—who now tower over me (and lord that over me): I love you guys.

To Sharon Mazel, the best writing partner and friend a girl could have—who eats, breathes, and (when she has the chance, which isn't often) sleeps *What to Expect*, and still somehow manages to don her Supermom cape and fly off to Mommy & Me class and car pool. You're half of our one-two, and I love you. To "the girls," Daniella, Arianne, Kira, and especially Sophia (who provided endless inspiration—and waves of nausea—during her perfectly timed stay in Sharon's uterus), and who were unwitting but cooperative guinea pigs when it came to recipe testing. And to their ever-patient doctor father, Jay, for always being on call when we needed medical questions answered, and for never begrudging Sharon those sixteen-hour days (I hope).

To Suzanne Rafer, my editor-for-life (or does it just seem that way, Suz?) and friend forever, for your support, good humor, and endless efforts on behalf of everything *What to Expect*—and to her daughter, Zoë, for giving *Eating Well* a whirl while nurturing Suzanne's first grandchild(!). To Peter Workman, for being such a gifted publisher.

To everyone else at Workman who lent a hand (or two) this book around. To Lisa Hollander, who has the eye of an artist and the patience of a saint (she certainly needed both this time!); to Judith Cheng, for successfully bringing our beautiful cover mom into the twenty-first century; to Judy Francis for her always illustrious illustrations. To Anne Cherry and Barbara Peragine, for making sure the copy flowed and fit. Beth Doty and Robyn Schwartz, for keeping the *What to Expect* ship running smoothly—and for not running screaming when they see "re: another update" in my e-mails. To all my friends at Workman, including Suzie Bolotin, Jenny Mandel, Kim Cox Hicks, David Schiller, Saundra Pearson, Beth Svinarich, Pat Upton, and Lily Tilton. And thanks to everyone, especially Jim Eber and Kate Tyler, who have moved on—but will always be in my heart.

To Rena Coyle, our wonderful recipe consultant, for her dedication to all things delicious, for her fabulous recipe contributions, and for being a super sport about those endless e-mails and q's.

To Alan Nevins, of The Firm, for always going that extra mile (and then some), for your incomparable support and wise guidance, and for always being so much fun to hang out with (we'll always have La Brigada). To Marc Chamlin, for taking such good care of me, and more important, for caring so much about me—you're my friend and my lawyer, and that's an unlikely combination! To Lisa Bernstein, not only for making the What to Expect Foundation a reality, but for your friendship (and as always to Zoe, Oh-That-Teddy, and Dan Dubno). And to Ken Knabke—for always being Ken-do (and for tasting even when the tasting got tough).

To Victor Shargai and John Aniello, for your love and support. To Howard Eisenberg, my adorable dad, and to Sandee Hathaway, my beautiful (and strictly organic) sister. And to my cherished in-laws, Abby and Norman Murkoff, for always believing in me (though not always listening to me).

To Arlene Eisenberg, for everything you've given me, and continue to give to me every day. Your legacy lives on; you'll always be loved and never forgotten.

To ACOG (American College of Obstetricians and Gynecologists), for being champions of women and babies, and to all of the doctors, midwives, nurses, and nurse practitioners who work every day to make pregnancy safer and happier for expectant couples. Most of all, to my readers—the inspiration for everything that I do, and the reason why I keep doing it . . . and doing it . . . and doing it.

Thanks again, everybody!

—Heidi

Contents

▼ ▼ ▼

The Dish on Eating Well

Ever notice that when it comes to nutrition, the more things change, the more they stay the same? Sure, you can yo-yo with fad diets (low-carb? That's so last week . . . low-fat? Week before last . . . raw foods? . . . raw deal), but if you step off the diet treadmill and take stock, you'll notice that the basics of healthy eating haven't changed all that much over time. A balanced diet of lean protein, calcium-rich foods, whole grains, fruits and vegetables, and healthy fats is what nutritionists, doctors, and Mom herself have been quietly touting for years while the conflicting nutrition books duke it out on the bestseller lists, only to be forgotten the moment the newest diet craze makes headlines.

And what about for pregnant moms? Have the fundamentals of eating well when you're expecting changed much over the years? They haven't really—and mostly because eating well for two isn't all that much different from eating well for one. The proportions may shift a bit (to accommodate a growing baby's proportions), but the basics are still pretty basic.

So if eating well when you're expecting is really just a matter of sticking to a balanced diet, why would you need a book to show you how?

To answer that question, let me backtrack a few years. Make that twenty-two (gulp) years. Six weeks into my first pregnancy (due to some cycle wrinkles, it

was a little late in the game when I first got the news), I was determined to make up for lost time—and make the most of the rest of my seven-and-a-half months of baby growing. I was a healthy twenty-three year-old who lived a healthy lifestyle and ate a healthy diet—and I was pretty sure I knew what it took to feed myself and my baby healthfully. So I stocked our fridge and prepared our meals with nature's best baby-building materials: fresh chicken breasts, fish, dairy, whole grains, and a plethora of produce.

And then I ran to the bathroom to throw up.

The chicken breasts, my usual protein of choice, were the first to go—victim of a sudden aversion to flesh foods (funny, I'd never thought of chicken as flesh before). The salmon didn't stand a chance, of course—the smell (that's before I even took the fillets out of the wrapper) sent me reeling (and back to the bathroom). Got milk? I did, but definitely couldn't bear the thought of drinking it. The whole grains were welcome to stay (in bread form, toasted within an inch of their life, thank you very much), as was the fruit (with the possible exception of the honeydew, which had somehow become a honey-don't). But the broccoli I used to gobble with a rabbit's abandon turned my stomach.

I knew that I was supposed to eat a certain number of green vegetables a day, but nobody (not even my OB) could tell me how to eat them without turning greener than they were. I knew protein was the building block of human cells (which meant that building a baby would take protein aplenty), but I had no idea that cottage cheese could stand in for those dreaded flesh foods until the first-trimester aversions had worn off. Or that microwaving the salmon zapped its offensive odor. Or that calcium did not have to come with a white mustache (and a side of bloat). Or that dried apricots quelled the queasies while simultaneously satisfying my baby's requirement for vitamin A (turns out babies don't need broccoli after all) or that I could drink my vitamin C in a smoothie instead of a glass of tummy-churning OJ. Or that I could take my baby out to eat almost anywhere (except maybe that Italian place, where just a whiff of the scampi could inflict third-degree heartburn).

So I spent the rest of my pregnancy eating the best I could—gagging down the milk, choking down the chicken, and, most of the time, worrying that my best wasn't nearly good enough. If only I knew then what I know now. That eating well when you're expecting doesn't have to be torture—and that it doesn't even have to be challenging. It can be fun, easy, and, most of all, delicious—no matter what pregnancy symptom has got you down (or is keeping food from staying down). You can coddle your cravings, pander to your aversions, mol-lify your morning sickness, indulge your indigestion—and still feed yourself and your growing baby exceptionally well.

Enter (twenty-two years too late for me, but hopefully right on time for you) *Eating Well When You're Expecting*, everything you need to know to feed yourself and your baby well in the real world— the world where nausea dictates what's on the menu (even if that's two crackers and an extra-cold glass of ginger ale); where heartburn can burn a hole in your resolve to eat your vegetables; where temptations (glazed, iced, fried, chocolate-covered, creamed, or super-sized) lurk around every corner; where "lunch" meetings in the conference room are catered by Doughnuts-by-the-Dozen; where airline flights aren't catered at all. Everything you need to make eating for two half the effort and twice the pleasure—from savvy shopping to smart snacking, dining out strategies to pregnant party protocol, brown-bag lunches to breakfasts on the fly. Everything you need to put it all together, including 175 recipes that neatly package all your nutritional requirements into gourmet—yet quick and easy—dishes, while taking into account the special needs of your often tender tummy. In short, everything you need to eat well when you're expecting.

Wishing you a delicious and nutritious nine months of eating well!

—Heidi

PART ONE

EATING WELL

Eating Well for Two

CONGRATULATIONS! The line on that pregnancy test you brought home from the drugstore turned pink, your visit to the practitioner confirmed the results, and you've marked your due date on the calendar with a big red circle. And now as you sit back to take it all in, you're probably joyful, but somewhat staggered (make that floored) by the enormity of what has just happened and what is about to happen. (That and, more than likely, a little queasy.) Ready or not, you and your body are about to embark on life's most fantastic voyage—pregnancy. In the next eight months or so, your baby will grow from a single cell into billions, from a shapeless blob not yet visible to the human eye to pounds of dimpled, suitable-for-hugging newborn.

What can you do to make this voyage as safe as possible? How can you help that wildly dividing bundle of cells transform into the warm bundle of baby you'll one day hold in your arms? And how can you make sure that bundle will arrive as healthy as he or she can be?

There are many ways to give your baby a head start in life, even this early in the voyage—even while that little pink line (and, maybe, those bouts in the bathroom) remains the only concrete evidence that there actually is a baby along for the ride. Like getting good medical care, right from the beginning. Like giving up smoking, drinking, and other habits that can derail baby's chances of being born healthy. And like eating well during your pregnancy.

Of course, you probably already know that maintaining a healthy diet during pregnancy helps make a healthy baby. Chances are you've already decided that feeding your

baby well while you're expecting is a priority. Maybe you don't need any facts or figures to convince you.

But the connection between good nutrition and good pregnancy results is compelling—and more far reaching than you may realize. Almost daily, scientists make a stronger case, discovering just how many aspects of a baby's development and future well-being can be influenced by a mother's diet. And as luck would have it, what's good for baby has also turned out to be good for mom. Research continues to show that healthy eating can make pregnancy safer and more comfortable.

Eating Well: What's in It for Baby

THINK YOU'LL BE UNDERGOING A lot of changes during the nine months of pregnancy? Consider what's happening to your fetus during those 40 weeks. Cells are dividing at an unbelievable rate; organs are forming; the circulatory, digestive, urinary, and other systems are developing; the senses—hearing, sight, taste, and smell—are taking shape. And through your diet, your baby will have to receive all the vitamins, minerals, calories, protein, fluids, and other nutrients necessary for all that growth and development. Though most babies do grow and

develop even when their mothers eat a diet that's only so-so, study after study shows that, on average, healthier diets yield far healthier babies.

Think of healthy eating as one of the best gifts you can give your baby-to-be. And it's a gift that keeps on giving. Your diet can affect so many aspects of your baby-to-be's health, including the following:

Your baby's brain development. While the development of most organs is relatively complete midway through pregnancy, your baby's brain will have its greatest growth spurt during the last trimester. Since protein, calories, and omega-3 fatty acids are particularly crucial to optimal brain development, ensuring an adequate intake of these nutrients becomes even more important in the last months of pregnancy. Even if you find you've gained more weight than you would have liked in your first six months, the last trimester will not be the time to cut back. And even if you haven't been eating particularly well during the early months of pregnancy (many women find that the first trimester queasies keep them from eating anything, never mind eating anything healthy), making a concerted dietary effort in the last trimester will fuel that amazing brain expansion.

Your baby's personality. Believe it or not, much of your baby's personality is being formed in your uterus, partly owing to fetal DNA and partly, according to some studies, because of what you're eating. Researchers have found that babies born to malnourished mothers smile less and are drowsier compared with babies born to well-nourished mothers. There is also evidence that newborns whose mothers consume enough omega-3 fatty acid during the last trimester exhibit healthier sleep patterns than do other babies (something you'll definitely appreciate come 3 A.M.).

Your baby's eating habits. Research shows that what you eat during pregnancy (and while breastfeeding)

affects not only your baby's health—it also affects your baby's tastes. Because a fetus can taste and become accustomed to the flavors that make their way from its mother's meals into the amniotic fluid, a baby's food preferences can be formed before he or she ever takes a spoonful of solids. In one study, infants whose mothers drank carrot juice while pregnant eagerly lapped up cereal mixed with carrot juice, while infants of mothers who steered clear of the orange stuff were more likely to turn up their little noses at the carrot juice–cereal mixture. The moral of the study: If you'd like your child to eat his broccoli later, you might be well advised to eat yours now. (And since breast milk picks up flavors, too, influencing a nursing baby's future gastronomic preferences, the same principle holds true during breastfeeding.)

Your baby's birth weight. Eating too little (or not eating enough of the right foods) can keep your baby from growing well in the uterus; eating too much can make your baby grow too big, too fast. Babies who are born small for their gestational age stand greater chances of having health problems after delivery than do babies of normal weight. Babies born too large can complicate delivery, making it more likely that an instrument (forceps or vacuum) or surgical (cesarean) delivery will become necessary. Eating just the right amount to maintain a steady and moderate weight gain for you (see Chapter Three) can keep your baby's weight gain on target.

It's not only the quantity, but also the quality of the food you eat that can impact how baby weighs in. Inadequate zinc intake is linked to low-birth-weight babies. A diet deficient in folic acid can cause fetal growth restriction (among many other problems). Eating the right amounts of the right types of food can help give baby a good bottom line at delivery.

Your baby's organ development. With all those body parts developing from scratch (the heart, liver, lungs, kidneys, and nervous system, just to name a few), and only nine months in which to accomplish this phenomenal growth, the baby-making factory is working at full-steam, day and night. The raw materials needed to turn a fertilized egg into a fully equipped bouncing baby are supplied by you through what you eat.

Fortunately, those raw materials aren't hard to come by. Even the average American diet today provides enough of most nutrients to ensure a healthy bouncing baby—and extra-good nutrition can offer extra insurance that your fetus will receive everything it needs to develop well. On the other hand, a diet that's *severely* deficient in the right types of nutrients (and such a diet is thankfully rare during pregnancy in this country) increases the risk that a baby may not develop normally. For instance, a lack of vitamin D and calcium can interfere with proper bone and tooth growth. An inadequate intake of folic acid can result in neural tube defects, such as spina bifida (a condition that has become far less common since folic acid supplementation has become routinely recommended for women of childbearing age).

Possibly, your baby's long-term health. Though still in its infancy—and still somewhat controversial—the study of how maternal nutrition during pregnancy affects a baby's long-term health has provided researchers and mothers-to-be with plenty of food for thought. Some studies have found that a predisposition to certain diseases (such as cancers and schizophrenia) and chronic conditions (such as diabetes, hypertension, and heart disease) may be programmed while the baby is still developing in the womb, if it received inadequate nutrition during pregnancy. Scientists have found that both babies who are undernourished in the first trimester and those who are overfed in the third trimester may be at greater risk for obesity. Nutrition during pregnancy, say some researchers, not only influences a baby's health at birth, but also affects his or her health years later, even into adulthood.

Eating Well:
What's in It for You

Baby's not the only one who benefits each time you grab a piece of fruit, make time for breakfast, or opt for a grilled chicken salad over a greasy taco. Eating well while you're expecting isn't actually as selfless as it may seem. In fact, what many moms forget is that eating well for their baby affects them, too. What you eat will have a profound effect on how well your body copes with and recovers from the physical and emotional challenges of carrying and delivering a baby.

A nutritious, well-balanced diet during pregnancy will have an impact on:

Your comfort during pregnancy. Let's face it: Most pregnant women don't really walk around all nine months with a rosy glow. In fact, in the first few months, they're more likely to walk around with a greenish tint. And morning sickness is just the tip of the iceberg. Other pregnancy symptoms include fatigue, constipation, hemorrhoids, heartburn, varicose veins, complexion problems, gum problems, swelling, and leg cramps—and that's just naming a few. While some of these symptoms are par for the pregnancy course (influenced by hormones and other factors, such as fluid retention or genes), many pregnancy inevitables are not inevitable at all. And some that are inevitable don't have to be inevitably miserable. Good nutrition can minimize, eliminate, and even prevent many unpleasant side effects of pregnancy. A diet with adequate complex carbohydrates, for instance, can reduce fatigue. A diet low in fatty foods can decrease heartburn. One rich in fiber and fluids can relieve (or even prevent) constipation. A diet with enough vitamin B_6 can lessen nausea and vomiting. Even complexion problems can be flushed out by adequate fluids and overall good nutrition. For more on minimizing pregnancy discomforts through nutrition, see Chapter Two.

The safety of your pregnancy. No controversy here. It's really as simple and straightforward as this: Research shows that pregnant women who are well nourished are more likely to have a safe and uncomplicated pregnancy than women who are not well nourished. And studies continue to show strong links between deficiencies in diet and pregnancy complications. For instance, anemia, a common pregnancy complication characterized by low levels of red blood cells, is directly connected to iron deficiency. Some cases of another pregnancy complication, preeclampsia (high blood pressure), have been linked to a variety of deficiencies in a pregnant woman's diet. Researchers have found that high amounts of sugar and polyunsaturated fats increase the risk of preeclampsia. Others studies have found that women who have a low intake of vitamin C are twice as likely to develop preeclampsia. Still other research has linked some cases of preeclampsia to deficiencies in vitamin E and magnesium.

The flip side to this research is also the bright side: Eating a well-balanced nutritious diet—adequate in vitamins, minerals, and other nutrients—will reduce your risks of pregnancy complications, ensuring a healthier pregnancy. And that's something to toast your orange juice to.

Your labor and delivery. Not only will a good diet benefit you during the 40 weeks leading up to labor and delivery, it may benefit you *during* labor and delivery, too. First of all, a good pregnancy diet may help prevent labor from striking too early. Though all nutrients in a balanced diet are important in helping a woman carry to term, research links deficiencies in zinc, vitamin A, vitamin C, and magnesium to an increased risk of premature labor. Second, childbirth is labor intensive, so to speak, requiring a prodigious

wisdom of ☀ the ages?

If there's one thing that every culture and every generation shares—from the East to the West, from the ancient to the contemporary—it's the tradition of telling pregnant women what they should and shouldn't eat. And though pregnancy is fertile ground for superstitions, folklore, and tales from old (or just plain opinionated) wives from around the world and through the ages, few of them, thankfully, have made the cut to modern obstetrical practice. Among the myths you can definitely discount:

■ Eat salty or sour foods and your baby will be born with a sour disposition.

■ Chow down on chilies and other spicy foods and your baby will be born bald.

■ Not a fan of the cue-ball look in babies? Another tale proposes that a teaspoon each of honey and vinegar, taken each morning during pregnancy, will help your baby grow more hair.

■ Dark-colored foods will make a baby's skin darker; light-colored foods will turn a baby's skin lighter.

■ Eat fish and your baby could end up stupid as a salmon; eat rabbit and your baby might sleep with his or her eyes open.

Check out the chapters that follow for more fun, folklore, and not so wise old wives' tales.

amount of energy. Though a well-nourished woman won't necessarily experience a pain-free or shorter labor, she's likely to better cope with the labor she's dealt than the woman whose body lacks sufficient stores of nutrients—in much the same way

THE ABC's (AND DEF's) OF EATING WELL WHEN YOU'RE EXPECTING

▼ ▼ ▼

Keep these key words in mind when you're planning your meals, and you can't help but eat well:

ASSORTMENT. Variety is the spice of life and the key to a good pregnancy diet—ensuring that you and your baby won't get too much of one nutrient and not enough of another. So while turkey breast and cheese with lettuce and tomato on whole wheat makes a great lunch, it isn't so great if you eat it every single day. A daily assortment of healthy foods will provide your fetus with a daily assortment of necessary nutrients. (An exception to the assortment rule: when you're suffering from morning sickness, you'll need to eat whatever you can get down—even if it's the same sandwich three times a day, seven days a week.)

BALANCE. Balance and moderation are the foundation of any healthy diet. One chocolate-chip cookie won't rock the nutritional boat; a whole bag will—especially when it takes the place of dinner. Adequate intake of vitamin A (in the form of fruits and vegetables) is crucial for good health; too much vitamin A (in the form of supplements) can be toxic. Whole grains and lean protein are both good for you and baby—but eating one to the exclusion of the other isn't beneficial. Striking that balance—eating the appropriate amounts of foods (both the healthy and the less healthy foods)—is a cornerstone of eating well during pregnancy. Extremes in either direction are never smart.

COLOR. Paint your plate with a bold palette of colors (the naturally occurring ones, that is), and you'll be pleasing your senses while filling your nutritional requirements. Follow the rainbow through your market's produce department, sampling the spectrum of nature's bounty. From blushing red strawberries and tomatoes and watermelon to vibrant yellow peppers and squash and melons to deep crimson cherries and pomegranates and beets, vivid colors signal a cache of nutrients. Hues are hot, so color your world daily. See page 140 for more.

DIETING . . . IS OUT. Pregnancy is never the time for a weight-loss diet. Your baby needs a continuous supply of calories and nutrients throughout its nine-month stay in your uterine café. The weight that you gain (assuming it's gained on the right types of food) is there for a very important purpose:

a well-nourished athlete is able to perform better and endure longer than one who hasn't been eating well. (And when it comes to athletic events, there's none more challenging than childbirth. Just ask any Iron Woman who's also a mom.)

Your postpartum recovery. A baby's not the only thing you can

to nourish your baby and ensure optimum growth in the womb. There will be plenty of time after pregnancy to shed any leftover pounds. See Chapter Three for more on weight gain during pregnancy.

EXPERIMENT. Been stuck in a food rut? Think of pregnancy as a time to expand your eating horizons as you expand your waistband—to explore uncharted (at least to you) culinary territory (including fruits, vegetables, grains you've never sampled before). Try new foods and experiment with old favorites (with new recipes). See the tips in Chapters Five and Six and the recipes in Part Two for ways to make the foods you eat new and exciting.

FUN . . . IS WHAT EATING SHOULD BE. Nothing dooms an eating plan faster than boredom. That's why it's so important to make eating well during pregnancy a pleasant experience (at least once the nausea has passed). Whenever you can, add the little touches that make food fun—whether its a dip for your veggies or a baked-taco-chip garnish for your chili. Take time to savor your food (instead of gulping it down), which will help with heartburn, too. And leave guilt off the menu—even those times when you're treating yourself to something that's not-so-good for you (but that tastes oh-so-good), let yourself enjoy it!

expect after delivery, though it's definitely the best thing. Whether your labor and delivery turn out to be enviably effortless or disappointingly difficult, the effects of childbirth will be enormous. In the days, weeks, and even months postpartum, your body will need significant resources to recover from a variety of physical insults, ranging from stretching and tearing to blood loss and sleep deprivation—while simultaneously caring for a newborn. One of the best ways to speed that recovery (and find the energy you'll need to keep up with the endless demands and challenges of new motherhood) is to eat a nourishing diet throughout pregnancy and to continue to do so after delivery. (See Chapter Ten for more on eating during the postpartum period.)

Your long-term health. When it comes to most nutrients, nature first takes care of an expectant mom's nutritional needs from incoming food, then serves up the leftovers to her fetus. But that's not true when it comes to that essential bone-builder, calcium. If you don't take in enough calcium when you're pregnant, your body will drain this important mineral out of your own bones to help strengthen baby's—possibly setting you up for osteoporosis later on. That's yet another good reason to eat well for your own health, as well as for baby's well-being, when you're expecting. But keep in mind that good eating habits that continue even after your pregnancy ends can do even more to ensure you a healthier future—reducing your chances of developing a wide variety of diseases, from hypertension to diabetes to cancer. By setting up the groundwork for a lifetime of healthy eating, good nutrition during pregnancy offers you and your family benefits that extend far beyond delivery day.

So What Does Eating Well Really Mean?

JUST WHAT IS A HEALTHY PREGNANCY eating plan? What foods should you be eating? Which ones should you be avoiding? And how are you supposed to make sure your baby's getting all the vitamins, minerals, and other nutrients he or she needs to grow to potential and arrive in good health while you're experiencing nausea you never could have imagined, aversions to everything green and/or leafy, cravings for foods you never knew existed, and heartburn no greasy spoon could ever hope to dish out—even on Liver and Onions Night?

Actually, you may already know more than you think you do. Eating well during pregnancy isn't all that different from eating well during any other time in your life. Following general guidelines for the kind of healthy diet that's recommended for all adults, pregnant or not, is the way to start: eating a wide variety of fresh fruits and vegetables, choosing whole grains rather than refined ones, concentrating on lean sources of calcium and protein, and limiting fat (particularly the less healthy kinds), sugar, and junk foods. But there are some notable differences. First, though the same foods that nourish nearly every human being well nourish expectant mothers well, too, many nutrients are—not surprisingly—needed in far greater amounts during pregnancy. Second, foods that may provide perfectly healthy eating when you're not expecting—such as unpasteurized cheeses and sushi—may be harmful when you are pregnant. The red wine that may ordinarily cut the risk of heart disease may increase risks of complications and birth defects during pregnancy. And the biggest difference of all—when you're not pregnant, the only one who stands to lose is you; when you're pregnant, your baby can also lose out.

Eat well for two, and you're both winners.

Ready to Get Started?

IT'S ALL HERE IN THE PAGES THAT follow. Armed with the tips, advice, nutritional information, and recipes in this book, you'll be able to eat your way through a healthy and comfortable pregnancy, prepare meals that are nutritious and well balanced (not to mention tasty and easy to make), support the proper growth and development of your baby (both inside and outside the womb), maintain a steady and healthy weight gain (one that will be easier to shed postpartum), and feel great about doing what's best for you and your baby.

Because every pregnant woman is different (and because no one eating plan fits all) the guidelines in this book should be considered only that—guidelines. They aren't provided to dictate meals, but rather to help you design your own personal pregnancy eating plan. What's presented here is the ideal—what an ideal woman in an ideal world under ideal circumstances should do to eat well during pregnancy. Keeping that in mind, realize that not every day during your pregnancy will be ideal, and many will be far from it. (You're too queasy to stomach anything but gingersnaps one day or your older kids are clamoring for a fast-food dinner the next; later in the week between a meeting that ran over, a deadline that's looming, and a traffic jam that kept you locking bumpers for two hours, you're just too exhausted to think about balancing a meal.) And that's okay. As long as your overall pregnancy eating is healthful and well balanced, and as long as you strive for the ideal (even if you don't always get there), you're doing what's best for your baby.

So sit back, sip a fruit smoothie, and read on to learn how to eat well when you're expecting.

Eating Well for a Comfortable Pregnancy

IT'S A LITTLE IRONIC, and more than a little frustrating. The reason you want to eat healthy is because you're pregnant—and the reason you're having a hard time eating healthy is also because you're pregnant. Let's face it—between morning sickness, food aversions, constipation, and indigestion, there are plenty of appetite-disrupting pregnancy complaints that can make healthy eating less than a piece of (carrot) cake. If you're lucky, only one or two such symptoms will stand between you and the eating plan that's best for you and baby. If you're not so lucky—and much more typical—you'll experience all of them at some point.

Though some symptoms (like morning sickness) usually confine their miseries to the first trimester, others (such as heartburn) can continue to cramp a pregnant woman's eating style all the way to delivery. So it's not surprising that on some days (and this may seem like every day if the queasies have you down), you may be far more preoccupied with finding ways to spell "relief" for yourself than with thinking of ways to spell "nutrition" for your baby. Luckily, many of the pregnancy side effects that can dampen your appetite can actually be alleviated—sometimes even prevented—by eating healthy foods. Then everyone wins: Baby gets the nutrition that will give him or her the best start in life, and you start feeling well enough to get that nourishing food down—and maybe even enjoy it.

Morning Sickness

DOES THE SMELL OF TOMATO SAUCE send you running for the nearest toilet? Does the mere sight of a chicken breast have you heaving? Are you queasy just contemplating a bowl of your formerly favorite cereal? Are you looking greener than that salad you're supposed to be eating? Welcome to your first trimester of pregnancy, a time when, if you're like about 75 percent of all pregnant women, morning sickness will change the way you look at food (not to mention the way you smell it and taste it), taking a toll both on your tummy and your ability to fill it. Or, at least, to keep it filled.

As just about every veteran of morning sickness knows, the joker who coined this pregnancy symptom's name was clearly never a victim of it. Rare is the woman whose nausea and vomiting subside when the clock strikes noon. With morning sickness, you're as likely to feel sick in the afternoon or evening as you are to be queasy in the morning.

And there's no such thing as "textbook" morning sickness, either, since symptoms vary from woman to woman. Some may experience only occasional queasiness. Others may suffer through constant nausea and frequent bouts of vomiting, especially during the early weeks. While symptoms typically abate by the end of the third or fourth month, a small percentage of women (such as those carrying multiples) find they persist—at least to some extent—into the ninth month.

Those who have spent weeks hovering over the toilet, avoiding onions like the plague, and subsisting on ginger ale and saltines may find it hard to believe that there's a silver lining to the cloud of morning sickness. But, there actually is. Nausea and vomiting during the first trimester (or, perhaps, the abundance of hormones that seem to trigger them) appear to have a protective effect on pregnancy. What's more, while you're certainly suffering—your baby almost certainly isn't. Even if you can't keep anything down, and even if you lose a little weight during the first trimester, your baby is able to weather the storm of morning sickness far better than you.

Of course, while this good news may make you feel better about having morning sickness, it won't make you feel better while you have it. But there are many dietary steps you can take that may alleviate your discomfort:

▲ Follow your nose. Out the door, that is. Pregnancy hormones cause most women to become extra sensitive to odors, making mild smells strong, strong smells overwhelming, and many smells sickening. If the smell of cooking makes you feel like hugging the toilet, ask someone to help out in the kitchen—or better yet, let someone else do the cooking while you step outside for some fresh air. (And make sure your chef ventilates while you're gone.) If you don't have anyone around to help in the kitchen, use the microwave instead of the stove, and open the windows after meals to clear out cooking odors. Stick to foods that are easy to prepare and cook (or are ready to eat) so you won't have to chop pungent onions, dice smelly green peppers, and sauté garlic to the sounds of your stomach churning. And hold off on preparing odorous favorites until your digestive sensibilities can handle them. (Simple, spice-free dishes will be easier to get down, too.) For the duration, stay out of restaurants where you can smell what's on the menu before it's placed in front of you.

▲ Eat often. Empty tummies are tumultuous tummies. That's because when there's no food around to break down, digestive acids are left with only stomach lining to feast on—a process that, not surprisingly, produces nausea. To keep your tummy from running on empty, and to prevent hunger-triggered nausea, eat six mini-meals a day (see box, page 16). And sneak in plenty of between-meal snacks, like dried fruit, cheese, bread sticks, or crackers.

▲ But don't eat too much. An overfilled tummy is as likely to elicit the queasies as an empty one. During pregnancy, food travels at a snail's pace so that nutrients are better absorbed. Cram in the chow, and you'll end up with what amounts to a digestive traffic jam—potentially leading to nausea and vomiting.

▲ Eat often in bed. Before you settle down for the night, snuggle up with a snack that's high in both protein and carbs, such as a fruit bar and milk, a handful of nuts and raisins, yogurt and bread sticks, or a toasted cheese sandwich. Bedtime nibbles will keep your blood sugar elevated throughout the night while hopefully keeping nausea from creeping back with the dawn's early light. Open the bedside snack stand once more when you wake in the morning. Before you even swing your legs over the side of your bed, grab the

VARIETY AND THE MORNING-SICK MOM

▼ ▼ ▼

Heard (ad nauseum) that variety keeps a pregnant mom's diet healthier and safer, but you can only stomach the same one or two foods over and over again? Don't worry, and don't force-feed yourself for variety's sake. For now, eat what it takes to get through the day (and night)—even if it's a hamburger (or cereal or cinnamon toast) for breakfast, lunch, and dinner. Once morning sickness has passed, you'll have plenty of time to add variety back into your diet.

crackers (or other dry, bland food) you stashed within arm's length, and start crunching. Let that snack settle in before you attempt to start your day, and hopefully you won't start out as sick tomorrow morning.

▲ Nip nausea in the bud. Stay ahead of the nausea game by eating before it hits (if your nausea is on a schedule), when food is more likely to go down and stay down. And, if you're really lucky, filling up (a little) before an attack may actually help to ward it off.

▲ Concentrate on carbs. From the ubiquitous cracker to just about any fruit on the produce stand, carbs comfort most every pregnant woman in the first trimester. Whenever your tender taste buds permit, choose complex carbohydrates to satisfy your craving for the bland and starchy (whole-grain toast, pretzels, even saltines). Some morning sickness sufferers prefer fresh fruit (including melon, bananas, sometimes citrus); others find relief in the dried variety (especially raisins and apricots).

▲ Think protein. Though carbs are the first food group women usually turn to when they're green around the gills, adding a little cheese (or another protein food) to those crackers can fight nausea even more effectively. Studies show that pregnant women experience less nausea when eating high-protein snacks than indulging in high-fat ones. So pass up the chips, and reach for any protein your tummy finds tolerable (a cheese stick, some almonds, a hard-boiled egg, or a dish of yogurt, for instance).

▲ Forgo fatty foods. Steer clear of greasy, fried, and other high-fat foods, which are hard to digest and are loaded with oils that can send the nervous system into overdrive (aggravating your nausea).

THE SIX-MEAL SOLUTION

▼ ▼ ▼

When heartburn, nausea, gassiness, and other pregnancy symptoms make eating (and digesting) three square meals a day feel too much like hard work, turn to the six-meal solution instead. Eating half as much twice as often will keep your blood sugar steady, your appetite appeased, and your digestive tract running more smoothly (lending relief from pregnancy tummy troubles). Dividing your meals will also help you to conquer your nutritional requirements more easily.

There are two ways to tap into the six-meal solution. One is to split your normal hearty meals in half, eating each portion two or three hours apart. The other is to forget traditional meals altogether and graze through the day on mini-meals and hearty snacks. (See page 106 for some snack ideas.) Here are some mini-meal suggestions:

■ A cup of soup sprinkled with grated cheese and whole-grain croutons

■ Chicken salad on a whole wheat roll

■ A muffin, cheese wedge, and a bowl of cut-up fruit

■ Half a bagel and one scrambled egg

■ A baked potato filled with cheddar and broccoli

■ A small bowl of whole-grain cereal with milk, half a sliced banana

■ A small salad topped with nuts and slices of hard-cooked egg

■ A yogurt-and-fruit smoothie (see page 422 for recipes)

■ Turkey breast with sliced tomato and Swiss cheese wrapped in half a whole wheat pita

■ Half a grilled chicken breast and a peach

■ A cup of yogurt topped with granola and blueberries

▲ Fluids, fluids everywhere . . . with lots of drops to drink. Your body needs to stay hydrated, especially if you've been vomiting. In fact, in the short term, drinking enough is more important than eating enough. Aim for at least eight glasses of water, juice, or clear broth a day. Some experts recommend drinking between, rather than during, meals to avoid overtaxing the digestive system. If you can't manage to quench your quota, munch on some watermelon cubes (1 cup of watermelon provides you with ½ cup of liquid), suck on some ice chips, or slurp some fruit-juice Popsicles. If you're having trouble keeping solids down but not liquids, consider drinking as many meals as possible (in the form of smoothies and soups).

▲ Be dense. In your food selections, that is. If half of everything you eat comes up, the half that stays down should provide you with as many nutrients as possible. So choose foods that are packed densely with high-quality nutrients, such as avocados, sweet potatoes, carrots, red pepper, cantaloupe, dried apricots, beans, cheese, almonds, brown rice, and edamame.

▲ Let your appetite rule. If something doesn't appeal to you, don't eat it—no matter how healthy a food it is. If fish makes waves in your stomach, look beyond the sea for your entrée. If the smell of cheese sends shudders down your digestive tract, don't nibble on cheddar just because you've read it eases nausea. On the flip side, pregnancy is the time to cater to your cravings. If your taste buds cry out for sweets, pay attention. If you're yearning for something salty, grab that jar of pickles and get busy. Ultimately, if there are only a handful of foods that don't make you choke, get down what you can—even if it's not a particularly nutritious choice.

▲ Go for ginger. For generations, ginger—the spicy root that is used to flavor many exotic dishes—has also been used to settle an upset stomach, ease cramps, and combat indigestion. As it turns out, this is one home remedy that has actually made its way out of the kitchen and into the medical books. Already proved effective for alleviating motion sickness, ginger can also be good for what ails a queasy pregnant woman, according to research. Take it in capsule form (available from health-food stores; ask your practitioner to prescribe a safe amount), use it in cooking, make ginger tea by infusing gingerroot in boiling water, or try ginger-based foods and beverages: ginger biscuits, crystallized ginger, ginger sucking candy, and real ginger ale (see page 20). Some women even find comfort for their bouts of morning sickness by sniffing a piece of fresh-cut ginger.

▲ Up your vitamins. Scientists have long suspected that vitamin deficiency can play a role in morning sickness. Research has confirmed that taking vitamin B₆ in moderate dosages (50 to 100 milligrams per day) successfully relieves nausea for many women. Researchers also found that women who have adequate vitamin intake in general *before* getting pregnant experience less nausea than those who come into the pregnancy already deficient in some vitamins. And if there weren't enough good reasons for taking a prenatal vitamin during pregnancy, here's another: That one-a-day habit can decrease nausea symptoms.

▲ But keep them down. Okay, how are those vitamins supposed to relieve your morning sickness when you can't stomach those vitamins *because*

wisdom of the ages?

B.C (before crackers), there was a variety of other morning sickness cures far more exotic than the humble saltine. For centuries, medicine men to modern midwives, shamans to herbal healers, folklore to old wives' tales, have advised women on ways to combat morning sickness through diet. From wild yam to papaya, many foods have been passed down from generation to queasy generation as supposedly effective weapons in the fight against morning sickness. Even today, modern midwives continue to suggest at least one of those time-honored cures: cutting a fresh lemon and sucking on it to ward off nausea. (When life gives you morning sickness, make lemonade?) Try it; you might like it. You'll find more tips for the queasy on pages 14 and 15.

of your morning sickness? There are a number of tricks you can try to keep a good vitamin down: Some experts recommend taking your prenatal at night (or at the time of day when you're the least nauseated). Others say it's best to take the pill with a meal so it doesn't upset an empty stomach. Some women find chewable vitamins or coated ones are easier to take; others find relief when they switch brands. If you find your prenatal vitamin doesn't agree with you no matter what time of day you take it and no matter what form or brand you use, ask your practitioner about prescribing a prenatal vitamin that has a greater amount of vitamin B_6 than does a standard

prenatal vitamin, has a controlled formula that releases the vitamins in your body evenly throughout the day, and that contains no iron, which can upset the stomach.

▲ For a tough case, try a tough approach. If your morning sickness is on the severe side and is interfering with eating, working, sleeping, and other important activities, you might also want to ask your practitioner about prescribing a combination of vitamin B_6 and the antihistamine Unisom Sleep Tabs. This combination has been shown to be safe during pregnancy and is extremely effective in reducing symptoms of morning sickness. (Don't take any medication, extra vitamins, or herbal remedies for nausea and vomiting unless prescribed by a physician who knows you are pregnant and has checked on the safety of the drug and the dose.)

▲ ▲ ▲

Q *"I'm sick of chewing on those dry crackers every morning. Is there anything else I can eat when I wake up?"*

A You've discovered, as so many pregnant women eventually do, that crackers aren't always all they're cracked up to be—especially after you've munched your way through twenty-seven crates of them. Yet chances are, the only morning-sickness advice you've been getting from well-meaning practitioners and friends is, "Eat two crackers, and call me in the morning." Unfortunately, even a food with a well-earned reputation for being comforting can take a turn for the discomforting when it becomes deeply associated with nausea. Then it's definitely time for a switch. But when looking for some alternatives to that all-too-familiar rectangle, consider looking to different yet similarly dry and bland foods. Try nibbling on some dry cereal, bread sticks, rice cakes, unbuttered popcorn, graham crackers (instead of saltines), or pretzels—all of which can fill the bill at your bedside, though not necessarily at the same time. Other good items to stock your bedside snack stand with include ginger ale (the kind that's made with real ginger) and gingersnaps, a piece of whole wheat toast (wrapped in foil to keep it fresh for morning snacking), and a jar of mixed nuts and raisins.

QUICK F·I·X TO QUELL YOUR QUEASIES Need something in your stomach but can't stomach a solid meal? Try drinking your nutrients in the form of a delicious fruit smoothie. Rich in vitamins and minerals to nourish you and your baby, it'll also—because of its high water content—keep you hydrated. Smoothies go down easy, and because they're cold, there's no strong odor or taste to offend your sensitive tummy. And don't stop mixing smoothies after the morning sickness has passed. They make a refreshing nutrient-packed pick-me-up (or a great breakfast on the go) anytime during your pregnancy and after it. For great smoothie ideas, see the recipes starting on page 422.

But why stop at a smoothie? There are plenty of other ways to quell your queasies while filling your nutritional requirements. Dip into a bowl of Ginger and Carrot Soup (page 282). Soothing because it's a liquid, the soup has the added bonus of ginger to help ward off your nausea. Ready to tackle something solid? Munch on a Ginger and Carrot Muffin (page 260) or a slab of Gingerbread Mom cake (page 439).

Q *"I can't seem to get myself out of the vicious 'morning-sickness cycle.' I'm too nauseous to eat, but when I don't eat, I get more nauseous, making me less likely to eat. Help!"*

A Take it slow. Start off by drinking just a little. Even tiny sips of water (or another liquid you tolerate) every fifteen minutes can start making you feel well enough to attempt some solid (and bland) food. But even if you're hungry, don't jump in with a full plate the moment your stomach settles down; no sooner than you get the food down, you're likely to feel it coming back up, beginning the cycle all over again. Instead, take advantage of those windows of opportunity that open up between bouts of nausea to sneak in some healthy, but not-too-filling snacks, preferably ones that include both a complex carbohydrate and a protein.

Try Carrot and Ginger Muffins (page 260) or Carrot-Ginger Soup (page 282).

Q*"I'll do anything to get rid of this queasy feeling. I've heard about the benefits of ginger tea, but I'm not sure I can stomach it."*

AThere are sweeter ways to reap the benefits of ginger—including a wide variety of hard candies, soft chews, and lollipops made with ginger and other natural ingredients, specifically designed to ease morning sickness. Best of all, these ginger snacks seem to work wonders for some mildly queasy women—hopefully they will for you, too.

Cooking (or better still, having someone cook for you) with ginger is another comforting way to go.

Q*"I think I'm queasy because of all the excess saliva that seems to always be accumulating in my mouth. Or maybe it's accumulating because I'm queasy. Either way, what can I do about it?"*

ATry a little minty magic. Some women find mint—in sugarless gum or in candy form—dries that excess saliva (a common side effect in early pregnancy) right up. Others find that chewing gum only exacerbates the problem. Experiment, and see whether it works for you.

▼ ▼ ▼

Food Cravings

WAS THAT YOU FORAGING IN THE freezer last night for the cookies and cream, and in the fridge for some pickles to dip in it? Spending your whole lunch hour searching for a deli that would make you a peanut-butter-and-salami sandwich on raisin bread? Embarrassing your spouse at the buffet table during last week's cocktail party by dipping the melon balls into cocktail sauce?

Welcome to the cravings club. More than three-quarters of all women experience food cravings at some point in their pregnancy, usually in the first trimester. The most commonly reported cravings (not surprisingly, many women prefer to keep their cravings to themselves, rather than report them) are for sweets, dairy products, and salty foods—often in peculiar combina-

TRY THESE INSTEAD

▼ ▼ ▼

From salty to sweet, starchy to crunchy, hot to cold, there's a nutritious counterpart for just about every food you can crave. Will it be easy convincing your inner chocoholic that your cravings for fudge can be satisfied with a mouthwatering slice of melon? Realistically, not always. But with a little creativity—and some willpower—you may often be able to find wholesome substitutes that truly satisfy both body and soul. Do it frequently, and you may be surprised to find your tastes—and your cravings—adjusting, making that melon as tempting to reach for as that fudge. Well, almost.

INSTEAD OF	TRY
Chocolate bar	Hot chocolate, made with skim milk
Sugar-frosted cereal	Whole-grain cereal topped with chopped dates and raisins or fresh strawberries
A slice of cake	Any of the nutritious and delicious cakes, cookies, and muffins for which recipes begin on page 256.
Candy	Dried fruit, frozen grapes
Ice cream with toppings	Nonfat frozen yogurt or sorbet topped with fresh berries and nuts
Potato chips	Soy chips or crisps, natural baked cheese puffs, Pirate's Booty or Veggie Booty, baked potato or taco chips, air-popped popcorn (tossed with grated Parmesan cheese for extra flavor), pretzels, rice cakes, lightly salted edamame
Soda	Fruit juice mixed with sparkling water

tions. But few pregnant women go by the book, especially when it comes to their dietary urges. Cravings have been known to range from the ridiculous (black olives on cheesecake) to the sublime (fudgy brownies and milk), from the wholesome (citrus fruit, by the crateful) to the downright dangerous (such as dirt or clay; see box, next page); from the ordinary (cheese, by the wheel) to the truly bizarre (gherkins and green apples dipped in salsa).

DON'T EAT THIS AT HOME (OR ANYWHERE)

▼ ▼ ▼

Not all cravings are good for you, and some are downright dangerous. Women who experience pica crave non-food items such as dirt, clay, soap, chalk, or ashes. Indulging these desires can be harmful or even fatal. It's theorized that women who experience such cravings may be extremely deficient in iron or calcium. Whatever the reason, if you find yourself craving anything that isn't edible, don't indulge. Call your practitioner for advice.

Another eating compulsion that might signal a nutritional deficiency is ice chewing. Scientists have found that women who crave ice are more likely to be suffering from iron-deficiency anemia. Though sucking ice chips to relieve nausea is fine, if you're constantly craving that icy crunch, check with your practitioner.

Many experts believe that cravings are a result of the body's dramatically changing hormones. (After all, women often experience similar though usually less pronounced urges premenstrually, when their hormones are also in flux.) The hormonal factor is compounded by a pregnant woman's more acute sense of taste and smell—which drive her away from some foods, and have her (or her spouse) driving at 2 A.M. to the nearest convenience store for others.

Another popular theory is that cravings may be nutritionally based; in other words, a message from your body to step up intake of a nutrient it needs. For instance, crave salty foods? It may be because your body needs more sodium as your blood volume increases. Or it may indicate that your body's short on fluids;

if you listen to your body and break open the salted nuts, you'll be thirstier, sending you to the fridge for a bottle of water. Can't get enough grapefruit? Maybe it's your body's way of sending an SOS for vitamin C.

Of course, while this message system often works efficiently, these days it also gets scrambled. It probably worked best before humans departed so drastically from the food chain—definitely before the invention of convenience stores—when we were better able to interpret the signals our bodies sent us. When a pregnant cavewoman's craving for sweets sent her searching for berries full of vitamin C, she and her body had communicated well. When a modern pregnant woman's cravings for sweets send her searching for a Snickers bar void of vitamin C (and full of sugar), she and her body have clearly had a disconnect.

Most likely, food cravings are a complex mix of physiological, psychological, behavioral, and cultural factors. Handling them, however, doesn't have to be so complicated. Here are some tips that might make your cravings easier (and healthier) for you to deal with:

▲ Cave in. At least some of the time. Since cravings usually stop toying with your taste buds by the end of the first trimester (typically coming and going with morning sickness), they're not likely to wreak much nutritional havoc, especially if they're tempered by good sense (you submit to one brownie, not the whole pan). And if you're suffering from morning sickness, catering to your cravings may be the only way to get and keep anything down. So as long as they're not dangerous (such as dirt or clay; see box, facing page), give in to your cravings— especially if it'll make the difference between a queasy day and a comfortable one.

▲ Start the day right. Eating a good breakfast can prevent hunger-triggered cravings later in the day.

▲ Seek substitutes. Try to find nutritious foods that can pinch-hit for the less nutritious ones you crave. If you're longing for potato chips,

wisdom of ☼ the ages?

Old wives, not surprisingly, have their share of theories about pregnancy food cravings. Check out these tales:

■ If you crave sweets, you're having a girl.

■ If you crave meats or cheeses, you're having a boy.

■ If you crave something during pregnancy and don't get it, the baby will have a birthmark in the shape of the craving. (A good reason to give in to that chocolate-dipped dill pickle?)

reach for the baked variety—or substitute some soy crisps, which offer protein along with that salty crunch. If you're hankering for double mocha chip ice cream, dip into some frozen coffee yogurt instead. (See box, page 21, for more substitution ideas.) That's not to say that you can't sometimes indulge your cravings outright—eccentric excess and all. Humor them only in moderation, and nobody will lose out.

▲ Think small. If you're craving chocolate, go for a snack-size bar instead of a king-size one (freeze it first, and it'll satisfy even longer). If ice cream is what your heart (and stomach) desires, savor a few spoonfuls slowly instead of consuming an entire carton—or opt for a Fudgsicle (which takes longer to eat than a scoop of ice cream and builds in portion control).

Food Aversions

ONE MINUTE YOU CAN'T GET enough of the chicken nuggets your friend ordered at lunch, and the next minute, you're running for cover at the mere sight of a drumstick. You open the fridge and double over at the smell of the Swiss cheese your spouse left half-unwrapped. (But wait—something's wrong with this picture! You love cheese, or at least you *used to* love cheese.) The foamy, hot latte you've always lived for (or, at least, couldn't get through your morning without) now leaves you cold. And queasy.

It seems you've discovered what's on the flip side of food cravings: food aversions.

And, as with food cravings, you're in plentiful pregnant company. Up to 85 percent of expectant mothers experience at least one food aversion, and they can be as powerful as cravings—sometimes even stronger. Confusing, too. Many pregnant women find that they can no longer stand the sight or smell—never mind the taste—of a food that they normally crave. Other women find that a food that normally makes them cringe becomes even more repulsive. Multiple aversions are also common.

Some researchers say that food aversions, like cravings, are related to your hormone levels: they peak when your hormones are in their greatest period of flux, during the first trimester (which explains why most food aversions pass by the time you're midway through your pregnancy). They can also be closely tied to morning sickness. (Women who suffer the most with nausea and vomiting typically also have the hardest time with aversions.)

Another popular explanation parallels the your-body-craves-what-it-needs theory of food cravings: that food aversions are your body's way of preventing you from consuming anything that might be harmful to the baby. This might account for several aversions that are very common during early pregnancy—including alcohol and coffee. Some researchers suggest that this mechanism might also kick in to keep pregnant women (whose immune systems are naturally suppressed, making them more vulnerable to toxins in foods) from succumbing to food-borne illness. This might have made particular sense before refrigeration made eating safer, and might explain why so many pregnant women experience aversions to foods that in pre-fridge days were likely to carry harmful microorganisms and parasites, such as meat, fish, poultry, and eggs.

Yet another theory also has its roots in more primitive times: Nature ensured a pregnant woman's safety by steering her away from pungent plants that might have been toxic and toward bland or sweet grains or fruits that were more likely to be safe (which would explain why so many women turn green around such greens as broccoli and cabbage). Of course, since few women forage for their food these days—and since produce in modern markets is pre-screened for toxicity—it would seem that this instinct, too, is evolution-arily out of date. The argument that aversions are protective also fails when you consider that many preg-nant women are turned off to foods that are especially healthy for them and their babies.

Because food aversions are so interconnected with feelings of nau-sea and vomiting, some of the tips for dealing with morning sickness (pages 14 and 15) can help with aversions as well. Here are a few other things to keep in mind when you've got that aversion feeling:

▲ Don't fight a healthy aversion. If your aversion is to coffee or alcohol, consider yourself lucky. It'll never be easier to give them up than when they're turning your stomach.

▲ Work around unhealthy aversions. Never force yourself to eat a food you have an aversion to just because it's healthy. But whenever possible, find an acceptable substitute for it. For instance, even if your body won't

QUICK F·I·X FOR AVENGING AVERSIONS If it's meat, fish, and poultry that you're finding unappealing, a quick dish made with the "super" grain quinoa (see pages 133–34) can give you a leg up on your protein requirement. Quinoa has been dubbed one of the best sources of protein in the plant kingdom, so you can get your fill of protein without tapping into the animal kingdom. Try Quinoa Pearls with Wild Mushrooms (page 417), or Leek Tomato Quinoa (page 418)—or any of the other great grain recipes starting on page 414.

let you get within smelling distance of chicken, meat, or fish, you can still find ways to get a little closer to protein. (Read on for some substi-tuting examples.)

▲ Be bland. At least, in the foods you choose. If you stick with mild-tasting and mild-smelling foods dur-ing the time when the aversions are strongest, you'll accomplish two things. First, your body will be hap-pier. Second, you may avoid bring-ing on brand-new aversions.

▲ ▲ ▲

Q "I can't eat any fish, chicken, or meat recently. Even the smell of them sends me reeling. But I'm wor-ried that I'm not getting enough pro-tein to feed my baby."

A You never have to force-feed your-self to make sure you're feeding your baby well. Protein comes in all kinds of packages, not just in the standard steak-house favorites. Try, instead, such typically inoffensive protein equivalents as cottage cheese, yogurt, soy products (especially tofu and edamame), quinoa, or beans. Eggs are a wonderful protein source that some women find palatable, others objectionable. And since it's often the sight of that slab of meat that offends—even more so than the taste of it—you might also try hiding the offending food. For instance, use ground beef (extra lean will offer a milder flavor) or ground turkey in stews or soups instead of serving up a steak; chop cooked chicken breast into a casserole instead of confronting it on the bone; camouflage cut-up seafood in a pasta dish.

Q *"Before I was pregnant, I would eat a salad every day. Now that I'm in my first trimester, I can't look at anything green. What can I eat instead?"*

A It isn't easy being green, so until this aversion passes, steer clear of any vegetables (such as lettuce, broccoli, and spinach) that turn you into a Kermit look-alike. Opt for yellow vegetables instead, like carrots and yams, which are generally better tolerated but offer all the same important nutrients. Or get your veggie vitamins the sweet way—in such beta-carotene-rich fruits as cantaloupe, mango, yellow peaches, and apricots.

Q *"I'm in my first trimester and am experiencing a metallic taste in my mouth. Not only is it unpleasant, it's turning me off food altogether. Can I do anything about it?"*

A Does your mouth taste like you've been sucking on a penny? Blame your hormones, again. Called dysguesia (in case you need to know), that metallic taste is surprisingly common (though not talked about as often as morning sickness or heartburn). Usually, it disappears by the second trimester, when hormones begin to level off. In the meantime, combat heavy metal with acid. Focus on sour flavors (such as citrus juices, lemonade, or foods marinated in vinegar—assuming your tummy can handle them) that tend to increase saliva production, thus decreasing the bad taste in your mouth. Ask your practitioner, too, about changing your prenatal vitamin; some promote the metallic taste more than others. Brushing your tongue each time you brush your teeth can help minimize the metal, and rinsing with a baking soda solution (¼ teaspoon baking soda to 1 cup water), which neutralizes pH levels in your mouth, can keep your food from having that just minted flavor.

▼ ▼ ▼

Constipation

YOU'VE FINALLY FIGURED OUT A WAY to get enough food *into* your body without throwing it up. But, if you're like 50 percent of pregnant women, now you've got a problem getting it *out* of your body. That's right—you're constipated.

Like so many pregnancy discomforts, constipation is a lousy symptom that's around for a good reason. Here's why it happens: During pregnancy, progesterone (one of the hormones responsible for a healthy pregnancy) relaxes the muscles of the bowels and causes the digestive tract to move at a much slower pace. The positive result of this digestive relaxation: better absorption of nutrients earmarked for baby making. The not-so-positive result: stool that sticks around too long becomes harder (literally) to eliminate. As pregnancy progresses, mounting pressure on the bowels from the growing uterus often compounds constipation.

There are ways to fight back against constipation,* without interfering with the digestive tract's good intentions:

▲ Focus on fiber. A diet high in fiber will combat constipation by absorbing water, thus softening stools and

*Nondiet-related tips for fighting constipation and other pregnancy symptoms discussed in this chapter can be found in *What to Expect When You're Expecting.*

speeding their passage. Favor such high-fiber foods as whole-grain cereals, including oatmeal and oat bran cereals (or add some oat bran to your favorite cereal or fruit smoothie), whole-grain breads, crackers, and muffins (especially those made with whole wheat or bran; see recipes starting page 256), fresh fruits (such as plums and melons) and vegetables, and dried fruits (figs, dates, raisins, apricots, and of course, that geriatric favorite, prunes). You should aim for about 25 to 30 grams of fiber a day, but there's no need to count. You'll

FINE FUZZY FRIEND

▼ ▼ ▼

Eating prunes is definitely one way to combat constipation, but if you like your fruit fresh, look no further than the kiwi to get things moving. Besides providing that prune-like laxative effect (with no stewing required), this diminutive fruit packs plenty of nutrition within its fuzzy skin—ounce for ounce, its juicy flesh provides more vitamin C and E than any other of its produce peers. Peel kiwis, then slice them into salads, into yogurt or on top of cottage cheese, into cereal (they pair especially well with strawberries)—or simply split them in half and scoop out the mouthwatering fruit.

FOR CONQUERING CONSTIPATION

There's nothing like a tasty soup rich in fiber and fluid to help combat constipation. And you'll get a healthy serving of protein in the bargain. See Purée of Black Bean Soup on page 290 or any of the other delicious soup recipes starting on page 281). Or are beans the last thing your gassy tummy needs? Bake a batch of Raisin Bran Muffins (page 263) instead.

know you're fitting in enough fiber and fluid when your stools are large and soft. (Frequency is less important than bulk and consistency). But also know when enough of a good thing becomes too much; an excess of fiber in the diet can lead to diarrhea (and a loss of much-needed nutrients).

▲ Drink up. Fluids keep digestive by-products moving efficiently through your system. So drink plenty of water or fruit juice—at least six to eight glasses a day. Keep in mind that a greater consumption of fiber increases your requirement for water; if there isn't enough water for it to soak up, fiber itself can be constipating. Take a water bottle with you wherever you go so you can sip the day away. (See page 100 for more tips on how to increase your fluid intake; also see drink recipes starting on page 423.)

▲ Befriend bacteria. The good kind, that is. The acidophilus in yogurt will stimulate the intestinal bacteria to break down food better, aiding the digestive tract in its efforts to keep things moving.

▲ Pass on the pills. If you are taking iron pills, they could be contributing to your constipation. Talk to your practitioner about switching

THE SCOOP ON POOP

▼ ▼ ▼

MYTH: You are constipated if you don't have a bowel movement every day.

FACT: Constipation is defined as the passage of small amounts of hard, dry bowel movements, usually less than three times a week, and often with difficulty and pain. Comrades in constipation include gas, bloating, and that "sluggish" feeling. Infrequent elimination is, by itself, not a symptom of constipation—and, in fact, there is no "right" number of daily or weekly bowel movements. Normal is what's normal for you—whether that's three times a day or three times a week.

to a slow-release formula or, if that still doesn't do the trick, staying off iron pills for a short time. He or she might also advise you to switch to a prenatal vitamin that contains less iron.

▲ Don't clog up the works. Actively avoid any food that is constipating, including refined baked goods and cereal (white bread, corn flakes), white rice, and bananas (the only fruit that is constipating instead of regulating).

▲ Check first. Ask your practioner whether taking a little extra magnesium would be a move that might get things moving. (There's no need to ask permission before adding to your diet magnesium-rich, constipation-

A PAIN IN THE REAR

▼ ▼ ▼

Constipation in pregnancy can cause or exacerbate hemorrhoids (which occur when rectal veins swell, bulge, or bleed due to increased pressure from either the enlarging uterus or excessive straining while having a bowel movement). Keeping constipation at bay will also help keep hemorrhoids away.

fighting foods, such as nuts, dried apricots, prunes, wheat germ, beans, and green leafies.) Don't take over-the-counter laxatives or herbal or home remedies without first consulting your midwife or doctor.

Gassiness

WONDERING HOW THAT BULGE around your belly can be so big when your baby is still so small? Chances are you can blame another unfortunate (and often embarrassing) by-product of pregnancy constipation: gas. Gassiness—and its uncomfortable buddy, bloating—often appears early in pregnancy, keeping waistbands from buttoning while baby's still pea-size. For some women, it's blessedly short-lived. For others, it can linger through the entire nine months.

And once again, you can blame that digestive relaxation. As the system that processes your food slows down, gas production (resulting in

FAST FACT

☑ Did you know that pregnant moms sometimes describe early fetal movements as "gas bubbles"? So if you're feeling lots of gas that you can't attribute to something you've eaten—and if you've already passed the 16th to 18th week of pregnancy, you just might be feeling your baby move!

TRY THESE INSTEAD

▼ ▼ ▼

By now you've probably uncovered yet another irony of pregnancy eating: Many of the healthy, nutrient-rich foods that best nourish your baby also make you so gassy that you feel too full to eat them. Don't give up. Not all healthy foods produce gas—and in most cases, you can find a substitute that gives you and your baby a nutritional edge, without bringing on the bloat.

INSTEAD OF	TRY
Baked beans for protein	¾ cup cooked couscous
Broccoli for vitamin A	¼ cup mango or cantaloupe
Coleslaw for vitamin C	½ cup cooked asparagus
Green pepper for vitamin C	6 strawberries

Fatty, fried foods and carbonated drinks also produce gas. Here are some substitutes:

Fried chicken fingers	Poached chicken breast
Potato chips	Soy chips, baked potato or taco chips, bagel chips
Sparkling water	Still water

flatulence) steps up. Constipation (and resultant bowel distention) compounds the bloating problem by keeping both stool and gas trapped inside the digestive tract.

Gas production won't harm you or your baby physically. (Socially is another matter.) But to diminish the discomfort and beat the bloat, you can try to do the following:

▲ Go slow. A slow digestive system calls for slower eating. Taking meals on the run (one hand filled with a breakfast burrito, the other with car keys as you dash out the door), tossing down snacks (trying to beat your nausea by chomping on some crackers while preparing supper and helping older children with homework), or mixing business with food pleasure (negotiating a crucial deal on a conference call while simultaneously negotiating a chicken sub) can lead to air swallowing. The gulped air forms pockets in the intestines that cause pressure, worsening your gas pains. Instead, make time for your meals and snacks (even if that means getting up ten minutes earlier in the morning or signing out for an actual lunch break) and take them sitting down. Chew well (to give your sluggish digestive system a head start), and try not to gulp.

▲ Avoid overload. Stuffing yourself will—obviously—only make you feel fuller and more bloated, while leaving your digestive system with too much to tackle. Eat small, frequent meals; try six meals over a day instead of three large ones.

▲ Keep it moving. By taking steps to keep your bowels moving (see tips, page 27), you'll also be helping your body stay gas-free.

▲ Phase in fiber. It's possible you're doing too much too soon in the fiber department, overtaxing your digestive system before it has a chance to adjust. Cut back a bit on high-fiber foods, and then gradually reintroduce them as your tummy acclimates.

▲ Ban the beans. At least until the gas eases up, steer clear of foods commonly associated with flatulence, such as onions, broccoli, cabbage, brussels sprouts, cauliflower, green pepper, fried fatty foods, and beans. (See tips on page 135 for making beans less gassy.) Avoid carbonated drinks, as well.

Heartburn

TO HEAR THE ANTACID COMMERCIALS tell it, you'd think heartburn was the exclusive territory of chili eaters and overstressed executives. But no one does heartburn like a pregnant woman (except, of course, a chili-eating, overstressed pregnant woman).

Despite its name, heartburn has nothing to do with your heart—though that's approximately the area where you'll feel that burning sensation when acid from the stomach leaks up into the esophagus. Normally, the esophagus acts as a one-way valve—allowing food to enter the stomach, but not letting anything back up. During pregnancy, however, the muscle at the top of the stomach that usually prevents digestive acids from splashing up relaxes (like all those other muscles in the tract), causing heartburn and indigestion.

More than one in four women experience heartburn at one time or another during pregnancy, most often (though not exclusively) in the third trimester. That's because as

HOW CAN YOU SPELL RELIEF?

▼ ▼ ▼

Don't feel like reaching for over-the-counter antacids? Here are some natural ways to prevent and alleviate heartburn:

■ Almonds have been touted throughout time as a stomach set-tler. (If nothing else, they'll provide you with a healthy dose of protein and calcium as well as baby-friendly fatty acids.)

■ A tablespoon of honey, mixed in a glass of warm milk, is an old-fashioned favorite for preventing heartburn. Some say dairy products in general, such as yogurt or milk, can also help; others claim these only exacerbate the problem. (Again, at the very worst, you'll still have the heartburn, but at least you'll have filled your calcium requirement.)

the baby grows, the uterus puts pressure on the stomach, crowding the digestive tract and allowing acids to travel back up where they don't belong.

Heartburn, like so many other pregnancy symptoms that bother you, will not hurt your baby. And as with so many other pregnancy symptoms, the best cure for heartburn is prevention. Taking these steps can help banish the burn:

▲ Take it slow. Eating quickly may save you time, but you'll pay in heartburn. So take a tip from your digestive system, and relax. Don't rush through your meals, and chew thoroughly (so that the stomach doesn't have to work so hard digesting your food).

▲ Take it early. Try to eat at least two hours before going to bed at night so your body has time to digest the meal. (An easy-to-digest light bedtime snack is fine, though.)

▲ Take it easy. Though heartburn is technically caused by a relaxed digestive tract, it's often related to stress; avoiding tension while you're eating may help prevent heartburn. Don't eat on the run, and try to make mealtimes as tranquil as possible.

▲ Keep it small. Large meals will stuff up your stomach, making it more likely that some of the food (and accompanying stomach acid) will find its way back up the esophagus. Yet another reason to eat small meals more frequently.

▲ Keep fluids separate. There's a place for fluids and a place for solids, but when you're suffering from pregnancy heartburn, there may not be a place for both at the same sitting. Drink before and after meals instead of with them, or just drink a little. Too much fluid mixed with too much food will distend the stomach, aggravating heartburn.

▲ Keep your head up. Sit in a comfortable upright position while you're eating. Don't eat while lying down (eat that bedtime snack propped up well with pillows) and avoid lying down, slumping, or stooping immediately after meals.

▲ Keep your weight on track. The heavier you are, the more pressure you place on your esophageal sphincter, the gatekeeper of the stomach. So try to gain your pregnancy pounds at the recommended pace (see Chapter Three).

▲ Don't pull the heartburn triggers. It doesn't take long to figure out which foods fire up the worst burn; once you do, you can eliminate them (at least temporarily) from your diet. Common culprits include highly seasoned spicy foods, alcohol (which you should be staying away from anyway), caffeinated drinks such as coffee, tea, and cola (because they also relax

wisdom of ☀ the ages?

If old wives are correct (and let's face it, they rarely are), a lot of heartburn during pregnancy means your baby will be born with a full head of hair. (And a taste for Tums?)

the esophageal sphincter), chocolate, mint, and citrus. A diet high in fat can also contribute to heartburn, so keep greasy foods to a minimum.

▲ Chew it away. Chew some sugarless gum for a half hour after meals to increase saliva production. Naturally alkaline, saliva helps neutralize the acid in the esophagus.

▲ Look for relief. An over-the-counter antacid that contains calcium (such as Tums or Rolaids) is safe to take during pregnancy and may keep the burn at bay while upping your intake of that important mineral. If your heartburn is severe, do check with your practitioner to see if there are other safe medications that might help.

Fatigue

USED TO BE, YOU NEVER MISSED *The Late Show,* but these nights you find yourself struggling to stay up for an eight o'clock sitcom. You used to breeze through your afternoon schedule of high-powered meetings; now your eyelids are drooping and your shoulders sagging before the clock strikes two. Your weekends were always packed with activities; now they're packed with catnaps. And like most pregnant

ABC's (AND DEF's) FOR FIGHTING FATIGUE

▼ ▼ ▼

Not only does *what* you eat have an effect on your energy level during pregnancy, so does *how* you eat. Here are some tried-and-true tips for the tired:

ADJUST THE SIZE OF MEALS. Filling your stomach to the brim at each meal will force much of your body's energy toward digestion, leaving the rest of you sluggish. Instead, eat smaller meals more often.

BREAKFAST LIKE A CHAMPION. Before you hit the starting gate, refuel your body after a foodless night with a good, complete breakfast that would make mom herself happy. Stay away from quick fixes that don't last (like sugar and caffeine) and stick to complex carbohydrates and proteins (whole-grain cereal and skim milk topped with banana; a whole wheat bread, tomato, and cheese melt) that will stay with you, keeping your blood-sugar level up and your body revved all morning.

CHEW ON LUNCH. You need lunch to refuel and prevent afternoon slumps. But don't lunch on just anything. As with your breakfast, your midday meal will last longer if it's filled with protein, whole grains, and healthy produce (whole-grain

pita stuffed with chicken salad, with a side of grapes; turkey and cheese on whole-grain bread with a cup of vegetable soup). See pages 265 to 279 for sandwich ideas.

DAYTIME EATING. Plan to consume most of your calories during the day instead of saving the biggest meal for dinner. Your body needs the most energy (and therefore the most food) when you're up and about, not when you're about to go to sleep. By stocking up on food when you're most active, you'll find your body reaps the most energy when it needs it most. Plus, you'll sleep better if you're not stuffed.

EAT BETWEEN MEALS. Snacks can give you an extra boost when you're starting to droop. Once again, snack sensibly, avoiding sugary treats and concentrating on those with protein and complex carbohydrates (yogurt and fruit; whole-grain crackers with cheese, nuts and dried fruit; see page 106 for more snack ideas).

FILL UP WITH FLUIDS. Fatigue has been linked to dehydration, so be sure you are getting enough fluids (but not the caffeinated kind) throughout the day.

women, especially in the first and last trimester, you're wondering where your "get up and go" has gotten up and gone.

The answer is simple. The energy you used to take for granted is now

being taken up with the monumental physical challenge of baby-making. Your body is working harder at rest these days than it used to work while you were on the go. In addition to nurturing a baby, you're fueling its factory. Your heart rate and metabolism are up. You're producing more blood. You're using up more water and nutrients. And if that's not enough to knock you down, higher levels of the hormone progesterone are circulating in your system, increasing fatigue.

Though the best cure for fatigue is getting more sleep (by both turning in earlier at night, and napping, if possible, during the day), there are also some dietary measures you can take to help pump up your energy levels during pregnancy:

▲ Extra calories. You need about 300 extra calories each day during the second and third trimesters (fewer during the first trimester) to help your body grow a baby. If you undercut this amount, your body will lack the strength it needs to do its job (see page 81).

▲ Extra nutrition. As important as making sure you get those extra calories is making sure they're packed with nutrients. It may sound obvious, but a healthy diet can be energizing. Being faithful about taking your prenatal vitamin will also help revive you.

▲ Extra sense. Don't fall for the candy-bar commercials that promise an "energy boost" to help you through those afternoon slumps. Though you might get a momentary lift from a candy bar, it'll soon be followed by a blood-sugar crash that will leave you

THE FLIP SIDE OF FATIGUE

▼ ▼ ▼

Could this be another pregnant paradox? You're so tired all day, you can hardly keep your eyes open; then you fall into bed and can't sleep? Ideas for the expectant insomniac include:

■ Take a light snack before turning in at night, such as warm milk (it contains the amino acid L-tryptophan, a sleep inducer) and oatmeal cookies. Another strange yet effective bedtime snack—turkey—contains the same supposedly soporific substance.

■ Limit fluids after 6 P.M. so you aren't being kept awake by frequent bathroom runs.

■ Avoid caffeine (in tea, coffee, or sodas) and chocolate in the afternoon so you're not all wound up when you're trying to wind down.

■ If your practitioner has prescribed a magnesium supplement for constipation, take it before bed. Magnesium has relaxing properties that can help you drift off (while warding off the leg cramps that can stand between you and a good night's sleep). Plus that laxative effect you're seeking will kick in just when you need it to . . . in the morning.

feeling more drained than ever. Caffeine, too, provides only a temporary pickup that can trick you into thinking your body doesn't need rest, when it really does. For a lift that lasts, turn instead to high-protein snacks, such as cheese and hard-cooked eggs (teamed up with a complex carb, such as an apple or a whole wheat roll for a mini-meal).

▲ Extra iron. Occasionally, extreme fatigue (as opposed to run-of-the-mill pregnancy fatigue) is related to iron-deficiency anemia. Your practitioner will recommend an iron supplement if blood tests show you are suffering from anemia. (Most practitioners advise that women begin taking iron supplements after twenty weeks as a precaution.) In the meantime, be sure your diet contains foods rich in iron, such as iron-fortified cereals, spinach, and lean red meat.

What's Eating You?
Maybe It's What You're Eating

EATING WELL ISN'T THE ANSWER TO every pregnancy complaint, but it can have a positive effect on a surprising number of aches, pains, and more pains. Here's a sampling of symptoms and how diet can help:*

Tooth and gum problems. Besides the obvious (see your dentist, brush your teeth at least twice a day, and floss regularly), making sure you get enough calcium and vitamin C will strengthen your own teeth and gums, and ultimately, your baby's, as well. When you're nowhere near a brush, munching on some cheese or nuts, or chewing on some sugarless gum, can do a good stand-in cleanup.

Dizziness. Going on empty for long stretches (something you're more liable to do in the afternoon, when many dizzy spells strike) can cause your blood sugar to dip, leaving your knees weak and your head spinning. So can dehydration. Snacking and drinking regularly to boost your blood sugar and keep yourself hydrated can ward off those woozy moments.

Leg cramps. Nothing cramps a good night's sleep like leg cramps, which keep many pregnant women tossing and turning in the second and third trimesters. And some say diet's at least partially to blame. One theory suggests that an excess of phosphorus and a shortage of calcium circulating in the blood trigger leg cramps. Another implicates a shortage of magnesium.

---

*Check out *What to Expect When You're Expecting* for nonfood remedies for these pregnancy symptoms.

Yet another indicts dehydration. To get a leg up on leg cramps, be sure your diet includes adequate calcium (see page 67) and magnesium (see page 69), as well as your eight daily glasses of fluids.

Swelling. A certain amount of swelling (also called edema) is normal and healthy during pregnancy; 75 percent of all expectant moms experience some. But too much water retention, especially when your shoes don't fit by the end of each day and you can barely stand on those puffy ankles, can prove uncomfortable, not to mention unsightly. Strangely enough, drinking extra water can keep you from retaining too much, by helping you flush out waste products.

Skin troubles. No matter what's wrong with the skin you're in, it's possible that diet has at least something to do with the cause or the cure. Dry skin? Maybe you're short on fluids; increase your intake to increase moisture. Flaky skin? Perhaps you're low on linoleic acid, an essential fatty acid (found in seeds, nuts, and legumes), or omega-3's (see page 98). Skin discoloration? A certain amount's normal during pregnancy, but too much blotchiness may be due to a folic-acid deficiency; make sure you're taking your prenatal supplement faithfully,

as well as eating plenty of green vegetables and whole-grain breads and cereals. Teenage-style breakouts? Hormones are the culprit (as they were when you were fifteen), and a vitamin B_6 supplement—which seems to help treat hormonally induced skin problems—may be the answer; check with your practitioner. Skin that's paler than usual? It could be a sign of iron-deficiency anemia; ask your practitioner, and make sure you're getting enough iron-rich foods. All-over skin blahs? Turn to sources of vitamin C, known to promote elasticity (and that glow you're supposed to be having).

Lackluster hair. Okay, it's not a physical pain—but it can definitely contribute to psychological discomfort. Though most women find their locks thicker than usual (pregnancy hormones prevent hair from falling out at its normal rate), some find it also lacks its usual luster. Others have trouble with flaky scalp issues. Maintaining an adequate intake of vitamins can help restore hair's shine: Vitamin A keeps hair supple and scalp healthy; the B vitamins are responsible for hair growth and color; and vitamin C is essential for strength (in other words, hair that doesn't break or split easily). Omega-3 fatty acids nourish hair and scalp. And since moisture is crucial for a healthy head of hair, be sure your fluid intake is adequate.

CHAPTER THREE

Healthy Weight Gain for Baby and You

IN TODAY'S THIN-OBSESSED SOCIETY, bestselling diet books fly off bookstore shelves so fast, the scientific research that supports their contents can't keep up. To many women, just the thought of "weight gain" is enough to send them running to the nearest gym.

But there is a time in a woman's life when weight gain isn't a dirty phrase—when putting on 30 pounds is something to be proud of, not depressed about. And that time, of course, is pregnancy. Achieving the recommended weight gain (between 25 and 35 pounds for the average woman) is important to ensure optimum fetal development, ward off pregnancy complications, and maintain maternal comfort. So pack away those weight-loss books (when was the last time they worked, anyway?) and get ready to embrace the next nine months of expansion.

How Much Should You Gain?

So, MAYBE YOU'RE UNNERVED watching the numbers on the scale creep upward. Or maybe you're overjoyed at finally having a legitimate reason to pile on the pounds. Either way, you're probably wondering just how much weight you'll be expected to gain over the next nine months. After all, you've heard of women gaining as few as 20, and as much as 70 . . . or even more. What's the right gain for you?

Since every pregnant woman—and every pregnancy—is different, one answer to that question doesn't fit all. Just how many pounds *you* should put on during pregnancy depends on a number of factors, including your height and your weight before you conceived. Your practitioner will probably recommend an ideal weight gain, possibly based on your body mass index (BMI, see next page). If your BMI is average—or close enough—he or she will probably suggest that you try to keep your weight gain between 25 and 35 pounds (the weight-gain total recommended for most pregnant women). If your BMI is well below average, meaning that you're considerably underweight, you may be advised to gain a little—or a lot—extra, about 28 to 40 pounds, which will compensate for the fat stores you don't have. If your BMI classifies you

as overweight, your doctor may advise that you gain somewhere between 15 and 25 pounds (because you'll have some extra fat stores to tap into); if you're obese, you may be told to limit your gain to about 11 to 20 pounds. If you're carrying multiples, the weight recommendations differ, too (see page 204).

Ideal recommendations aside, how much you actually gain—and how quickly you gain it—will depend on your metabolism, a little bit of genetics, and your level of activity. If you're very active and exercise often (or if you're blessed with a speedy metabolism), you'll need more calories to make up for the ones you burn—otherwise, you might end up gaining too little or too slowly. If you're more the sedentary type (you get most of your exercise from opening up the car door) or if you inherited a sluggish metabolism, you'll likely have the opposite problem—keeping too much weight from piling on too fast. In that unhappy case, you'll have to adjust calories downward, (or adjust activity upward, or both) to keep your gain on target.

Gaining Weight at the Right Rate

NOW YOU KNOW ABOUT HOW MUCH weight (give or take five or ten pounds) you should be planning to gain over the next nine months. But how quickly should you plan on gaining it?

Slow and steady wins this race, hands down. A gradual weight gain—

CALCULATING YOUR BMI

▼ ▼ ▼

The formula for calculating your BMI is:

[Weight (in lbs) ÷ height (in inches)^2] x 703

For example, a woman who is 5 feet 5 inches tall and weighs 145 pounds will have the following BMI equation:

First, figure out the inches: 5 feet 5 inches = 65 inches
Next, square 65 (multiply it by itself):
65 x 65 = 4,225 inches
Then divide the weight by the inches:
145 ÷ 4,225 = 0.0343
And multiply the result by 703: .0343 x 703 = 24.1

BMI	19	20	21	22	23	24	25	26	27
Height (in.)					Weight (lbs.)				
58	91	96	100	105	110	115	119	124	129
59	94	99	104	109	114	119	124	128	133
60	97	102	107	112	118	123	128	133	138
61	100	106	111	116	122	127	132	137	143
62	104	109	115	120	126	131	136	142	147
63	107	113	118	124	130	135	141	146	152
64	110	116	122	128	134	140	145	151	157
65	114	120	126	132	138	144	150	156	162
66	118	124	130	136	142	148	155	161	167
67	121	127	134	140	146	153	159	166	172
68	125	131	138	144	151	158	164	171	177
69	128	135	142	149	155	162	169	176	182
70	132	139	146	153	160	167	174	181	188
71	136	143	150	157	165	172	179	186	193
72	140	147	154	162	169	177	184	191	199
73	144	151	159	166	174	182	189	197	204
74	148	155	163	171	179	186	194	202	210
75	152	160	168	176	184	192	200	208	216
76	156	164	172	180	189	197	205	213	221

Once you've calculated your BMI (or, if you don't want to do the math, just check the chart below), you can determine what category you fall into:

■ If your BMI is less than 18.5, you're considered underweight.

■ If your BMI is between 18.5 and 26, you're considered average weight.

■ If your BMI is between 26 and 29, you're considered overweight.

■ If your BMI is greater than 29, you're considered obese.

28	29	30	35	40
134	138	143	167	191
138	143	148	173	198
143	148	153	179	204
148	153	158	185	211
153	158	164	191	218
158	163	169	197	225
163	169	174	204	232
168	174	180	210	240
173	179	186	216	247
178	185	191	223	255
184	190	197	230`	262
189	196	203	236	270
195	202	207	243	278
200	208	215	250	286
206	213	221	258	294
212	219	227	265	302
218	225	233	272	311
224	232	240	279	319
230	238	246	287	328

without any sudden drops or jumps—is best for both baby and you. In fact, the rate at which weight is gained is just as important as the total number of pounds put on. For that fetus of yours, which is growing constantly during its stay in the uterus, a continuous supply of nutrients and energy (in the form of calories) will guarantee the fuel needed for that growth. A significantly uneven weight gain pattern for you might mean an uneven supply of nourishment for baby—not an issue in the first trimester when baby is tiny, but definitely an issue in the second and third trimesters, when baby begins doing some serious growing.

But it's not just your baby who will benefit from a well-paced weight gain; you will, too. Your body will enjoy an easier adjustment to the increased poundage—and the physical strains that come with it—if those pounds are added gradually. And for those who hope to unpack the tight jeans and bikinis postpartum before they gather too much dust in the attic, there's another reason to make slow and steady their weight-gain motto: Pounds put on at a reasonable rate will result in fewer stretch marks, less flab, and better weight distribution (in other words, more inches in the baby-making belly, and fewer inches in the hips and thighs), and a speedier post-delivery return to prepregnancy shape.

It's important to understand that a steady pace doesn't mean that you'll need to spread your recommended

RATE OF WEIGHT GAIN

▼ ▼ ▼

BMI	First Trimester (Weeks 2 to 13)	Weekly Weight Gain for Weeks 14 to 40	Total Weight Gain
Underweight (BMI less than 18.5)	5 pounds	Slightly greater than 1 pound per week	28 to 40 pounds
Normal weight (BMI 18.5 to 26)	3.5 pounds	Approximately 1 pound per week	25 to 35 pounds
Overweight (BMI 26 to 29)	2 pounds	Approximately 2/3 pound per week	15 to 25 pounds
Obese (BMI greater than 29)	2 pounds	Approximately 1/2 pound per week	11 to 20 pounds

30-pound weight gain evenly over your 40 weeks of pregnancy. Early on in the pregnancy game, with baby as small and light as a grain of rice, weight gain should be minimal. In the first trimester, most women need to gain no more than a total of two to four pounds. (Some, particularly those who are suffering from morning sickness, may not gain at all, or may even lose some weight, while those who are underweight—or are just plain overeating—may gain considerably more.) As baby grows, so should mom. In the average pregnancy, weight gain should pick up to a rate of about one to 1½ pounds per week in months four through six (for a total of about 12 to 14 pounds), then drop

off again in the last three months to a pound or even less per week (for a total of about 8 to 10 pounds). In the home stretch of the ninth month, however, gain often slacks off (as baby's weight gain slows, and as mom reaches the beached-whale stage of pregnancy that makes eating—or doing anything comfortably—impossible). Some women gain only a pound or two during the last month, while others even lose weight during the last two weeks of their terms.

Will every pregnant woman follow this "model" formula precisely? Far from it. A woman who gets off to an enthusiastic start, with a substantial weight gain in the first few months, may slow down as the weeks

---

F A S T   F A C T

✔ Did you know that while much of the weight gained during your second trimester is caused by expanding tissues (including the growing placenta, maternal fat stores, breast tissues, and blood volume), during the third trimester it's your baby that's causing those numbers to inch up? After all, baby will double in size during the last trimester. At least now you have something (or someone) else to blame besides the ice cream.

---

to run out). And you'll have periods of above-average appetite (typically spurred on by baby's growth spurts). Women often enter the "hunger zone" as they transition from week 12 to week 14; as nausea suddenly lifts, appetite suddenly soars. But take care with this newfound appetite. Though it may be a relief to enjoy food again after so many weeks of avoiding it,

pass (and as she realizes that she's taking the phrase "eating for two" just a little too literally). Another may be too queasy to add an ounce, but do a good job of catching up once meals start staying down. Even a woman who minds her eating habits—and her scale—carefully from day one may find her gain fluctuating a little, from ½ pound one week in the second trimester, to 1½ the next. As long as your overall gain is on target and your rate averages out close to the model (without any huge dips or giant jumps), you're doing fine.

One reason why weight gain tends to fluctuate so much during pregnancy is that appetite varies. You'll find that hunger will come in peaks, valleys, and plateaus, and consequently, so will your food intake. You'll have periods of below-average appetite (most common in the first trimester, when nausea nips hunger in the bud, and in the last trimester, when tummy room starts

WEIGHT CHECK DO'S AND DON'TS

▼ ▼ ▼

DO check with your practitioner if you gain more than 3 pounds in any one week in the second trimester or if you gain more than 2 pounds in any week in the third trimester, especially if it doesn't seem related to overeating. Too much sudden and unexplained weight gain can indicate a pregnancy problem, such as preeclampsia.

DO check with your practitioner if you gain no weight for more than two weeks in a row during the fourth through eighth months.

DON'T obsess too much about your weight gain. If your practitioner is not concerned, you shouldn't be either. As long as you stick to a healthy diet, keeping efficiency in mind when choosing foods (see page 77), your weight gain will probably fall well within the recommended range.

proceed with caution. While it's extremely important to eat enough to nourish your baby—which is why nature has wisely presented you with hunger pangs—too much eating can lead to too many pounds.

The Downside of Too Little Weight Gain

MOST WOMEN WORRY MORE ABOUT gaining too much weight during pregnancy than too little. But actually, a weight gain that's too low is potentially more harmful to your baby and your pregnancy than a weight gain that's too high. Women who don't gain enough weight during pregnancy have an increased risk of:

**WEIGHT,
ME WORRY?**

▼ ▼ ▼

Does the thought of gaining weight during pregnancy (even if it's for the good of your baby-to-be) make you shudder—and then reach for the celery sticks? You're not alone. Many women become unnerved (or even physically ill) at the thought of adding any pounds anywhere. It's extremely important to work through weight-phobia before it can have a negative impact on your pregnancy and your growing baby, so remind yourself often: Pregnancy weight is both healthy and beautiful.

Preterm delivery. Women with low pregnancy weight gain are at an increased risk of delivering prematurely, particularly if they start out underweight or at average weight before pregnancy.

Babies with low birth weight. If you gain too little, your baby is at risk for slowed growth in the uterus and for being born small. Calorie restriction and inadequate weight gain during pregnancy are second only to smoking as risk factors for infant low birth weight. Low birth weight babies have a greater chance of health concerns and developmental problems.

Pregnancy complications. Low maternal weight gain is associated with an increased risk of amniotic fluid infections, abruptio placenta (separation of the placenta from the uterus before delivery), premature rupture of the membranes, damage to the placenta, and placenta previa (abnormal location of the placenta). These complications can lead to preterm labor and other serious complications.

The Downside of Too Much Weight Gain

IT'S CLEAR WHY GAINING TOO LITTLE weight while you're pregnant can be harmful to your baby's health and development. But going to the opposite extreme—piling on far too many pounds—presents its own problems. Most of the problems are mommy-centric, affecting the expectant mother, her health, and her comfort (though they can affect baby at least indirectly). Women who gain much more than the recommended amount of weight during pregnancy are at risk for:

An uncomfortable pregnancy. Pregnancy complaints multiply with the pounds. Excessive weight gain can contribute to just about every discomfort of pregnancy, from backaches to fatigue, leg pain to varicose veins, heartburn to hemorrhoids, breathlessness to joint pain.

Pregnancy complications. Gaining too much weight puts you at increased risk for developing hypertension and diabetes during pregnancy, as well as heartburn, chest infections, headaches, carpal tunnel syndrome, and symphysis pubis dysfunction. It also makes it hard to measure the fetus.

Labor and delivery complications. The heavier mom gets, the heavier (often) baby gets. Not surprisingly, bigger babies have a harder time exiting the traditional way than do ones of average size, increasing the chance that delivery will require instruments (forceps or vacuum) or that a cesarean will prove necessary.

Breastfeeding difficulties. One study found that women who gained more than the recommended 25 to 35 pounds during pregnancy were nearly 75 percent more likely to have breastfeeding difficulties. The more extra weight, the harder time they had.

Future obesity. Moms-to-be who gain more weight than recommended tend to retain twice as much weight after delivery as those who stay within the weight-gain guidelines. More weighty issues—researchers found that women who gain excessively and then fail to lose the extra weight within six months after giving birth are at a much higher risk of being obese a decade later.

Future health problems. Women who gain too much weight during pregnancy and don't take it off afterwards may be setting themselves up for a variety of potential health problems, including hypertension, diabetes, stroke, and heart disease.

So Where Does All the Weight Go?

AT THIS POINT YOU MAY BE ASKING yourself, If the average baby is born weighing between 7 and 8 pounds, and I'm supposed to gain 25 to 35 pounds, where will the rest of the weight be headed? Will I be wearing it on my arms? Padding my hips and thighs with it? Sporting it around my waist long after I have a pregnant belly to blame for it?

Not to worry. While some of those extra pounds are slated to end up in places you'd rather they didn't (you'll need to store up some reserves for labor and delivery, as well as for lactation), there's a lot more than maternal fat that goes into the making of a baby.

Although it varies from woman to woman, this is how those pounds may add up:

Average baby's weight: ...... 7½ pounds

Breast enlargement: .... 2 pounds

Placenta: .... 1½ pounds

Enlargement of uterus: .... 2 pounds

Amniotic fluid: .... 2 pounds

Your extra blood: .... 4 pounds

Your body's extra fat: .... 7 pounds

Your body's extra fluids: .... 4 pounds

Average total weight: .... 30 pounds

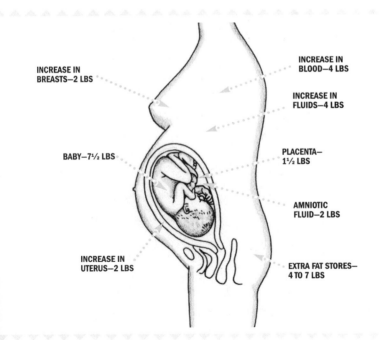

INCREASE IN BREASTS—2 LBS

INCREASE IN BLOOD—4 LBS

INCREASE IN FLUIDS—4 LBS

BABY—7½ LBS

PLACENTA— 1½ LBS

AMNIOTIC FLUID—2 LBS

INCREASE IN UTERUS—2 LBS

EXTRA FAT STORES— 4 TO 7 LBS

Weighing In

MOST WOMEN HAVE AN AMBIVALENT relationship (and that's being polite) with their scale; few look forward to weigh-ins, whether in the privacy of their bathroom or in front of a practitioner. Fortunately, weighing yourself daily during pregnancy isn't necessary. In fact, a once-a-week (or once-every-other-week) weigh-in will be a much more reliable tool in monitoring your gain than a daily one (weight can fluctuate too much from day to day, depending on a number of factors—from what you've eaten, to how much of it has come out). On the other hand, if you're not sure whether you're eating right, waiting until your practitioner's appointment for a monthly tally may be asking for trouble. (You might gain 10 pounds in a month—or none at all—without realizing it, throwing your total off target.)

If you feel compelled to step on the scales daily, write down what you weigh each day and at the end of the week, add the daily weights and then divide by seven to get a weekly average. This figure will give you a more accurate picture of your progress. And no matter how often you weigh yourself, make sure you do it at about the same time and approximately under the same conditions each day (before breakfast, for instance—naked, or with the same amount of clothing).

It's also best to weigh yourself consistently before or after having a bowel movement, if regularity permits. Also, be sure to compare weights only from the same scale. In other words, don't compare your weight on your home scale to your weight on the practitioner's scale. If you weighed in at home this morning at 135, but tipped the practitioner's scale at 140 by afternoon, don't panic—it's unlikely you put on 5 pounds in six hours. Keep that in mind before you fall off the scale in horror.

To get the most out of a partnership with your scale, you have to understand the eccentricities of the weight gain it registers. Don't expect to gain one-seventh of a pound daily in order to gain one pound a week, or exactly one pound per week to gain four per month. Small fluctuations, or even larger, short-term fluctuations are a normal part of the weight-gain process of pregnancy. A salty meal, or one especially high in bulk and water, can move the scale up a shocking two pounds overnight; a bout of diarrhea or an active day in the sun can make it slide back a pound or more. Both reactions are temporary, and are likely to disappear in a day or two, once normal fluid balance returns or once a full bowel empties out. When it comes to pregnancy weight gain, it's the big picture that counts.

PLOT YOUR WEIGHT GAIN

▼ ▼ ▼

As you'll find out, keeping track of anything when you're expecting becomes a challenge. That's why it may help to write down your weight gain as you go. Weigh yourself every week or two if you have a scale at home (or use your monthly weight check from your prenatal appointment). Then plot your gain on this graph. First, locate the number of weeks along you are in your pregnancy at the bottom of the graph. Then find your weight gain in pounds along the left side of the graph. Make a dot where the pounds meet the weeks. Play "connect the dots" to watch your rate of change.

	1st trimester	2nd trimester	3rd trimester
44			
42			
40			
38			
36			
34			
32			
30			
28			
26			
24			
22			
20			
18			
16			
14			
12			
10			
8			
6			
4			
2			
0			
-2			
-4			

WEIGHT GAIN

0 2 4 6 8 10 12 14 16 18 20 22 24 26 28 30 32 34 36 38 40 42

WEEKS

If You're Gaining Too Fast

HOW CAN YOU TELL IF YOU'RE gaining too much or too fast? Some research suggests that the first trimester gain is key: If you find you've piled on more than 3½ pounds at that 12-week milestone (2 pounds if you're overweight, 5 pounds if you're underweight), you may need to watch your diet (and your scale) more closely to keep those numbers from soaring out of the recommended range. But even a woman who ends her first trimester with a considerably higher net—and many women do, often because nausea leads them to scarf down comforting carbohydrates by the bag and boxful—can finish up her pregnancy well within healthy weight-gain limits. Which is why most practitioners won't worry about a slightly greater weight gain in the first trimester, especially if it has been gained largely on nutritious foods.

If you and your practitioner do decide that your first trimester (or any trimester) weight gain is on the fast track, following these tips can help slow it down a bit:

▲ Cut those calories. Though you should never try to actually lose weight while you're pregnant, you will need to slow the rate at which you're gaining. Apply some simple calorie-cutting strategies, aimed at delivering the most nutrition for the fewest calories. For instance, substitute skim milk for whole or low-fat milk; opt for fresh melon or strawberries instead of dried apricots or raisins; bake your fries; take the skin off your chicken, choosing a breast over a leg and roasting, poaching, or grilling it instead of frying or sautéing.

▲ Cut that fat. Some fat is essential in your pregnancy diet, but too much can add on those pounds faster than you can say, "Extra Value Meal." Try

POINTERS FOR THE PLUS-SIZED

▼ ▼ ▼

Some overweight women who are chronic dieters or who lost a substantial amount of weight close to becoming pregnant may actually gain excessive amounts of weight during pregnancy, even if they don't overeat. Some experts speculate that a body that's been through a recent weight loss may feel "starved" and may overcompensate during pregnancy for that earlier loss of fat by piling on the pounds. Tell your practitioner or a nutritionist about any prepregnancy weight loss and discuss with them a game plan for keeping pregnancy weight gain under control.

FIGHTING THE FAT WITH FACT

▼ ▼ ▼

MYTH: Cookies, muffins, chips, and frozen yogurts that are labeled "fat-free" won't make you gain weight.

FACT: Just because a bag of food is labeled "fat-free" doesn't give you the green light to reach the bottom of that bag in one sitting. Too many servings of fat-free foods can still add up to too many calories (from the sugar and the refined carbs often found in these items), causing you to gain too much weight too quickly. For a moderate weight gain, eat all foods—even the "fat-free" ones—in moderation.

MYTH: "Low-carb" foods aren't fattening, so you can eat as many as you like.

FACT: Turns out there really is no such thing as a free lunch—or, in this case, a free bag of chips, candy bar, or cheesecake. According to nutritionists, most low-carb products are still highly processed, non-nutritious foods that are often high in fat and, consequently, high in calories—definitely not a dieter's dream come true. What's more, low-carb products aren't designed for pregnant women (who actually need the carbs). So (low) carb your enthusiasm. If you do decide to indulge in an occasional low-carb treat, do so with your eyes (and not just your mouth) wide open to the facts (see page 78).

trimming a full fat-serving off your Daily Dozen requirement (see page 95) to see if that puts the brakes on your runaway gain. If it doesn't, trim another serving. Keep in mind that fat takes a variety of forms besides oil, margarine, and butter. Pay attention to those that may slip by unnoticed (those in the salad dressing, the gravy, the sautéed scampi, the fried eggs).

▲ Get active. Those extra pounds may be due less to your food intake and more to lifestyle. If you're a member in good standing (or sitting) of the couch potato club, you may need to get up (off the couch) and go. With your practitioner's approval, take several brisk walks around the block each day, join a prenatal exercise class, or follow the exercises described in *What to Expect When You're Expecting.*

▲ Keep your eyes open at the table. Paying attention *while* you're eating will help you keep track of *what* you're eating. It's too easy for one muffin to lead to another when you're munching them with your head in the morning paper, or for a few chips to lead to the whole bag when you're catching up on e-mail, or for that second portion of pasta to find its way to your plate when you're engrossed in a TV show. That's because when there's something on your mind other than what's going into your mouth, more is liable to end up in your mouth. Distracted eating leads to overeating. Slowly savor your food (taking the time to actually taste what you're chewing), and you'll feel satisfied with less.

▲ Check in with your practitioner. If you're eating sensibly, getting plenty of exercise, and still packing pounds on too quickly, it's possible you have a medical reason. Your practitioner may want to assess your thyroid function to determine if an imbalance in your metabolism is at the root of your weight-gain problem. Sudden rapid

QUICK F·I·X **WHEN YOU'RE FILLING OUT TOO FAST** If you're gaining weight too quickly, aim for dishes that pack few calories and a wallop of nutrition—while filling you up enough so you won't hunger for seconds.

weight gain (more than 3 pounds in a week in the second trimester or 2 pounds a week in the third trimester), especially when accompanied by swelling of hands and face, headaches, blurring of vision, or any combination of these, should be reported to your practitioner at once.

If You're Gaining Too Slowly

MORNING SICKNESS (HOW AM I supposed to get food down?) and early pregnancy bloating (if I do get it down, where am I supposed to fit it in my bloated tummy?) may have left your weight gain at a standstill or even dipping into the negative zone. That's nothing to worry about in the first trimester, when baby (and baby's needs) are still relatively tiny. Once you pass the first trimester milestone, though, it's essential that you start putting on the pounds. To get your weight gain going:

▲ Fatten up your diet. Since pure fat is the most concentrated source of food energy, increasing your intake by a serving or two a day will significantly increase your calorie intake without significantly decreasing your appetite. Don't increase your intake further, however; because fat supplies little but calories, there are more nutritious ways to step up weight gain.

▲ Don't be too efficient. Most pregnant women benefit from eating foods that supply them with the most nutrients for the fewest calories because most pregnant women don't have trouble gaining weight. If you're among the envied few to whom pounds don't come easy, such efficient eating may be counterproductive. To keep your scale on the upswing, favor foods with

IF YOU'VE GOT A LOT TO GAIN

Sure, you're the envy of all your pregnant friends who can't look at a bagel without putting on two pounds. But catching up on pregnancy gain when you've fallen behind isn't always as easy as it seems—especially for the weight-challenged. Serving up dishes that offer plenty of calories and plenty of nutrients (plus a little extra fat) can help. Try any of the following tasty dishes: Breakfast Burritos (page 244), Ginger Blueberry Whole Wheat Pancakes (page 251), Cozy at Home Macaroni and Cheese (page 306), Black Bean Quesadillas (page 275), Turkey Trio Sandwich (page 271), or Pork Quesadillas (page 346). Better still, add (or add extra) cheese, avocado, nuts, beans, or oil to any of them.

a more balanced ratio of nutrients to calories. Focus on concentrated sources of both, such as avocados, nuts, hard cheeses, beans, and split peas.

▲ Sneak in some snacks. Build snack breaks (one midmorning, one mid-afternoon, and one before bedtime)

into your schedule. Make the snack substantial in caloric content, but not substantial enough in volume to sabotage your appetite for the next meal. (See page 106 for some ideas).

▲ Slow down. If you're working out too much or too hard, you may be burning up the calories you eat instead of using them to nourish your body and your baby. So cut your exercise time down, and don't forget to compensate for the calories you do burn, by heaping your plate extra high with healthy foods. If a stressful job is keeping you on the run, make sure you slow down long enough for lunch and snacks.

▲ Check with your practitioner. This is important, especially if your slow weight gain doesn't seem related to undereating. A thyroid condition or some other undiagnosed medical problem may be keeping you from achieving your weight-gain goals and needs prompt attention.

If You're Gaining for Three … or More

MORE THAN ONE BABY ON BOARD? Then you'll be gaining faster than the typical expectant mother-of-one, right from the start—not only because you're housing two (or more) growing babies, but also because you're toting two placentas (unless your identical twins are sharing a large one). You'll also be carrying additional blood and fluid supplies, a larger (and heavier) uterus, and more amniotic fluid.

Your recommended weight gain will, not surprisingly, be substantially higher than that for a singleton pregnancy. If you're carrying twins and your prepregnancy weight (and BMI) was normal, it's recommended that you gain 37 to 54 pounds. If you started pregnancy overweight, aim to gain between 31 to 50 pounds. If you have triplets on board, your weight gain recommendations will be a little higher.

THE LONG ROAD BACK

▼ ▼ ▼

Gaining the weight is (usually) the easy part. It's losing all that weight after the baby is born that's often hard. Check out Chapter Ten for tips on how to shed the pounds postpartum.

wisdom of the ages?

Who needs sophisticated technology to distinguish the baby's sex? Old wives telling tales out of medical school have long held that how a pregnant woman's weight gain is distributed offers just as accurate an answer, and without filling out any insurance forms. According to their system, if the pregnancy weight gain ends up in your belly (and all out in front), you're carrying a boy. If it's spread out all over your body (with special mention to those X-chromosome favorites: hips, buttocks, and thighs), then you're carrying a girl, on her way to womanly proportions of her own.

But though such speculation is fun to pass around at parties, planning your nursery colors around it is risky business. The fact is that how you carry has far more to do with a variety of other factors (including your size, shape, genetics, diet, and rate of weight gain) than it does with the sex of your unborn baby. Like all unscientific methods of predicting a baby's sex used by old wives and others, this one has just about a 50 percent chance of being correct.

Loving Your Pregnant Body

WOULDN'T IT BE NICE IF EVERY pregnant woman gained just the right amount of weight—and each and every pound went directly to her cute little belly? Nice—but not realistic. For most women, the reality of pregnancy weight gain is that it ends up everywhere. Yes, plenty of the pounds you gain will go to rounding out your belly and your baby. But many will also end up rounding out your hips, thighs, cheeks (both kinds), and bust.

Some women make peace early on with their new Rubenesque full figures (complete with dimpled thighs), realizing that the extra inches they and others can pinch are there to ensure the health of their baby. Others, especially those who have struggled with weight issues before, might have a hard time adjusting to the Renaissance body image—feeling less beautiful and more bloated. For some women, pregnancy provides a welcome respite from constant weight worries—a time when it's actually okay to weigh more on Monday than they did on Friday. For others, pregnancy only exacerbates their weight-gain phobia; as the numbers on the scale climb, their self-esteem plummets.

Even if you have trouble welcoming weight gain, you can learn how to be proud of your pregnant body—dimpled thighs and all. Keeping these tips in mind may help prevent body-image struggles:

▲ Look the other way. If you're the type to obsess about your new curves (and you know who you are), make a conscious effort not to do so. Don't weigh yourself every week. Don't plot your weight gain on the graph in this chapter. Don't even peek at the scale at practitioner's visits—and should the nurse say the number out loud, hum loudly so you can't hear. If your doctor or midwife is satisfied with your weight progress, you should be, too. And if the wider view from

BOYS WILL BE BOYS

▼ ▼ ▼

Are you eating like a teenage boy? It could be you're carrying one—or at least, a baby boy on his way to becoming a teenage boy. According to researchers, women pregnant with boys tend to eat 10 percent more calories (approximately 200 calories), 8 percent more protein, and more carbohydrates and fat per day than those carrying girls. And the bonus—piling on those extra calories doesn't necessarily mean you'll be piling on extra pounds. Boy-carrying women don't gain more weight, on average, than girl-carrying ones do.

These findings may explain, in part, why boys are typically heavier than girls at birth. It also suggests a fascinating prenatal premise—that the fetus sends signals to its mother that drives her appetite during pregnancy (as in "Feed me, Mom—I'm hungry again!"). In other words, male fetuses require more calories for their optimal in-utero growth, so they send their moms to the refrigerator more often. Interesting science, and perhaps, a glimpse of refrigerator raids to come during those teenage years?

behind sends shudders down your spine, avoid the two-way mirrors in the maternity store.

▲ Eat right, and enjoy. For once in your life, take pleasure—not guilt—in your meals. Look at pregnancy as a chance not only to enjoy eating, but to enjoy eating healthily, too. Instead of counting every calorie, count your nutrients. And if you're concerned about the long-term effects on your figure, consider this: If your weight is gained on a diet of quality food, the pounds will be distributed far more efficiently—with more reaching the baby-making factory and fewer reaching your thighs. A win-win situation for you and your baby.

▲ Celebrate the shape you're in. Find ways to feel good about your changing body. Take a prenatal exercise class; not only will you be able to stay toned (which will help you feel better about your figure), but you'll also be able to share your feelings about your body image with other pregnant women. Look for maternity clothes that hug your pregnant curves, instead of trying to hide them. (Belly-flaunting outfits are more flattering—and slimming—than tents, anyway.) Take monthly snapshots of your growing silhouette to document your pregnant progress.

▲ Remember who you're gaining for. Your gain, literally, is baby's gain.

As long as you stay within the recommended guidelines, each and every ounce you put on has a purpose in pregnancy—nourishing that beautiful baby of yours. And that's something to cheer.

▲ Remember it's not forever. Pregnancy may sometimes seem like it's going to last a lifetime (especially when you're midway through the ninth month), but it's only a temporary state. With the birth of your baby (and a few postpartum months later) will come the return of your old body.

▲ Seek support. Let your spouse know that you could use some help feeling better about your figure. (Men almost always find the pregnant shape incredibly sensuous, yet often forget to mention that to the very person who's yearning to hear it.) Swap feelings with other pregnant women or with women who've been pregnant before. If that doesn't help you conquer your negative feelings about weight gain, consider talking to a therapist who deals with body-image issues.

▲ ▲ ▲

Q *"My midwife told me I should gain 3 to 4 pounds by the end of the third month. I'm 12 weeks pregnant now and not only have I not gained the right amount, but I've actually lost 5 pounds. I'm worried for my baby."*

A For many women, gaining weight in the first trimester is a piece of cake (make that many pieces of cake). For others, particularly those suffering from food aversions and morning sickness, it's a struggle. In fact, some, like you, find the numbers on the scale slipping back when they should be inching forward.

Lucky for you and your still very tiny baby, the fetal need for calories isn't as great during the first three months of pregnancy as it is during the next six months. So no harm done. That said, now that you've passed the 12-week mark, you'll need to work hard at compensating for your early weight loss by gaining weight at a slightly faster clip (which will become easier as baby gets bigger and you get hungrier). A diet rich in nutritionally dense foods should help, especially if your appetite is still tender. (Follow the tips on page 51.)

Q *"I'm 34 weeks pregnant, and I've already gained the recommended amount of weight. Can I start dieting now to get a jump start on getting my body back to my prepregnancy shape?"*

A There's no time in pregnancy that's the right time for dieting. Though you may have reached your weight gain goal, your baby hasn't— and he or she will continue to need a steady flow of calories and other nutrients until delivery day, courtesy of what you eat. Keep in mind, too, that while you're winding down pregnancy-wise, baby has plenty more to do to get ready for birth. Calcium is being laid down in his or her bones (which means you need to keep drinking that milk or eating that cheese and yogurt). Eye, brain, and nerve development are being completed—work that requires plenty of healthy fats, especially omega-3 fatty acids (see page 98). Baby is also putting on the pounds in the last trimester; cut back on those calories now, and he or she might not gain enough.

But that doesn't mean you can't slow down your weight gain some (especially if it has been a little on the swift side). Eat efficiently, to ensure you're getting the most nutrients for the calories you take in, and follow the other tips on page 49.

▼ ▼ ▼

The Nutrients That Make a Baby

YOU SEE THEM ON FOOD LABELS EVERYWHERE: Daily Value (DV) or Dietary Reference Intake (DRI)—formerly known as Recommended Dietary Allowances (RDAs). The fine print that lets you know (if you can read it) what a product's made of nutritionally—how much protein, fat, carbohydrates, and sodium it contains, as well as which vitamins and minerals it provides.

Just about every food on supermarket shelves has some nutrients naturally occurring, and many these days (from bread to pasta to cereal) are heavily fortified in the factory. On top of all those you'll be consuming through your diet, there's the long list posted on the side of the prenatal vitamin supplement your practitioner recommended (try reading that one without a magnifying glass). But as you toss that box of granola bars (2 grams of protein, 25 percent

of the DV of thiamin, 10 percent of iron) and that bag of frozen strawberries (35 percent of the vitamin C, 15 percent of the vitamin A) into your shopping cart, you might be wondering, what, exactly, all these nutrients you're eating every day do for you. And, more important, what do they do for you and your baby when you're pregnant?

The Pregnancy Diet outlined in Chapter Five details how many servings of each food group you'll need to net the nutrients necessary to ensure the healthy progress of your pregnancy. But for those curious about what's behind those nutrients, about what makes them so vital to the growth and development of a fetus—about the role they play in the making of a baby-to-be—read on for all the details.*

A Baby in the Making

IN APPROXIMATELY 266 DAYS, YOUR baby transforms from a single cell to a complete human being. During that time, miraculous changes are occurring, sometimes on an hourly basis, from the formation of crucial organs (heart, lungs, stomach) to the formation of vital systems (digestive system, urinary system, circulatory system), from the development of arms and legs (including those tiny fingers and toes!) to the development of the central nervous system and brain. Here are some highlights of that transformation:

The First Trimester. Soon after sperm meets egg, the fertilized ovum begins dividing rapidly as it moves down your fallopian tube. Approximately seven to ten days post-conception, the bundle of cells (already more than 100), implants in your uterus. The outer cells will form the placenta; the inner cells (made up of three layers) will form your baby.

The newly implanted embryo is already starting to specialize. The outer layer (the ectoderm) will develop into the brain, nervous system, hair, and skin. The middle layer (the mesoderm) develops into the muscle, bones, cardiovascular, and excretory systems. The inner layer (endoderm) will develop into the digestive tract, lungs, and glands. As your pregnancy progresses, your baby develops a rudimentary brain and the beginnings of a spinal column. The heart starts to beat somewhere around the middle of the fifth week. Arm buds and leg buds begin to form. As the embryo grows to the size of a grain of rice, the liver, kidneys, and thyroid gland become visible. The eyelids begin to appear and the nose, ears, lips, teeth, gums, and jaws are taking shape. Toward the middle of the first trimester, the kidneys begin to function, blood forms in the liver, and the stomach begins to produce some digestive juices. By the time the fetus has reached the size of a coffee bean, your baby's skeleton has already

---

*For more on DRIs, check out the USDA's Food and Nutrition Information Center: fnic.nal.usda.gov; or the Institute of Medicine of the National Academies: www.iom.edu.

THE PLACENTA AT WORK

▼ ▼ ▼

The placenta is what makes the making-of-a-baby possible—sort of the mission control of the baby factory. A complex network of blood vessels and tissues attached to the uterine lining and to the baby via the umbilical cord, the placenta contains two blood supplies: yours and baby's. These blood supplies communicate but never touch.

The placenta takes on several important roles, including producing several of the hormones that regulate growth and development. But its most significant function is as a vital pipeline, shipping nutrients from you to your baby and waste products from your baby back to you for disposal. Here's how that pipeline works.

When you eat something, your body digests it, taking available nutrients and transferring them into your bloodstream.

Once your body takes what it needs, it sends the rest of the nutrients to the placenta, where the fetus's blood vessels distribute them, along with fluids, oxygen, and other important substances. After baby's been fed, the placenta deposits waste products that are eventually shipped back for excretion via your kidneys.

As baby grows, the placenta grows, but not without help from you. The growth of your baby's placenta is directly related to your food intake. A better-nourished mother produces a bigger, more productive placenta.

Remember, too, that wholesome nutrients aren't the only thing that can be shared between mother and baby through the placenta. Harmful substances, such as alcohol, tobacco, and drugs, travel the same route.

---

formed, and the fingers and toes are taking shape. Fingerprints appear, and internal organs continue to mature. By the end of the first trimester, your baby, looking more like a human being now, can make facial expressions. Vocal cords are developing, bones are beginning to calcify, nails are forming, and the beginnings of teeth are present. Sexual organs are also developing.

The Second Trimester. Bones continue to develop and harden, causing the fetus to straighten from its curled position. Hair is beginning to grow, and muscles are more developed. (You'll probably begin feeling those first kicks sometime around the sixteenth to twentieth week.) Your baby can hear by the sixth month, and will react to loud noises with a startle. Lanugo (a downy coat of hair) appears on the skin, as does vernix caseosa, a waxy covering that protects the baby's skin during its long soak in an amniotic bath. By the end of the second trimester, the fetus has regular periods of wakeful-ness and sleep and is making more coordinated movements; its eyes open and close, reacting to light. A baby boy's testicles begin their descent from the abdominal cavity and into the scrotum.

The Third Trimester. Your baby will gain an average of one-half to three-quarters of a pound each week during this trimester (almost as much as you're gaining). As the ounces accumulate, baby fat develops under the skin, filling out that cute little form and ironing out that wrinkled look. Head hair is starting to fill in (more in some babies than in oth-ers), eyebrows and eyelashes are pre-sent, and nails are already set for a manicure, having grown beyond the tips of the fingers and toes. The lungs and the digestive tract are reaching the final stages of maturity, but the most remarkable growth is in the brain, which is working overtime on its development. Your baby's immune system is also get-ting stronger. And 40 weeks or so after the amazing transformation began, it's showtime: Baby is ready to be born.

From A to Zinc: Encyclopedia of Vitamins and Minerals

FEW PEOPLE DIGGING INTO THEIR morning oatmeal or tucking into their lunchtime sandwich give a first—never mind a second—thought to the vitamins and minerals they're about to absorb. But every food you eat contains at least some of these essential elements (some foods obvi-ously contain more than others), each of them so vital to sustaining your health and your life. During preg-nancy, their mission becomes even more important, as they fuel the needs of two bodies, including one rapidly growing one. As a result, you'll need to take in more of these vita-mins and minerals than ever before. You'll get a good supply from your prenatal vitamin-mineral supplement, but you'll benefit even more from get-ting plenty of each from their natural sources. Being more conscious of where vitamins and minerals come from can help you meet that goal. And knowing how each vitamin and mineral contributes to making a healthy baby can make you a more educated consumer—and diner. Here's a guide to the most important nutrients your body needs.

Vitamins

YOU ALREADY KNOW that, as a pregnant woman nourishing a growing baby, you have a higher vitamin requirement than other adults do. But where are they all supposed to come from? Since only three kinds (D, K, and the B vitamin biotin) can be manufactured in the body from nondietary sources, most vitamins must be provided by your diet or by supplements. That's why you'll have to eat well while you're expecting, and why you'll also have to take a prenatal vitamin-mineral supplement.

Vitamins get around in your body, and your baby's, playing numerous important roles. They're active in metabolism, in cell production, in tissue repair, and in a variety of other vital processes. They also help convert carbohydrates, fats, and proteins that you eat into energy. (Vitamins themselves are not sources of energy.) Quite simply, you can't live without them, and neither can your baby.

Vitamins are either fat-soluble or water-soluble. Fat-soluble vitamins (A, D, E, and K) can be stored in the body; a buildup of these vitamins, especially vitamins A and D (which might occur if you take these as megadose supplements), can be dangerous. Water-soluble vitamins (B and C) dissolve in water and therefore cannot be stored in the body. Your body uses what it needs for the day and then eliminates the rest via urine. So, water-soluble vitamins must be replenished daily.

Vitamin A. Vitamin A is a powerhouse of a nutrient—essential to so many aspects of baby-making, including the growth and development of cells, bones, skin, eyes (especially important for night vision), teeth, and immunities. Too little vitamin A in a mom's diet has been linked to premature delivery and to slow growth in her baby, as well as to skin disorders and eye damage. But as with other fat-soluble vitamins, too much of a good thing can also present a problem. When taken in extremely high doses for long periods of time, vitamin A can be toxic; pregnant women who take very high doses of vitamin A (beyond what is included in a prenatal supplement) may increase the risk of birth defects in their unborn babies. But don't worry if you're a big eater of broccoli, carrots, and other vitamin A–rich foods—you can't get too much vitamin A from your diet.

The DRI for vitamin A during pregnancy is 770 ug—and it's easy to obtain what you need from a well-balanced diet, though your prenatal supplement will offer a safe bonus. Good sources include dairy and other animal products, spinach, kale, green leafies, orange and yellow vegetables (such as carrots, winter squash, sweet potatoes, and pumpkins), red pepper, oatmeal and other whole

WHAT'S AN UG?

▼ ▼ ▼

Maybe you're wondering how many bananas you'll need to eat to reach your goal of 1.9 mg of vitamin B₆ or how many carrots equal 770 ug of vitamin A. And now you're also probably wondering, What the heck is an "ug"?

Food labels (see page 146) give you a lot of the information you need to ensure you're filling your mg and ug requirements—if you're willing to struggle through the fine print. Better still, the Daily Dozen (page 81) lets you dispense with all the ug, mg, and mcg measurements and makes meeting your nutritional needs much easier—not to mention easier on your eyes.

But, if you're still curious, this chart should help make sense of what all these measurements mean:

g	gram	A unit of weight equal to about 0.03 ounces.
mg	milligram	One-thousandth of a gram
mcg	microgram	One-millionth of a gram
ug	same as mcg	One-millionth of a gram

Now for some perspective: A paper clip weighs one gram. A single grain of salt is equal to approximately 120 mcg or 120 ug. (770 ug isn't looking so daunting after all, is it?)

So when you read that the DRI for vitamin B₆ in pregnancy is 1.9 mcg, it's reassuring to know that all you need to meet your requirement are one banana and a bowl of cereal. See, that's not so bad (especially after you factor in all the other nutritional requirements you've met with that same bowl of cereal and banana).

grains, wheat germ, cantaloupe, mangoes, and apricots.

Vitamin B₁ (thiamin). Thiamin is essential for converting carbohydrates into energy, is responsible for regulating the supply of carbohydrates to your baby (critical for brain development), is involved in the pro- duction of red blood cells (which you and your baby need plenty of), and helps in the normal functioning of the nervous system. It also pro- motes normal appetite—something that can definitely come in handy when you're trying to eat healthily and heartily for two. Deficiencies can cause fatigue and weakness in the mother and impaired growth and heart irregularities in the baby.

The DRI for thiamin during pregnancy is 1.4 mg. Good sources include oatmeal, wheat germ, dried beans, peas, peanuts, raisins, cauliflower, corn, nuts, and sunflower seeds.

Vitamin B₂ (riboflavin). Riboflavin helps release energy (something every pregnant woman can always use more of) from fats, proteins, and carbohydrates. Adequate intake of riboflavin aids in cell division (remember, baby's cells are dividing at a remarkable rate), and in the growth and repair of tissues. It also stabilizes appetite and promotes healthy skin and eyes for you (and the development of healthy skin and eyes for baby), while boosting brain growth (making a steady supply especially important in the third trimester). Deficiencies of this vitamin can cause poor bone formation, anemia, poor digestive function, and a suppressed immune system in the fetus as well as poor appetite and mouth sores for mom.

The DRI for riboflavin during pregnancy is 1.4 mg. You'll find it in liver, milk, yogurt, cottage cheese, eggs, chicken, mushrooms, peas, and beans.

Vitamin B₃ (niacin). Not only is niacin involved in releasing much-needed energy from the foods you eat, but it's also a factor in increasing blood flow—and thus the circulation of nutrients to your baby—by widening blood vessels. Adequate intake of niacin fosters a healthy nervous system and digestive tract for the fetus and promotes healthy skin. But beware of overdoses, which can cause mom to suffer itchy skin (something pregnant women definitely don't need more of) and stomach problems (something else pregnant women don't need more of).

The DRI for niacin during pregnancy is 18 mg. Good sources include: meats, fish, chicken, veal, lamb, salmon, peanuts, and mushrooms.

> **F A S T   F A C T**
>
> ✓ Exposure to light and air can destroy riboflavin, so make sure foods filled with riboflavin (like yogurt and milk) are kept tightly sealed.

Vitamin B₆ (pyridoxine). Pyridoxine helps the body use protein to build tissue—a very good thing when there's so much tissue to build. Because it specifically has an effect on those proteins that play a role in the brain and nervous system, adequate intake of pyridoxine reduces the risk of neural tube defects. It also helps form red and white blood cells. And an added bonus: B₆ has been shown to reduce morning sickness symptoms, as well as help clear up skin unsettled by pregnancy hormones. Deficiencies may cause skin problems in the newborn.

DON'T DO THE MATH

▼ ▼ ▼

Just skimming through this chapter, you can clearly see how vitamins, minerals, and other nutrients help build a healthier baby. But remember that good nutrition is not just about numbers; it's about food. So before you whip out your calculator to see if your DRIs for this mineral or that vitamin add up—sit back and continue reading. The Pregnancy Diet in Chapter Five does all the calculating for you. Follow the guidelines there (no need to do the math), and you and your baby will get your share of every nutrient, from A to zinc. Use the recipes in Part Two, and you'll get more eating enjoyment in the bargain, too.

The DRI for pyridoxine during pregnancy is 1.9 mg. Feasting on many of your favorites will ensure that intake: bananas, avocado, wheat germ, brown rice, bran, soybeans, oatmeal, chicken, beef, veal, lamb, potatoes, tomatoes, spinach, and watermelon.

Vitamin B₇ (biotin). Biotin is involved in the production of amino acids and helps digest fats, carbohydrates, and proteins. The rapidly dividing cells of the developing fetus require biotin for DNA replication. Deficiencies can exacerbate several pregnancy symptoms, including fatigue, nausea, skin problems, and muscle pain. It can also trigger something that isn't common during pregnancy: hair loss.

The DRI for biotin during pregnancy is 30 ug. You'll find biotin aplenty in many favorites, including peanuts, nuts, eggs, soybeans, mushrooms, peas, avocados, cauliflower, milk, bananas, tomatoes, and whole grains.

Vitamin B₁₂. Vitamin B₁₂ is important for the formation of red blood cells, for building genetic material, and for the proper development and functioning of the nervous system —in other words, for the making of a healthy baby. It also partners with folate (see next page) to help with proper fetal development. Deficiencies can cause neural tube defects (spina bifida), digestive tract disorders, or neurological disorders in the fetus and fatigue in the mother.

The DRI for pregnant women is 2.6 ug. The only natural dietary sources are animal products, including meat, eggs, dairy products, and fish. If you're a vegan you'll need to get your vitamin B₁₂ from supplements or sources like nutritional yeast or B₁₂-fortified soy milk.

Choline. Part of the family of B vitamins, choline is essential for fetal brain and neural tube development and for learning and memory. (You'll appreciate this most when pregnancy forgetfulness kicks in.) Low levels of choline during pregnancy increase the risk of birth defects in the newborn. Excessive doses can cause intestinal problems.

The pregnancy DRI for choline is 450 mg. Sources include peanuts, eggs, broccoli, cauliflower, wheat germ, soy beans, and meats.

Folate (folic acid). Here's the one that's been making headlines. Another B vitamin, folic acid is crucial in preventing neural tube defects in the fetus during early pregnancy. In fact, studies show that low levels of folate in the first months of pregnancy are responsible for about 70 percent of all neural tube defects (which is why your prepregnancy diet is important, too). But an adequate intake of folate during pregnancy does more than prevent birth defects. It also aids in cell division and in the formation of red blood cells (yours and baby's), and in later pregnancy is associated with a lower risk of growth restriction and an increased birth weight, as well as a lowered risk of premature birth, and possibly preeclampsia. Some research has suggested that adequate folate intake might help prevent Down syndrome. Other research suggests that too little folate during pregnancy may be linked to ADHD in the child later on. A deficiency in folate can also cause anemia in the mother, leaving you tired and rundown. (Aren't you tired enough already?)

Aim to consume 600 mcg of folic acid daily both before (if possible) and during pregnancy. Sources include avocados, bananas, orange and grapefruit juice, asparagus, most fruits and leafy green vegetables, lentils, black-eyed peas, beans, peas, and spinach. Most grain products are also fortified with folic acid.

Pantothenic acid. Pantothenic acid is important for the metabolism of fats, carbohydrates, and proteins and the production of steroid hormones. It also regulates the body's adrenal activity, is involved in the production of antibodies, and stimulates wound healing. Deficiencies can cause impaired coordination and sleep disturbances in the mom and slow growth in the baby.

The pregnancy DRI for pantothenic acid is 6 mg. Sources include meats, milk, eggs, oranges, potatoes, broccoli, whole grains, mushrooms, and green leafies.

Vitamin C. It's probably the first vitamin you ever heard of (as your mother urged you to finish your orange juice), and possibly the most important one, too. Vitamin C's list of accomplishments is long. For one thing, it's essential to the production of collagen. This protein is what gives structure and strength to a developing baby's cartilage, muscles, blood vessels, and bones; it's also found in skin and eyes. For another, it's needed (by both you and baby) for tissue repair, wound healing, and various other metabolic processes. And if that's not enough, vitamin C also helps in the absorption of iron and may help you to resist infection. Adequate doses of vitamin C have been linked to a healthy birth weight and a decreased risk of premature rupture of the membranes. Deficiencies of vitamin C can cause scurvy (rare these days) and periodontal disease (which pregnant women are more susceptible to anyway, and which can trigger preterm labor). Low intake may also lead to premature delivery and a higher risk of preeclampsia.

The DRI for vitamin C during pregnancy is 85 mg. Besides the obvious orange, sources include other citrus fruits, asparagus, broccoli, brussels sprouts, raw cabbage, cauliflower, kale, red and green peppers, snow peas, sweet potatoes, tomatoes, apples, cantaloupe, cranberries, honeydew, kiwifruit, mangoes, papayas, peaches, strawberries, and watermelon.

Vitamin D. Essential for maintaining healthy teeth and bone structure, vitamin D helps in the absorption of calcium and is especially important during pregnancy. A deficiency of vitamin D can lead to rickets (a softening of bones), muscle disease, and seizures in the newborn, as well

as to preeclampsia and an increased risk for a C-section. Women who get enough D are less likely to go into preterm labor, deliver prematurely, or develop infections.

The current daily DRI for vitamin D is 200 to 400 IU, but many experts say that's far from high enough—and that most pregnant women should be getting much more of this vital vitamin. While the body produces vitamin D when exposed to sunlight, making enough can be challenging—especially for those with darker skin and those who live in less-sunny climates, don't get outdoors enough, or who wear sunscreen. Can you eat (or drink) your D? Not easily, since it isn't found in large amounts in any food. Fortified milk and juices contain some, as do sardines and egg yolks, but not nearly enough to prevent a D deficit. Your best bet is to ask your practitioner about testing your vitamin D levels to see if you're deficient, and filling in any shortfall with a supplement.

Vitamin E. Vitamin E helps ward off cell-membrane damage. Research shows that pregnant women who take enough vitamin E are less likely to experience premature rupture of the membranes. There is also evidence that adequate intake of vitamin E during pregnancy may help prevent allergies in the developing child (though more study needs to be done). Too much vitamin E from

much vitamin E from supplements can be dangerous, so be sure to get your E from food sources and from your prenatal supplement only.

The DRI for vitamin E during pregnancy is 15 mg. Get your fill from vegetable oils, sweet potatoes, avocados, spinach, asparagus, mangoes, prunes, almonds, peanuts, hazelnuts, and sunflower seeds.

Vitamin K. Vitamin K is essential for blood clotting and prevents excess blood loss after injuries (and after childbirth). It also maintains healthy bones and helps to heal bone fractures. Lack of sufficient vitamin K can cause easy bleeding and bruising in both you and the baby. Too much vitamin K (which you could only get from oversupplementation) can be toxic. Because little vitamin K gets transferred from mom to fetus during pregnancy, newborn babies receive a vitamin K injection soon after birth.

The DRI for vitamin K during pregnancy is 90 ug. Good sources include canola oil, olive oil, beef, broccoli, turnip greens, green leafies, oatmeal, bran, green apples, asparagus, avocado, blueberries, and bananas.

Minerals

VITAMINS MAY GET ALL the media buzz. But you wouldn't get very far without minerals—elements that are necessary for the health and proper functioning of so many systems in

wisdom of ☼ the ages?

Here's a tart tall tale from the old wives' club: Drinking limewater frequently while you're pregnant builds strong teeth in the unborn baby. There's only one problem with that one. Even if it did strengthen baby's teeth (and it does not), it might weaken yours. (The acid from the limes can wear away enamel over time, unless, of course, you brush after drinking.) For a drink that's good for baby's teeth and yours, pour yourself a glass of milk instead.

your body. Though they tend to get lumped together with vitamins (did your mother ever tell you to "take your minerals"?), minerals are different, and they're important in different ways. The body (including your baby's body) contains about twenty-five essential minerals. Not surprisingly, the need for certain minerals increases when you're pregnant.

Calcium. Calcium is best known for its contribution to strong bones and teeth (including tiny baby bones and teeth). But this vital mineral is also necessary for muscle contraction, blood clotting, and normal heart rhythm, as well as nerve development and enzyme activity. While mom gets priority when it comes to most vitamins and minerals, when calcium intake is inadequate, her bones will be drained to supply calcium to the growing fetus. Still, deficiencies can cause bone problems for both mother and baby. Another reason to get milk while you're expecting—optimal calcium intake has been associated with a decreased risk of preeclampsia and lower blood pressure in the baby.

The DRI for calcium during pregnancy is 1,000 mg. Besides that glass of the white stuff, you can claim calcium from yogurt and other dairy products, sesame seeds, tofu, almonds, fortified fruit juice, dried figs, green leafies, sardines, canned salmon with bones, and broccoli.

Chromium. Chromium works with other substances to control insulin and maintain the normal regulation of blood sugar—a process that's so important during pregnancy, when baby needs a steady supply of fuel for growth and development. This versatile mineral also stimulates the synthesis of protein in the fetus's tissues and is necessary for baby's muscle strength, brain function, and immunity. Deficiencies can lead to weight loss and poor blood glucose control in the mother (which can then lead to gestational diabetes) and glucose intolerance in the baby.

The DRI during pregnancy is 30 ug. Sources include cheese, whole grains, chicken, meat, spinach, mushrooms, peas, and beans.

Copper. Copper allies with iron to form red blood cells (though iron usually gets all the credit). It also aids tissue growth, glucose metabolism, and growth of healthy hair and

is essential for the development of the fetus's heart, arteries, blood vessels, skeletal system, brain, and nervous system. Deficiencies can cause seizures and neurological abnormalities in the baby.

The DRI for copper during pregnancy is 1,000 ug. You can cash in on copper by eating potatoes, dark leafy greens, mushrooms, prunes, lobster, crab, barley, dried beans, brown rice, nuts, and seeds.

Fluoride. Everyone knows that fluoride is important for maintaining good dental health and for preventing tooth decay. What you may not know is that it's good for bones, too. Fluoride doesn't work alone; it acts as a bonding agent for calcium and phosphorus. Since baby is busy building both bone and teeth during pregnancy, getting enough fluoride is important for him or her. It's also important for you; deficiencies can cause tooth decay. Too much fluoride can cause fluorosis, especially in young children.

The DRI for fluoride during pregnancy is 3 mg. And you won't just find it in your toothpaste. It also shows up in tea, kale, spinach, milk, canned fish with bones (but only if you eat the bones), and treated tap water.

Iodine. Iodine is a component of the hormone thyroxine (which regulates the body's metabolism). It is needed for the proper function-ing of the thyroid gland and for reg-ulating maternal basal metabolic rate, and is necessary for nervous system development in the baby. Deficiencies can cause thyroxine lev-els to drop, causing a condition called goiter in the mother and pos-sibly in the fetus, as well. Some evi-dence also links low iodine intake with a decline in IQ for baby or learning problems later on.

The DRI for iodine during pregnancy is 220 ug. Most people get what they need from iodized salt, but the mineral is also available in seafood and some milk products.

Iron. Getting enough of this min-eral—so vital to the production of red blood cells and the distribution of oxygen throughout the body—is one of the greatest nutritional chal-lenges known to women during their childbearing years. A good supply is always essential, but it's particularly important during pregnancy, when blood production steps up so dra-matically. A mother with low iron supplies is more likely to deliver a low-birthweight or a premature baby. Deficiencies can also cause fatigue and eventually, iron-deficiency anemia; too much iron can cause constipation.

The DRI for iron during preg-nancy is 27 mg. You can get iron the Popeye way (by eating your spinach), or opt for other sources, such as beef, turkey dark meat, dried beans, peas,

dried apricots, potatoes, prunes, lentils, and oatmeal. Most women should also take an iron supplement during pregnancy.

Magnesium. Another mineral that helps calcium out in the bone-build-ing department, magnesium is also needed for nerve and muscle func-tion, as well as for helping the body process carbohydrates. What's more, it's essential in the regulation of insulin and blood-sugar levels (so important to baby) and needed for the removal of toxins from the body (so important during pregnancy). Because magnesium relaxes muscles (as opposed to calcium, which stim-ulates muscles to contract), adequate levels of magnesium during preg-nancy can prevent premature con-tractions of the uterus (otherwise known as premature labor). Getting enough magnesium can help ward off leg cramps and constipation. Severe deficiencies can cause pre-eclampsia in the mom and stunted growth, muscle spasms, and con-genital malformations in the baby.

The pregnancy DRI for magne-sium is 350 mg. Tasty ways to fill it include eating peanuts, nuts, beans, tofu, yogurt, milk, wheat germ, dried apricots, bananas, prunes, and leafy vegetables.

Manganese. Not on many people's mineral radar (and often confused with magnesium) manganese is vital

FOOD FORTIFICATION FRENZY

▼ ▼ ▼

Food enrichment and fortification were introduced in the United States during the first half of the twentieth century to prevent the thousands of deaths caused each year by severe vitamin and mineral deficiencies. It worked, big-time; such deficiencies have been virtually eradicated. Today, fortification of foods is being brought to a whole new level, as a new generation of "superfoods" is being brought to the marketplace—and to a store near you. You can now find calcium (not to mention vitamins A to E, plus zinc) in orange juice and phytochemicals in gummy candies; antioxidants in carbonated drinks and protein in pasta; vitamins and electrolytes in water (water!). Even foods that always had plenty of naturally occurring vitamins and minerals, such as peanut butter, fruit juice, tomato sauce, and yogurt, are being beefed up with extra nutrients by manufacturers eager to cash in on this fortification frenzy.

Some of the fortification in foods is extremely helpful even in today's more healthful society: iodine added to salt to prevent goiter, vitamin D added to milk to prevent rickets, calcium, as well as vitamins A and D, added to fruit juice (for those who can't or won't eat dairy products), and folic acid added to grains to prevent neural tube defects in developing babies. But it's important to bring a little perspective with you as you stroll down the supermarket shelves. A few phytochemicals thrown into a processed food (especially gummy candies) cannot take the place of fresh fruits and vegetables in your diet. A handful of vitamins added to an otherwise nutritionally deficient cereal doesn't make it equal to a whole-grain one that comes by its bounty naturally. Even a diet high in enriched processed foods but low in fresh foods might leave you short on important minerals that many manufacturers don't include, but that nature wisely does, such as magnesium, copper, and zinc.

There's no harm in eating enriched or fortified foods, even if you're also taking a prenatal vitamin supplement (it's unlikely you'll ever reach toxic levels of nutrients, unless you take megadoses of vitamin supplements in a single sitting—something no pregnant woman should do). And there's also no harm in taking comfort knowing that your bowl of Total in the morning or that nutrition bar you wolfed down midafternoon has supplied you and your baby with your daily quota of vitamins and minerals. But it's important to remember that processed foods—no matter how many vitamins and minerals have been tossed in—should never take the place of wholesome natural foods. Enrichment and fortification can help compensate for poor nutrition, but can never substitute for a healthy diet.

for the development of baby's bone, cartilage, and hearing mechanism. It's also necessary for good repro-

ductive function. Deficiencies can cause growth restriction for the fetus.

The DRI for manganese is 2 mg. Sources include spinach, carrots, broccoli, whole grains, nuts, brown rice, strawberries, bananas, and raisins.

Molybdenum. You probably haven't heard of this mineral before (and you almost certainly can't pronounce it), but humble molybdenum is thought to help in a monumentally important task: the transfer of oxygen from one molecule to another. It is also required for protein and fat metabolism, and it helps the baby to mobilize and use iron.

The DRI for molybdenum during pregnancy is 50 ug. You can find it in dried beans, grains, leafy greens, milk, and liver.

Phosphorus. Another comrade of calcium, phosphorus is a component of healthy teeth and bones. It's also needed to maintain the right balance of body fluids and is essential for muscle contractions, normal heart rhythm, and blood clotting. Deficiencies can cause a loss of appetite (no good when you're pregnant), weakness (you're tired enough), and a loss of calcium from bones (your bones). Too much phosphorus (as you might get from drinking too much soda, see box this page) can interfere with your body's ability to properly use calcium and iron.

The DRI for phosphorus during pregnancy is 700 mg. Look for it in yogurt (where you'll also find your

> **F A S T   F A C T**
>
> ✓ Need yet another reason to limit your intake of soft drinks during pregnancy? Most sodas are loaded with phosphorus (listed as phosphoric acid; with drinks offering up to 500 mg of phosphorus per serving), which lowers the level of calcium in the blood. So not only does drinking too much cola prevent you from reaching for healthier liquids (like calcium-loaded milk), it also impedes the absorption of whatever calcium you do get from other sources.

calcium), fish, meats, poultry, cheese, eggs, oatmeal, and lima beans.

Potassium. Potassium works with sodium to maintain fluid balance in cells (so important during pregnancy, when fluid levels must increase significantly) and regulate blood pressure (possibly helping to prevent preeclampsia). It also maintains proper muscle tone (which can help prevent pregnancy aches and pains, aid in delivery, and speed postpartum recovery).

Pregnant women need 2,000 mg of potassium a day. There are many delicious sources of potassium, including bananas, bran, avocados, dried apricots, oranges, peaches, pears, prunes, carrots, lentils, lima beans, peanuts, peas, potatoes, pumpkin, spinach, squash, tomatoes, meat, fish, poultry, and dairy products.

Selenium. Selenium is important for your body's defense against disease—

preventing cell damage, working with vitamin E as an antioxidant, and binding with toxins in the body, rendering them harmless (and protecting baby from them). Deficiencies can cause preeclampsia and possibly have negative effects on a fetus's development and growth.

The pregnancy DRI for selenium is 60 ug. Sources include Brazil nuts (a whopping supplier), fish, meats, chicken, eggs, and whole grains.

Sodium. Sodium is needed to maintain the right balance of acids and bases in body fluids and helps nutrients cross cell membranes. It also maintains an appropriate amount of water in blood and body tissue— always important, but especially essential during pregnancy, when blood and fluid volumes increase.

Though your need for sodium during pregnancy increases slightly, most people get plenty of sodium from their diet. You should aim to get approximately 2,400 mg of sodium per day. You'll find sodium in almost every food in some amount, and in plentiful quantity in foods processed with salt, in cured foods, and, of course, in table salt.

Zinc. Zinc is one of a developing baby's best friends, essential for cell division and tissue growth, as well as for hair, skin, and proper bone growth. It also helps in the perception of taste and works with insulin to regulate blood sugar (important in the prevention of gestational diabetes). Zinc has garnered a great deal of attention from researchers, who have discovered that deficiencies in this vital mineral can increase the risk of miscarriage, low-birth-weight infants, preterm delivery, and possibly defects in the fetus such as spina bifida, cleft lip or palate (or both), and visual impairment.

The DRI for zinc during pregnancy is 11 mg. Good sources include turkey, beef, wheat germ, yogurt, oatmeal, corn, cooked oysters and shellfish, and eggs.

wisdom of ☼ the ages?

Old wives in Indonesia seem to love pouring salt on a pregnant woman's wounds. A superstition there advises expectant mothers to avoid putting a spoon in the salt container. According to the tale, failure to keep their salt shaken, not stirred, may cause them to have difficulties during labor.

Beyond Vitamins and Minerals

YOU TOOK YOUR PRENATAL SUPPLE-ment and ate your fill of every vitamin and mineral known to scientists (and maybe a few they haven't even discovered yet). Think your job in nourishing baby is done? Think again. There are many other nutrients you'll need to ensure you and baby a healthy pregnancy. Some are detailed in The Pregnancy Diet's Daily Dozen (see page 81), but you'll find some nutritional superstars below:

Fiber. Fiber lowers cholesterol and blood-sugar levels, helps move waste through the intestines (which is why it's a constipated pregnant woman's finest friend), and may reduce the risk of heart disease, some cancers, diabetes, and preeclampsia. Sources of fiber include fruit, vegetables, beans, and whole grains.

Omega-3 fatty acids. These good fats are needed to make cell membranes, hormones, and prostaglandins. But they've received the most kudos for their important work in fetal brain and eye development. Research also shows that eating foods rich in omega-3 can help boost your mood—and may even prevent postpartum depression. Sources include fish, nuts and nut oil, and DHA eggs. Read more on page 98.

Phytochemicals. They've been around since the first sprout, but they've been big news lately, and for good reason. Phytochemicals (literally "plant chemicals") are found in all plants (fruits, vegetables, grains) and are the plant's natural protection against disease, damage from the sun, and bugs. Research has shown that phytochemicals are good for the humans who eat plants, too; they reduce disease risk (including heart disease), inhibit the production of bad cholesterol (LDL), strengthen blood vessel walls, and stimulate immunities. Some phytochemicals are said to prevent or slow cancer growth. Every day, researchers are uncovering more and more benefits to these and other natural components of plants—all the more reason to eat a healthful diet and not rely on supplements. (Supplements do not contain phytochemicals.) Fruits and vegetables are superb sources of phytochemicals (see page 140).

The Pregnancy Diet

NOW YOU KNOW WHAT IT TAKES to make a healthy baby—from the vitamin A that'll help those little eyes see you for the first time to the manganese that'll help those little ears hear you, from the calcium that will build strong bones and teeth (and make those tiny finger- and toenails grow!) to the omega-3 fatty acids that will boost the development of a brain that has so many things to learn in a lifetime.

The next step is taking all the nutrients you and your baby need during the next nine months and putting them together in an eating plan that makes sense, one that's easy to follow, practical to live and work with—that makes eating during pregnancy pleasurable (at least once morning sickness has passed), as nourishing as possible (allowing you to get the biggest nutritional bang for your diet buck), and, hopefully, guilt-free (because feeding yourself and your baby well should feel good).

Welcome to The Pregnancy Diet.

Nine Basic Principles for Nine Months of Healthy Eating

THESE GUIDELINES SUM UP WHAT eating well when you're expecting means. But they're also pretty good tenets for eating well in general. Following them as best as you can will give your baby the best possible start in life, make your pregnancy safer and more comfortable, and if you stick with them once your nine months are over, give you and your family health benefits that can last a lifetime.

Bites count. In a typical day, you're likely to take hundreds of bites that will eventually, in one form or another, find their way to you and your baby. Thinking about those bites before you take them is a practice that will benefit you both. Sure, one bite of chocolate layer cake won't hurt your baby. But take a few bites of that cake in midmorning followed by several more bites from that pile of cookies the last meeting left in the conference room after the lunch meeting, topped off with a whole bunch of bites from your spouse's fast-food fries at dinner—and you'll find those worthless bites are adding up fast.

Each bite during the day is an opportunity to give that growing baby inside you vital nutrients. With an allowance of only about 300 extra calories a day during your pregnancy, you'll want to make many, if not most, of those bites count.

All calories are not created equal. A calorie is a calorie, whether it comes from a carbohydrate, protein, or fat. But the package that calorie comes in is important. Your baby will be better nourished by a diet in which calories are carefully selected for their nutritional content, and not as well nourished when those calories are furnished by fats and sugars. So try to spend your calories accordingly. Here's an illustration from the coffee cart: The 200 calories in a doughnut are not equal to the 200 calories in a raisin bran muffin. One from the cafeteria line— the 300 calories you'd squander on a hot dog with ketchup on a white bun is far better spent on a grilled chicken sandwich on whole wheat, with lettuce, tomato, and mustard. And here's a bonus you'll get from smart calorie spending: Not only will your baby benefit from nutrition-packed calories, but your postpartum body will, too. Calories accumulated from fats and sugar are a lot harder to take off than calories gathered from protein and produce and whole grains.

MY BABY, THE PARASITE?

▼ ▼ ▼

MYTH: The baby takes what it needs for growth and development from the mother, regardless of her diet.

FACT: The fetus is not a parasite, able to live off its mother no matter what she eats. A mother's diet and nutritional stores need to be adequate to meet both her and her fetus's needs. If the supply is low, mom gets first dibs. In order to ensure the survival of the species, Mother Nature swings in favor of the mother (who, if she's healthy and well-fed, can live to reproduce again)—not in favor of her baby. In fact, babies can be born with vitamin deficiencies to moms who show no signs of deficiency.

Starve yourself—starve your baby. Would you ever consider leaving your newborn crying for food because you're too busy to feed him or her? Or skip your infant's breakfast because you're just not in the mood to prepare it? Of course not. But when you miss a meal while you're expecting—whether it's because you're busy at work, preoccupied at home, or just not up to fixing it or eating it—keep in mind that baby's missing it, too. And while you may be able to weather missed meals occasionally (especially when food aversions send you flying

out the door faster than your spouse can yell "Breakfast!"), your baby counts on a steady supply of building materials from you through the placenta—every single day. A late brunch may be just the ticket for you on Sundays (who needs to make breakfast *and* lunch?), but not for baby, who doesn't like to be kept waiting for the next nutritional shipment. Skipping lunch because a meeting ran over might leave you with only a headache and a few hunger pangs, but will leave your fetus running on empty for many hours of growing time. (Fetuses are growing around the clock.)

In fact, scientists agree that frequent eating by the mother may be the best route to a well-nourished full-term fetus. Research has shown that mothers-to-be who eat at least five times a day (three meals plus two snacks, or six small meals, for instance) are more likely to carry to term.

Easy to say (especially by scientists who aren't pregnant), but not always easy to do. What about all those pregnancy symptoms that often make eating seem like too much hard—and uncomfortable—work, and make skipping a meal welcome? What about the fact that you're either too busy throwing up to keep anything down, your heartburn's keeping your heart (and appetite) out of the kitchen, or your uterus has practically lodged itself in your stomach, leaving you feeling so full that the words *extra* and *calories* are not allowed to be spoken in your presence. Rather than give in to these biologic obstacles to regular eating, try to find ways around them. For help in doing this, see Chapter Two.

Efficiency is effective. Packing all your nutritional needs (summed up by the Daily Dozen beginning on page 81) into three meals and a few snacks each day may seem daunting—even impossible. How can you possibly fill so many requirements without overstuffing your stomach—and spending more time each day chewing than breathing?

The answer? Efficiency. Becoming an efficiency expert will keep you from being a pregnant heavyweight. Learning how to choose foods that take you the furthest nutritionally for the fewest calories and that fill two or even more requirements at the same time will help you feed your baby well, without overfeeding yourself.

First, look to foods that are good nutrition buys. For example, you'll get the same protein serving from a cup of low-fat cottage cheese (weighing in at 180 calories) as you would from a cup of the full-fat variety (240 calories), but you'll save yourself 60 calories (which could buy you an extra slice of whole wheat bread or a large peach). You'll bank even more calories (enough practically to buy yourself lunch) if you choose to find your calcium in a dessert of frozen yogurt (about 300 calories per calcium serving) instead of in one of premium ice cream (about 500 calories per calcium serving).

Second, try as often as possible to fill two or more requirements for the price of one. Broccoli will fill a vitamin C and a green leafy requirement (plus a calcium bonus) in one serving. Calcium-fortified orange juice offers up a vitamin C food, a calcium serving, and a fluid, all neatly and tastily packaged in one glass. Dried apricots double as both an iron source and a yellow fruit (with a side of fiber).

If you're having trouble gaining weight, being an efficiency expert will come in handy as well, with a switch in strategy: Choose foods that are dense both nutritionally and in calories (see page 51).

Carbohydrates are a complex issue. Refined or simple carbohydrates (such as white bread, white rice, cakes, cookies, and sugars) are nutritionally weak and heavy on empty calories. But, despite what the low-carb diet hype might lead you to believe, that's not the whole carbohydrate story. First, it's never smart for a pregnant woman to shun any food group entirely (except for junk food). A fully balanced diet, which is rich in both protein and carbohydrates, is what your baby needs.

Second, like all calories, all carbo-hydrates are not created equal. Complex and unrefined carbohy-drates (such as whole-grain breads and cereals, brown rice, fruits and vegeta-bles, and dried beans and peas) con-tain energy-yielding and -sustaining nutrients that the pregnant body needs. They provide not only essential B vitamins and minerals, but the all-important fiber (which keeps consti-pation at bay and may reduce the risk

THE LOW-DOWN ON LOW-CARB

▼ ▼ ▼

When it comes to carbs, low isn't the way to go when you're expecting. A diet short on carbs (especially the complex variety) may be short on vital baby-making ingre-dients, such as the folic acid and other vitamins and minerals found in grains, fruits, and vegetables. It can also be sky-high in protein—and too much protein is a definite no-no as far as developing fetuses are con-cerned. And what's bad for baby can also be bad for mom: Skimp on car-bohydrates, and you'll be skimping on constipation-fighting fiber—plus on the B vitamins known to battle morning sickness and pregnancy-unsettled skin. Balanced diets may not generate the media buzz, but they do generate the healthiest envi-ronment for growing babies.

of developing gestational diabetes). And that's a happy ending.

Sweet nothings are exactly that. Do you have a sweet tooth that just won't quit? Join the club. Americans, on average, consume about 150 pounds of refined sugar a year, adding up to about 500 to 600 empty calories a day.

Certainly, no one benefits from socking away so many empty calories a day (and most Americans have the extra pounds to prove it). But preg-nant women—and their babies—stand to benefit the least (and lose the most) from a diet that's high in sugar. After all, with so many nutri-ents to eat—and so few extra calories to spend on them—a lot of sugary foods can easily interfere with opti-mum nourishment.

Sure, it's fine to have a sugary treat every once in a while. (After all, you're entitled to some eating that's just for fun.) And, in fact, denying yourself your occasional desserts can lead you to crave them even more (and lead you to demolish the whole bag of cookies, instead of stopping at one or two). But a diet packed with too much sugar will leave you with little room for food with real nutritional value. Sugary foods (like candies and soft drinks), after all, are usually poor sources of vitamins, minerals, and other nutrients.

But cutting back on your sugar intake doesn't mean you'll have to deprive that sweet tooth. Sweet foods

SHORT ON SUGAR

▼ ▼ ▼

Some sugar-addicted folks have an easier time quitting completely than cutting down. But for other sugarholics, cold-turkey tactics just make them crave the stuff more—and doom any new pregnancy eating plan to failure. Remember, pregnancy is a time to eat right, but it's also a time to enjoy what you eat. If you can't (or don't want to) cut sugar out of your diet entirely, there are ways to cut back on your intake:

■ Choose a lower-sugar cereal (5 or 6 grams per serving) and add a teaspoon of sugar to it instead of buying supersweetened cereals (those with 12 or more grams per serving). *Even better:* Eat a whole-grain, very-low-sugar cereal (1 to 3 grams per serving) with only a sprinkling of sugar on top. *Better still:* Top your cereal with sliced bananas, strawberries, blueberries, or raisins to get your sweet-

tooth fix without the sugar. Or satisfy your craving with sucralose (Splenda) instead of sugar.

■ If the only way you can drink milk is to sip it alongside some cookies (the better to dunk them with), try chasing the glass down with two cookies instead of six. *Even better:* Dunk fat-free oatmeal raisin cookies instead of chocolate chip. *Better still:* Make those cookies whole-grain and sweetened with fruit juice.

■ Drink real fruit juice instead of sugar-loaded fruit "drinks." *Even better:* Squeeze your own juice.

■ Bake blueberry pie or peach crisp for dessert instead of tunnel-of-fudge cake. *Even better:* Bake with whole grains. *Better still:* Substitute fruit juice concentrate for some or all of the sugar.

don't always come in sugary packages. Fresh fruits (a mouthwatering summer peach, a slice of ripe melon, a perfect banana) are deliciously sweet and nutritious. So is a cranberry spritzer (fruit-only cranberry juice and sparkling water). Cookies and cakes made with whole grains can satisfy your cravings and your nutritional requirements (see recipes starting on page 431). And don't forget that some low-calorie sugar sub-

stitutes such as sucralose (Splenda) appear to be safe for pregnancy use (see page 172), which means you can sweeten the pot (or the coffee, or the yogurt, or even the candy and cookies) without adding empty calories.

Good foods remember where they came from. It make sense that nature would know a thing or two about nutrition. And, sure enough, the best sources of vitamins and nutrients are foods in their natural state. A prime example of nature's finest and most nourishing foods are the freshest fruits and vegetables—the ones that haven't had to travel far or long from the field or the orchard to your table or your lunch bag. In looking for produce, try to follow descriptions of freshness, color, firmness, and overall condition: Broccoli that feels soft and seems pale and anemic from its journey across country or from its lengthy layover in a refrigerated warehouse isn't a good nutritional bet. Neither are carrots that have softened, split, or lost their vibrant orange hue, asparagus that's limp and gray, or prematurely picked strawberries or tomatoes that weren't given the vine time they needed to develop a deep red blush. When you can't find produce that's as fresh as nature intended, don't change your menu, just head to the frozen-food aisle. Quick-freezing is done almost immediately after harvesting, when produce is at the height of its nutritive value, so most frozen fruits and vegetables have as much to offer as their "fresh" counterparts, or even more nutritive value. (Be careful, however, to pick frozens that are as close to their natural states as possible, with no added sauces, salt, sugar, butter, or chemicals; avoid packages that are covered with frost or otherwise look as though they have been refrozen.) Unadulterated canned fruits and vegetables (no added sugar, salt, or preservatives) can also be nutrition packed and are handy when time for shopping and cooking are short.

Carry the freshness principle over to the other aisles of the market, too. When possible, select rolled oats over instant oatmeal, fresh potatoes over dehydrated instant, natural cheese over those cellophane-wrapped squares, fresh turkey over smoked.

Healthful eating should be a family affair. While what your family eats during your pregnancy would seem less significant than what you eat, enlisting them as allies in healthy eating will make it much easier on you. (It's not easy to sit by with a plate of carrot sticks while your spouse plows through a bag of chips.) But wait, there's more. Not only will your good eating habits result in a healthier baby and a relatively slimmer you, but there will also be the postpartum bonus of a fitter and trimmer spouse and older children (if you have them) with better eating habits. And The Pregnancy Diet, when used as a foundation for permanent improvement in your family's nutritional profile, gives all of them the best chances of longer and healthier lives—with a lowered risk of such diet-influenced diseases as cancer, diabetes, and high blood pressure.

Bad habits can sabotage a good diet. Good diet makes a big difference in your pregnancy outcome, but not all the difference. Your child's health can be thwarted by other baby-unfriendly lifestyle choices. By taking a glass of wine with each well-balanced dinner, or lighting up a cigarette after a nutritionally sound snack, you're offsetting the benefits excellent nutrition ordinarily offers your pregnancy and your baby. To ensure your baby the healthiest possible start in life, team your dietary efforts with other good choices, avoiding alcohol, tobacco, and all recreational drugs during pregnancy. (See Chapter Seven for more.)

The Pregnancy Daily Dozen

NO NEED TO KEEP TRACK OF YOUR K, add up your A, chart your chromium, monitor your manganese, or follow your fiber. The Pregnancy Diet Daily Dozen serves up all the vitamins, minerals, and nutrients you and baby need in twelve easy food groups. Just eat the prescribed number of portions from each of the twelve categories (keeping in mind that many foods overlap in two or more categories, cutting down on the number of portions you'll have to eat from each), and you're done for the day.

Calories: approximately 300 extra daily. If you've ever had to count them—and cut down on them—in order to diet, chances are you don't have anything good to say about calories. After all, aren't they just those things they put in candy bars and french fries that make people gain weight?

Actually, that's not what calories are about at all (though too many can make people gain weight). And they don't deserve the bad rap diets (and dieters) have given them, especially during pregnancy. Calories represent the amount of energy supplied by the carbohydrates, protein, and fats in foods. They're essential to life, but especially essential to pregnant women, who need energy for so many things, from just staying on their feet (no easy task when fatigue sets in), to keeping their baby-making factory running smoothly.

But the need for energy from calories during pregnancy isn't a license to eat everything in sight—

F A S T   F A C T

☑ Over the course of forty weeks, it takes an estimated 75,000 calories to make a baby. Just don't try to eat them all at one sitting.

your license has a limit. Believe it or not, you need only about 300 extra calories (added to the number of calories required to maintain prepregnancy weight*) a day to make a baby, and fewer than that during early pregnancy. Mothers carrying multiples need more calories; see page 204. And that's not much of a bonus. After all, 300 calories doesn't go such a long way. Consider—one banana, or a glass of low-fat milk represents 100 calories; a slice of whole wheat bread, an ounce of cheddar cheese, and a half cup of grapes equals 200 calories. So while you'll need the extra energy those extra calories buy you, spending sprees at the doughnut shop or the candy store will almost certainly send you over your limit—and if they take the place of sensible food choices on a daily basis, such habits leave baby short on needed nutrients.

Now that you know how many calories you'll need every day for the rest of your pregnancy, forget it. Besides being a tedious chore, counting your calories is not an effective way of determining whether your baby is getting his or hers. Since multiple factors go into whether a person loses or gains weight—for example, the level of activity and exercise, individual

metabolism (which increases in pregnancy), the amount of fiber in the diet (fiber pushes some calories through the system before they can be burned for fuel)—that 300 number can only be used as a very rough guide. Monitoring your weight gain, keeping it within the limits of the steady and moderate pattern described on page 39, is a much more efficient way to keep track of your calories. Bottom line—if you're not gaining weight quickly enough, then you're not getting your Daily Dozen of calories. If you're gaining too quickly, you're getting more than you need.

Protein: three servings daily. No one material is more essential to the making of a baby than protein's amino acids, the building blocks of human tissue. Though a growing fetus doesn't require much of an increase in calories, it does need you to consume significantly more protein. Aim for about 75 grams of protein a day (three protein servings). Not only does adequate protein intake serve to protect against some pregnancy complications such as preeclampsia or poor placental function, it also helps maximize fetal brain development, particularly in the last trimester.

These days, most people get at least that much protein without even trying (and those on high-protein diets take in much more). So filling up those three servings a day probably won't be much of a struggle. Have just

---

*To determine how many calories you need in order to maintain your prepregnancy weight, multiply that weight by 12 if you're sedentary, 15 if you're moderately active, and up to 22 if you're extremely active. Because the rate at which calories are burned varies from person to person even during pregnancy, calorie requirements vary, too, so the figure you arrive at is just an estimate.

THE TRUTH ABOUT EATING FOR TWO

▼ ▼ ▼

MYTH: You're eating for two during pregnancy. So that means you should take everything you usually eat and then double it.

FACT: While it's true you're eating for two people—you and your baby—you need to remember that one of those two is pea-size at the beginning, and never (thankfully) gets close to your size during its stay in your uterus. You'll only need about 100 extra calories a day during the first trimester (when the fetus's caloric needs are not that great). As your pregnancy progresses (your body is working harder and your baby getting bigger), you'll be working your way up to about 300 more calories a day. But unless you're very active, you probably won't need more than that. To tell if you're eating enough for both of you throughout your pregnancy, don't count calories, just watch the scale.

one serving at each meal (for example, a cheese omelet for breakfast, a salad topped with grilled chicken for lunch, and a fish fillet for dinner), and you're there. If you're having six meals a day, six half servings will substitute nicely. Or, if you prefer cereal (not a full-protein portion) for breakfast, you can have a double portion of poultry or fish (just 8 ounces) for lunch or dinner to compensate.

Remember, too, that you can get additional protein from whole-grain breads, pastas, and cereals. And don't forget to tally the substantial amount of protein found in most calcium foods you're eating, too: a glass of milk and an ounce of cheese provide a third of a protein serving; a cup of yogurt equals half a serving.

Every day, have three of the following (or a combination equal to three servings). Remember, if you're using dairy sources for protein, you can count the same servings for calcium:

24 ounces (three 8-ounce glasses) milk or buttermilk

1 cup cottage cheese

2 cups yogurt

3 ounces cheese (¾ cup grated)

4 large whole eggs

7 large egg whites

3½ ounces (drained) canned tuna or sardines**

4 ounces (drained) canned salmon

4 ounces cooked seafood (shelled shrimp, lobster, clams, etc.)

4 ounces (before cooking) fresh fish

**See page 169 for information on safe fish eating during pregnancy.

4 ounces (before cooking) chicken, turkey, duck, or other poultry without skin

4 ounces (before cooking) lean beef, lamb, veal, pork, or buffalo

Vegetarian proteins are considered incomplete proteins because they are deficient in at least one amino acid. (Complete proteins—such as those listed above—come from animal products and contain all the essential amino acids needed for tissue growth.) Although it is no longer considered necessary for vegetarians who consume no animal products to combine

DIVIDE, COMBINE, AND CONQUER

▼ ▼ ▼

Can't drain the whole glass of milk? Had your fill halfway through your cup of yogurt? Just because they don't add up to a full serving doesn't mean they can't be added onto your daily total. When a full serving is just too much, combine half (or third, or quarter) servings together instead. For instance, that 1 egg (¼ protein serving), plus 1 slice of whole-grain toast (¼ protein serving), plus ½ cup of soy milk (½ protein serving) equals a full protein serving—and you don't even have to eat them all in the same sitting (just in the same day). Divide, combine, and conquer—and you'll have to do a lot less eating to finish up your Daily Dozen.

two types of vegetarian proteins at the same meal, vegetarians should still combine complementary vegetable source proteins within the same day (grains and legumes, for instance). To be sure you are getting a full protein serving at each meal, double or choose two half servings of the following. Remember that some of these will also contribute to whole-grain and fat servings—and nonvegetarians, feel free to select from this group, too:

Legumes (half protein servings)

¾ cup cooked beans, lentils, split peas, or chickpeas (garbanzos)

½ cup cooked soybeans (edamame)

¾ cup green garden peas

1½ ounces peanuts

3 tablespoons peanut butter

¼ cup miso

4 ounces tofu (bean curd)

3 ounces tempeh

1½ cups soy milk*

3 ounces soy cheese*

½ cup vegetarian "ground beef"*

1 large vegetarian "hot dog"*

1 large vegetarian "burger"*

1 ounce (before cooking) soy pasta

Grains (half protein servings)

3 ounces (before cooking) whole wheat pasta

⅓ cup wheat germ

---

* Protein contents of soy products vary widely, so check labels. you're looking for about 12–15 grams of protein for a half serving.

¾ cup oat bran

1 cup uncooked (2 cups cooked) oats

2 cups (approximately) whole-grain
ready-to-eat cereal

½ cup uncooked (1½ cups cooked)
couscous, bulgur, buckwheat

½ cup quinoa

4 slices whole-grain bread

2 whole wheat pitas

2 whole wheat English muffins

Nuts and Seeds (half protein servings)

3 ounces nuts, such as walnuts, pecans,
and almonds

2 ounces sunflower, sesame, or pumpkin
seeds

½ cup ground flaxseed

▲ ▲ ▲

Q *"Can I use a protein supplement to make sure I'm getting
enough protein?"*

A As with the rest of your nutrients, nature—not a supplement
maker—is the best protein provider.
And for a few reasons. First, supplements—which contain whopping
amounts of protein—can easily give
you too much of a good thing.
Second, supplements don't just offer
protein; they may also contain ingredients (such as sugar substitutes,
extra vitamins, and even herbs) that
may be unsafe during pregnancy.
Third, they're pretty expensive to
buy. A better choice for your baby?

wisdom of ☼ the ages?

I n ancient Rome, pregnant women were
advised that if they wanted their baby to
be born with dark eyes, they should eat mice
often. While a mouse might be an interesting protein choice (if you're a pregnant
snake, that is), this is clearly a case where
you wouldn't want to do as the Romans did—
even if you did happen to be in Rome.

Protein the way nature intended it—
in the form of any of the foods listed
on this and the previous page.

▼ ▼ ▼

Calcium: four servings daily. Make
no bones about it; calcium intake is
crucial during pregnancy, not only for
your baby's bones (approximately 200
mg of calcium per day is deposited
into your baby's skeleton during the
last trimester of pregnancy), but also
for yours. Women begin to lose bone
mass in their thirties, and they'll lose
it faster if calcium is drained from
their own bones to help build baby's.
Getting adequate calcium daily (especially during pregnancy) will ensure
continued bone health and prevent
osteoporosis later in life. Adequate
calcium is also believed to prevent
preeclampsia during pregnancy. So it's
clear that calcium does a mom-to-be
and her baby good.
　Milk is the most well-known
source of calcium, and a very efficient one, too. So if you "got milk,"
and you love drinking it, great—

SHAKE IT UP, BABY

▼ ▼ ▼

Much of the calcium in calcium-fortified beverages (juice, soy milk, and calcium-added milk) tends to settle at the bottom of a container—good if you're getting the last sip, not so good if you're getting the first. To make sure the calcium is evenly distributed from first sip to last, shake these beverages thoroughly before each use.

you'll have no problem meeting your calcium requirement. If your tummy can tolerate milk, but you can't stand its taste, also no problem—it's easily disguised. It can be downed in delicious milk shakes, smoothies, soups, skim milk decaf latte, or low-fat chocolate milk; it can be eaten in puddings, breads, cereals (hot and cold), meat, fish, or vegetable loaves, pancakes, homemade frozen desserts, pancakes, casseroles, sauces, and more. (See page 88 for alternatives if you don't like milk.)

But should you think milk holds the monopoly on calcium, check out the list below. From yogurt to cheese, there are plenty of dairy sources of this marvelous mineral. For the lactose intolerant or the vegan, there's no shortage of nondairy sources.

Protect your calcium intake by avoiding or limiting those things that may interfere with absorption (most are not recommended in pregnancy anyway): alcohol, caffeine, laxatives, diuretic pills, excessive salt, and excessive phosphorus (as from too much soda). And, since dietary fiber can rob your body of the calcium you eat before it has been absorbed, try not to take the bulk of your fiber along with the bulk of your calcium foods (in other words, avoid chasing down your bran muffin with your milk).

Choose four servings daily from the following list. And don't forget that many of the dairy sources (and the seafood ones) also provide protein; many of the nondairy provide vitamin C and green leafies.

¼ cup grated or shredded cheese

1 ounce cheese

½ cup pasteurized ricotta cheese

1 cup milk or buttermilk

5 ounces calcium-added milk*

1 cup yogurt

1½ cups frozen yogurt

½ cup evaporated skim milk

⅓ cup nonfat dry milk
   (enough to make 1 cup liquid)

1 cup calcium-fortified orange juice*

1 cup calcium-fortified soy milk*

1½ ounces calcium-fortified soy cheese

4 ounces canned salmon with bones

3 ounces canned sardines with bones

3 tablespoons sesame seeds

*Shake before serving.

VISUAL REALITY

▼ ▼ ▼

Do your eyes deceive you when you're judging the serving of food on your plate? Chances are, yes. Most Americans, weaned on supersize fast-food portions, extra-large dinner plates (and the extra-large steaks served on them), and all-you-can-eat buffets, are actually eating two to three times the recommended serving amount per food item. A plateful of spaghetti at a typical restaurant, for instance, is closer to three grain servings than it is to one. The hunk-of-chicken special, closer to two protein servings.

So before you decide that you're going to turn into a blimp trying to keep up with The Pregnancy Diet's Daily Dozen, keep these visual aids in mind: A serving of meat, poultry, or fish is equivalent to a computer mouse; a serving of fruit or vegetables is about the size of a light-bulb; a serving of pasta would fill an ice-cream scoop; and a serving of butter or oil would just cover the tip of your thumb. In other words, you may find that your requirements aren't quite as filling as you thought.

1 cup cooked greens, such as collard

1½ cups cooked bok choy

1½ cups cooked edamame

1¾ tablespoons blackstrap molasses

Spinach: ½ cup cooked = ¼ serving

Cooked dried beans: 1 cup = ½ serving

Flaxseed: ¼ cup ground = ¼ serving

▲ ▲ ▲

Other Calcium Foods

Cream cheese: ¼ cup = ¼ serving

Cottage cheese: 1 cup = ½ serving

Tofu: 8 ounces = ½ serving**

Sour cream: 3 tablespoons = ¼ serving

Dried figs: 6 = ¼ serving

Almonds: 1 ounces = ¼ serving

Almond butter: 2 tablespoons = ⅓ serving

Broccoli: 3 cups = ⅓ serving

**Some varieties of tofu and tempeh have considerably more calcium than others. Check the label—you're looking for about 30 percent of the DRI for calcium in a calcium serving.

Q *"I hate milk. Do I have to drink four glasses of it a day to make sure I meet my calcium requirement?"*

A If milk leaves a sour taste in your mouth, there are plenty of ways to sneak your calcium in without drinking milk straight up (or even at all). Cook up a low-fat cheese sauce to pour over your steamed vegetables (or just sprinkle on a heaping handful of shredded cheese); blend dips and salad dressings out of low-fat yogurt; you can coat your chicken with ground almonds or sesame seeds (both contain calcium); opt for calcium-fortified juice. Best of all, many milk substitutes also fulfill another Daily Dozen requirement, for extra efficiency. If you can't drink milk because you're lactose intolerant, see page 208. If you don't because you're a vegan, see page 207. (Look for dozens of other high-calcium recipes in the recipe section beginning on page 238. Among many others, they include Broccoli and Cheese Soup, page 281; Hearty Fish and Potato Chowder, page 296; Mexican Lasagna, page 344; Tomato Chicken Parmesan, page 352; Tomato-Layered Mini Meatloaves, page 343; Alotta Broccoli with Chicken and Penne, page 302; and Tomato and Roasted Red Pepper Frittata, page 243.)

▼ ▼ ▼

COUNT 'EM ONCE, COUNT 'EM TWICE

▼ ▼ ▼

Sometimes, you'll even be able to count them thrice. Many of your favorite foods fill more than one Daily Dozen requirement in each serving. Case in delicious point—a slice of cantaloupe fills a green and yellow plus a C. Same goes for a tangerine. Broccoli covers green and yellow and C with a calcium bonus. And so on. So don't forget to give yourself credit where credit is due. Count 'em once, count 'em twice.

Vitamin C: three servings daily. Because the body doesn't store vitamin C, you and baby will need a fresh supply every day. Which shouldn't be too much of a chore, considering that vitamin C comes in a wide range of foods that naturally taste good.

As vitamins go, C is fairly fragile. Exposure to heat, light, and air destroys it over time. So it's best to get at least some of your vitamin C from foods that haven't been cooked, prepeeled, or precut. Whenever you can, section your grapefruit, squeeze your orange, slice your peppers, or blend your frozen juice just before serving to preserve the maximum vitamin C.

Another great thing about vitamin C foods (besides their terrific taste): they're efficient. Many of them also fill the requirement for green leafy and yellow vegetables and yellow fruit. Especially fond of C produce? Help yourself to extra servings, if you'd like:

$1/3$ cup fresh strawberries

$2/3$ cup fresh blackberries or raspberries

$1/8$ small cantaloupe or $1/2$ cup cubed

$1/8$ small honeydew or $1/2$ cup cubed

$1/2$ medium-size grapefruit

$1/2$ cup grapefruit juice

$1/2$ medium-size orange

$1/2$ cup orange juice

$1/4$ cup fresh lemon juice

2 tablespoons orange juice
   concentrate

2 tablespoons white grape juice concentrate

1 large tangerine

1/2 large guava

1/2 medium-size kiwifruit

1/2 medium-size mango

1/4 medium-size papaya

1/2 cup diced fresh pineapple

3/4 cup canned juice-packed pineapple, drained

1 medium-size plantain

1 wedge (4 x 8 inches) watermelon or 2 cups diced

11/2 cups red or green grapes

1/2 cup raw or cooked broccoli

1/2 cup cooked brussels sprouts

1 cup shredded raw green cabbage

3/4 cup coleslaw mix

1/2 cup broccoli slaw

2/3 cup cooked bok choy

3/4 cup raw red cabbage

1/2 cup raw daikon (Chinese radish)

1/2 cup raw or cooked cauliflower

1/2 cup cooked kohlrabi

12 spears asparagus

3/4 cup cooked greens, such as collards, mustard, or turnip greens

1/2 cup cooked kale

1 packed cup raw spinach, or 1/2 cup cooked

1 cup watercress

3 cups arugula

2 cups romaine

1/2 medium-size green bell pepper

ONE SERVING SIZE DOESN'T FIT ALL

▼ ▼ ▼

When serving yourself up your Daily Dozen of fruits and vegetables, keep a couple of points in mind. First, since the serving sizes are approximate, you can approximate, too, when counting them up (rather than driving yourself crazy with cups and tablespoons). Second, they're based on average servings—some (such as orange juice, melon, carrots, and sweet potatoes) will actually give off-the-chart nutritional stats in much smaller servings. And third, if you ever find yourself hankering for more than an average serving of a fruit or vegetable, go for it. You can take "all-you-can-eat" literally at the lunchtime salad bar; nibble your way through two carrots instead of just half of one; don't stop at a single slice of a sweet and juicy cantaloupe. Enough is like a feast, but more is definitely not less when it comes to baby-friendly produce.

1/4 medium-size red, yellow, or orange bell pepper

1 medium-size tomato

3/4 cup canned tomatoes

11/2 cups tomato sauce

3/4 cup tomato juice

1/2 cup vegetable juice

1/2 cup snap peas

2/3 cup green garden peas

QUICK F·I·X

FOR GETTING THOSE VITAL VEGETABLES Don't like to eat your vegetables? Drink them instead, in nutritious and delicious soups. See recipes starting on page 281.

1 sweet potato, baked in skin

1 baking potato, baked in skin

1 cup cooked soybeans (edamame)

Green leafy and yellow vegetables and yellow fruits: three to four servings daily. These are the powerhouses of the produce section—superstar vegetables and fruits that serve up some of nature's finest nutrients, often in whopping quantity. They're a rich source of a class of phytochemicals called carotenoids (including alpha-carotene, beta-carotene, lutein, zeaxanthin, and beta-cryptoxanthin), the importance of which scientists are researching in labs—and we're reading more about in newspapers—daily. The biggest headline-maker of these is beta-carotene, which is crucial for fetal development (see page 140). Since some carotenoids are more plentiful in yellow vegetables and fruits, others in green vegetables, adding a good mix to your diet makes sense.

And there are more good reasons to make green and deep yellow your Baby Team colors. The greens and deep yellows are also excellent suppliers of vitamin E, riboflavin, B_6, folic acid, magnesium, and a host of other essential minerals. And, as a bonus, when eaten raw or cooked only lightly, greens and yellows (particularly the vegetables) supply plenty of constipation-countering fiber. Need another reason to up your veggie intake? Researchers have found that children born to women who ate plenty of vegetables during pregnancy have a lower risk of developing type 1 diabetes.

Even if you've never been a vegetable lover, or if early pregnancy aversions are temporarily turning you off green, you're sure to find at least a few palatable veggie choices among those listed below (carrots and sweet potatoes, for instance, often score points with those who shun spinach). Or, cleverly conceal offending produce under sauces (such as a high-calcium cheese sauce over steamed broccoli); in soups (minestrone, pumpkin, or ginger-carrot); in casseroles (you'll never notice the chopped cauliflower in your tuna-noodle favorite) and stuffings; and grated into fish cakes or meat loaves and burgers. Most of the recipes in the recipe section starting on page 238 feature fruits and vegetables. Among them, Glazed Carrots and Pineapple, page 399; Spicy Greens with Ginger Dressing, page 404; Stove Top Brown Rice Pilaf, page 414; Tomato Soup with Avocado, page 285; Sweet Potato Vichyssoise, page 284; Salmon Cakes with Tropical Salsa, page 382; and Red Snapper with Mango Salsa, page 373.

And there's sweet revenge for those who just refuse to eat their vegetables. Though mother probably wouldn't want you to hear this, the right fruit can stand in for just about any vegetable. Which means you can bypass the broccoli entirely for a slice of sweet cantaloupe, or eschew the escarole in favor of a nice, juicy nectarine. Or, if you're just not in the mood to chew—have a V-8 to help fill your daily requirements.

Use color as your key to selecting the most nutritious green and yellow vegetables: the deeper green or yellow (on the inside—cucumbers don't count), the higher the vitamin levels. Deep green romaine or chicory, for example, is a much better choice for your salad than the paler iceberg. Deep orange-yellow sweet potatoes will provide more carotenoids than paler varieties, and yellow peaches far more than white ones.

Try to have at least three to four servings (preferably one raw) from the following every day, ideally including at least one green and one yellow (and help yourself to more, if you'd like). Keep in mind that in the case of many, you'll also be fulfilling your vitamin C in the same serving:

2 fresh apricots

6 dried apricot halves

1/2 cup juice-packed canned apricots

1/8 cantaloupe, or 1/2 cup cubed

1/2 medium-size mango

1/4 medium-size papaya

1 nectarine

1 large yellow peach

3/4 cup pink grapefruit juice

1 pink or ruby red grapefruit

1 clementine

2 small tangerines

1 small persimmon

1/4 cup cooked bok choy

1 cup shredded raw green cabbage

1/2 cup broccoli slaw

1 cup coleslaw mix

1/2 cup raw or cooked broccoli

1 packed cup raw spinach, or
   1/2 cup cooked spinach

1/4 cup cooked greens, such as
   Swiss chard, kale, or collards

1 packed cup green leafy lettuce,
   such as romaine, arugula, red or
   green leaf, or field greens

1/4 cup chopped parsley

1/2 carrot, or 1/4 cup grated

1/4 cup carrot juice

1/2 medium-size red bell pepper

1/4 cup cooked winter squash

1/2 small sweet potato or yam

2 medium-size tomatoes

6 ounces vegetable juice

Other fruits and vegetables: one to two servings daily. So they're not as nutritionally glamorous because they don't offer significant quantities of any single nutrient. But these "other" fruits and vegetables—the ones that aren't known for their A or their C—

AN APPLE (AND TWO CARROTS AND A CUP OF BROCCOLI) A DAY

▼ ▼ ▼

For salad bar buffs and fruit fanatics, filling the various produce requirements of pregnancy may be a challenge they can't wait to sink their teeth into. However, for those who have always found managing even that one apple a day a struggle, the task may seem daunting—to say the least. And even confirmed produce lovers occasionally run out of ideas for serving up their beloved bounty. Here are some tips for fitting more fruits and vegetables into anyone's day:

■ Start your day with 100 percent fruit or vegetable juice.

■ Top pancakes or waffles with fresh fruit.

■ Add mashed banana or blueberries to pancake batter.

■ Whip up some fruit smoothies and drinks (see recipes starting on page 423).

■ Add peaches, bananas, strawberries, or blueberries to your cereal.

■ Add mushrooms, peppers, broccoli, or tomato to your omelet (see page 241).

■ Stuff a baked potato with broccoli or wild mushrooms.

■ Bake carrot muffins or carrot cake (see pages 260 and 437).

■ Add chopped dried apricots into anything you're baking.

■ Grill vegetables on skewers. Fruit, too.

■ Add mandarin oranges, carrots, tomatoes, peppers, mangoes, or strawberries to your salad.

■ Add lettuce and tomatoes to your sandwiches.

■ Toss green peas, carrots, cauliflower, broccoli, or mushrooms into your casseroles and lasagnas.

■ Stir grated carrot into your meat loaf mix.

■ Add fresh vegetables to low-sodium canned soups.

■ Add peppers, zucchini, eggplant, or even grated carrot to your tomato sauce.

are actually great dabblers in many different categories. From that apple a day to those blueberries (making some headlines themselves for their antioxidant attributes), "others" supply vital fiber, as well as respectable doses of a wide range of other vitamins, minerals, and phytochemicals. Besides, with research putting new spins on vegetables and fruits almost daily, today's "others" may become tomorrow's superstars.

Aim for one to two of the following delicious choices every day:

1 medium apple

1/2 cup unsweetened applesauce

1/2 cup apple juice

2 tablespoons apple juice concentrate

1 medium-size banana

■ Top chicken or seafood with a mango salsa (see page 373).

■ Add peas, red peppers, asparagus, or other colorful vegetables to your rice or pasta dishes.

■ Take the fast track to nutrition—and dinner—by stirring up a veggie-filled stir-fry, such as Many Peppers Steak (see page 338).

■ Add dried fruit to stuffing.

■ Blend a bowl of gazpacho (see page 288).

■ Eat a fruit salad for dessert.

■ Dip carrot sticks, broccoli, celery, cauliflower, green beans, or peppers in vegetable salsa or guacamole. (three baby carrots, and you've filled your Green and Yellow requirement for the day.)

■ Enjoy some natural fruit sorbet, and top it with fresh berries.

■ Eat a poached pear (see page 451) or baked apple for dessert.

■ Have a virgin sea breeze (cranberry juice and grapefruit juice minus the vodka) or a virgin Mary (tomato or vegetable juice and spices, also minus the vodka) as a predinner mocktail.

½ cup blueberries

⅔ cup pitted fresh cherries

¼ cup cooked cranberries

2 small fresh or dried figs

1 medium-size white peach

1 medium-size fresh pear or
   2 dried halves

½ cup pomegranate juice

½ cup pomegranate seeds

2 small plums

½ cup sliced rhubarb

3 dried dates

3 large prunes

½ cup prune juice

¼ cup dried apple rings

¼ cup raisins

¼ cup dried fruit, such as blueberries,
   cranberries, and cherries

½ cup freeze-dried fruit

½ medium avocado

½ cup (drained) canned bamboo shoots

½ cup (drained) canned water
   chestnuts

½ cup cooked green beans

½ cup cooked beets

2 large ribs celery or 1 cup diced

1 small ear cooked sweet corn
   (yellow preferred)

½ small peeled cucumber, or
   ½ cup chopped

½ cup cooked eggplant

½ cup sliced Jerusalem artichoke
   (sunchoke)

1 cup shredded iceberg lettuce

½ cup fresh raw mushrooms

½ cup cooked okra

½ cup sliced onion

½ cup cooked parsnip

½ cup cooked turnip

½ cup green garden peas or
   snow peas

½ cup cooked zucchini

4 to 6 radishes

DON'T GO AGAINST THE GRAIN

▼ ▼ ▼

So what's so special about whole grains? What makes the white bread you may have been raised on—that sandwiched your peanut butter and jelly, that layered your BLT—less worthy of a space in your lunch bag, a place next to your eggs, a home in your dinner roll basket?

Understanding how white bread gets its color (or lack of it) may help you see why whole grains take the cake nutritionally. All grains start out whole (that's the way nature grows them). It's during their processing into refined bread, rolls, and cereals that the nutritious parts of the grains are removed (including the vitamin-and-mineral-packed germ and the fiber-packed bran). And though you may think that white bread and other refined grain products can duplicate nature's nutritional formula through enrichment and fortification, it isn't so. Enrichment merely tosses in a few of the vitamins and minerals found in the whole grain, but it leaves out about twenty more—along with the naturally occurring fiber. And since a number of trace minerals and phytochemicals were unknown when enrichment was first mandated, and others remain to be discovered, it's likely that laboratory re-creation of whole-grain nutrition in a loaf of white bread will remain a scientific impossibility. Keep in mind that products that are marked "wheat" are probably made largely with white flour (and some coloring to lend a wholesome dark hue); to make sure you're getting the *whole* wheat, and nothing but the whole wheat, read the label carefully. (For more, see box, page 133.)

Whole grains and legumes: six or more servings daily. Poor grains— served nobly as the staff of life for millennia, now widely shunned by a generation of carbo-phobes. But while refined grains may deserve the bad press they've received, whole grains (wheat, corn, rice, oats, rye, barley, millet, triticale, and so on) and the breads, cereals, pastas, and other dishes made from them, as well as legumes (dried beans and peas), certainly don't, especially where pregnant women are concerned. These complex carbohydrates contain a wealth of vitamins, particularly vitamin E and the B vitamins, so essential for every part of your baby's developing body. They're rich in trace minerals, such as zinc, selenium, chromium, and magnesium. And possibly most significant to some women in the early months of pregnancy, their starchiness can prove a comfort to queasy stomachs—and their fiber a relief to clogged-up colons.

Because certain vitamins and minerals, as well as constipation-fighting fiber, are found in plentiful supply only in *whole* grains, it's important that most of your daily servings come from these. (But that doesn't mean you can't choose a few items made from refined grains, especially when queasiness demands bland.) Here's another reason to stick with the whole grain: recent research has found that these foods may lower the risk of heart disease, type 2 diabetes, and certain types of cancers. Choose from the following:

½ cup cooked brown or wild rice

¼ cup whole-grain or soy flour

½ cup cooked millet, bulgur, couscous, kasha (buckwheat groats), barley, quinoa, wheat berries, or other cooked whole grains

¼ cup whole-grain (nondegerminated) cornmeal

1 cup cooked whole-grain cereal, such as oatmeal or Wheatena*

½ cup rolled or quick-cook oats

1 cup whole-grain, ready-to-eat cereal*

½ cup granola*

2 tablespoons wheat germ

¼ cup ground flaxseed or oat bran

1 slice whole wheat, whole rye, or other whole-grain or soy bread

½ whole wheat pita

½ large whole wheat roll

½ whole wheat bagel or English muffin

1 small corn tortilla, or ½ large

½ whole wheat tortilla or wrap (12-inch whole)

2 to 6 whole-grain crackers*

2 whole-grain crispbreads

2 brown rice cakes

½ cup cooked beans, lentils, or split peas

½ cup cooked soybeans (edamame)

1 ounce (before cooking) whole-grain or soy pasta

2 cups air-popped popcorn

1 tablespoon brewer's yeast

Iron-rich foods: some daily. Your body's demand for iron will never be greater than it is now, as it works overtime to generate enough red blood cells for baby-making. To make sure the demand is met—and that an iron deficiency, which could lead to anemia—doesn't develop, adequate iron intake is essential. Since the iron requirement in pregnancy is so high, it's often difficult to fill it through diet alone. Your practitioner will likely recommend you take a daily supplement of 30 to 50 milligrams of iron in addition to your regular pregnancy supplement from the twentieth week onward. (Taking your supplement with orange or tomato juice will help your body utilize the iron, since vitamin C enhances iron absorption.) Coffee and tea, antacids, bran, and other very high fiber foods can interfere with iron absorption, as can calcium-rich foods, so don't take an iron supplement along with these. And remember that iron from animal sources (meat, fish, poultry, but not milk or cheese) is much more absorbable by the body than iron from

---

*Serving size varies; check labels.

DIDN'T MAKE THE LIST?

▼ ▼ ▼

Can't find your favorite fruit, grain, or protein source on these food lists? Just because a food didn't make the cut doesn't mean it isn't worthy of your dietary attention. For reasons of space (and so you don't have to spend nine months flipping through pages to find the food you're looking for), only more common foods and beverages are listed in this chapter. If your enquiring mind wants to know more, you can check out the USDA's National Nutrient Database website at www.nal.usda.gov/fnic/foodcomp/search/.

plant sources (vegetables, fruits, legumes); eating an animal and a plant source at the same meal will enhance absorption.

Augment your supplement with these foods in which iron naturally occurs:

Beef or buffalo, lean cuts

Duck

Sardines (drained, if canned; with bones, for a calcium component)

Cooked clams, oysters, mussels, and shrimp

Cooked dried beans

Soy bean (edamame) and soy products

Oat bran

Barley

Pumpkin seeds

Dried fruit (raisins, apricots, prunes, peaches, or currants)

Jerusalem artichokes

Spinach

Seaweed

Blackstrap molasses

Fat and high-fat foods: approximately four servings daily (depending on your weight gain). Though some daily requirements may be a struggle to fill, this one is more likely a struggle not to overfill. One trip through those Golden Arches, for example, and you're done for the day.

Still, while a lower fat diet may be preferable for most adults, it isn't a good idea to eliminate or drastically reduce dietary fats in pregnancy. Your baby needs the essential fatty acids they provide (that's why they call them *essential*) for growth and development. Especially important in the last month of pregnancy and first month of breastfeeding are omega-3 fatty acids, since this form of fat is needed for optimum brain development (see page 98).

The following are foods composed completely (or mostly) of fat. Though they won't be the only source of fat in your diet (you'll get extra fat from dairy products, nuts, meat, poultry, and more), they're the only ones you'll need to keep track of on The Pregnancy Diet. Keeping track will be easier if you keep an eye out for the many places fat foods tend to show up (the mayonnaise on your chicken salad sandwich, the oil in your salad dressing, the butter on your roll).

If you're gaining weight too quickly, you can cut back by one or two fat servings. You might also want to consider cutting way back on foods that are prepared with a lot of fat (anything fried or swimming in butter or cream, particularly if they're not particularly nutritious). If you're gaining weight too slowly, you may want to add a fat serving—as well as some extra high-fat foods (preferable healthful ones, like nuts and avocados). But also make sure you're getting enough of the other daily eleven.

1 tablespoon oil, such as vegetable, olive, canola, and sesame

1 tablespoon regular margarine or butter

1 tablespoon regular mayonnaise

2 tablespoons regular salad dressing

3 tablespoons light cream

2 tablespoons heavy (or whipping) cream

$\frac{1}{4}$ cup whipped cream

$\frac{1}{4}$ cup sour cream

2 tablespoons cream cheese

2 tablespoons peanut butter

Other high-fat foods. These are high in fat. You don't have to officially count them in your total, but

FAT AND VEGGIES DO MIX

▼ ▼ ▼

Fat-phobics, it's time to confront your fears. Or, at least, start drizzling them on your salads and steamed vegetables. Turns out that a little fat actually brings out the best in broccoli (or romaine, or carrots). Though it's tempting to save yourself a few calories by pouring on the fat-free dressings or opting for a virtuous squeeze of lemon, new research has shown that sparing the fat spoils the nutrients. Scientists have found that many of the vital dietary properties in vegetables (like alpha-carotene, beta-carotene, or lycopene) aren't well absorbed without a side of fat. So order the salad, but don't hold the fat. Make a point of including a little fat in veggie-containing meals and snacks—whether it's in the form of dressing for your salad, dip for your carrot sticks, oil for your stir-fry, or just a side of meat, cheese, or nuts. Just keep in mind that a little fat goes a long way (think 1 tablespoon of oil in your stir-fry, not $\frac{1}{4}$ cup)—no need to drown your green leafies in Thousand Island in order to reap their nutritional benefits.

SALT SENSE

▼ ▼ ▼

Early pregnancy cravings have you reaching for the dills? The good news is that for most pregnant women, salt restriction isn't considered necessary. In fact, a certain amount of sodium is needed to allow for pregnancy's higher fluid volume. The bad news (if one dill tends to lead to another . . . and another) is that eating large quantities of foods and seasonings high in salt (besides the pickles, count chips, most fast food, and soy sauce in that category) isn't a healthy move for anyone, pregnant or not. And for some women, a high sodium intake during pregnancy may cause a variety of potential complications (high blood pressure, for instance).

Most women get plenty of sodium naturally in a typical diet and there is rarely a need for additional salt use. Americans typically consume 4,000 to 8,000 mg of sodium each day, well above their daily needs. A healthy goal for all adults, pregnant or not, is approximately 2,400 mg of sodium per day.

Keeping your sodium intake at a healthy level is as easy (or as difficult) as cutting back on foods that are high in sodium (nutritional labels on packaged foods will clue you in to the numbers). In general, that would include processed foods (like macaroni and cheese mix and luncheon meats), most canned soups and vegetables, most frozen entrees, and, of course, most fast foods. Also, watch the shaker in your kitchen and at your dinner table. Salt only lightly (or don't salt at all) during cooking. If you can trust yourself not to overdo it (or reach for the shaker without thinking or tasting first), salt foods to taste at the table. To be sure you meet the increased need for iodine during pregnancy, use only iodized salt (unless you have hyperthyroidism and your practitioner recommends avoiding iodized salt).

---

you should be aware that eating too many might pile on the extra pounds:

Cream sauces

Full-fat cheese

Whole-milk yogurt

Nuts and seeds

Fatty meats

Omega-3 fatty acids. Fat that you can actually feel good about eating? Yes, there is such a thing: omega-3 polyunsaturated fatty acids (such as docosahexaenoic acid, or DHA), have been shown to lower cholesterol and blood pressure, reducing the risk for heart disease. More important to pregnant women, DHA is a major component of the brain and retina and is essential for proper brain growth and eye development in fetuses and young babies. DHA fuels the rapid brain growth of the last trimester (when the brain's DHA content multiplies by three to five times) and the first three months of life (when the DHA content triples). Some studies show that maternal levels of DHA decrease considerably during pregnancy, so including DHA in your diet is essential for your baby's normal brain, eye, and vision development, especially during that last trimester and while you're breastfeeding. (Experts also suspect there may be a connection between low DHA and postpartum depression—all the more reason to increase your intake of DHA-rich foods while you're pregnant.)

There is no recommended daily intake of DHA yet; more research needs to be done to calculate it. Until then, your best bet is to consume a good amount of DHA, especially toward the end of your pregnancy. This fabulous fat is found in concentrated amounts in oily fish such as salmon, trout, herrings, anchovies, and sardines, as well as in walnuts and walnut oil. It's also found in other nuts (including almonds and Brazil nuts), seeds (such as pumpkin, sunflower, and flax), canned tuna (which should be limited; see page 169), crab, shrimp, chicken, eggs, and arugula. Omega-3-rich eggs are an especially good source; they come from hens fed a heart-healthy diet; look for them in your market. Also now available for pregnant women are DHA supplements derived from algae. Ask your practitioner if you should take one.

TAKE IT WITH A GRAIN OF SALT

▼ ▼ ▼

Not a fan of the puffy look when it comes to ankles? Think restricting your salt intake can decrease the chances you'll retain water—and increase the chances that your shoes will still fit come month nine?

The fact is that you retain fluid not because of salt, but because of pregnancy hormones. And a certain amount of swelling is normal and healthy in pregnancy. While too much sodium in your diet can aggravate this normal swelling, salt restriction can cause problems for you and your fetus by disrupting the delicate fluid balance needed to maintain a healthy pregnancy. So don't hide the salt shaker; just sprinkle within reason.

▲ ▲ ▲

"There is no way I can eat all the food that's suggested in the Daily Dozen and still keep my weight gain reasonable. Is there?"

Sure there is—especially if you choose foods that fill more than one Daily Dozen requirement at a time so you can double up, even triple up on nutrition without doubling or tripling up on calories. In other words, you need to become an efficiency expert. A cup of yogurt, for instance, yields a serving of protein and a serving of calcium for the

WATER, WATER EVERYWHERE

▼ ▼ ▼

Never been a big drinker—of water? Here are some tips to help you get you in the water habit:

■ Carry a small, refillable water bottle with you at all times. Drink while you're in the car, at the ATM, while checking your e-mail, waiting in line at the market, riding on the subway.

■ Fill a large container or water jug (24 ounces, for instance) with water and keep it with you all day, at your desk or at home. You'll need to fill it only one more time to get six of your Daily Dozen fluids. Top it off with a few fruits, vegetable juice, and a soup for dinner—and you've met your goal (plus covered a few other of your Daily Dozen needs).

■ Drink one glass of water every two hours during the day.

■ Use larger glasses or mugs, such as twelve-ounce size, so you can drink more at each sitting.

■ Drink two full glasses of liquid at each meal, one before and one after. (Stick with between-meal drinks, however, if you're still contending with nausea or if you're having trouble finding room in your tummy come mealtime.)

■ When eating out, down a glass of water before you leave for the restaurant. And down another one at the table while you're waiting for your food.

■ Look for other sources of fluids, besides the strictly liquid ones: 1 cup watermelon yields ½ cup liquid; a fruit juice Popsicle adds some, too, and so do soups.

---

broccoli nets both a vitamin C and a green leafy (while earning a bonus of calcium). Eat efficiently whenever you can, and you'll be able to pack in the nutrition without packing on the pounds. (See page 77 for more).

▼ ▼ ▼

Fluids: at least eight 8-ounce glasses daily. A person can survive for many days or even weeks without food, but only a few days without water. Water comprises one-half to three-fourths of the human body mass, is part of nearly

all cells, and is necessary for almost every bodily function. During pregnancy, it is particularly vital. Between amniotic fluid, augmented maternal blood volume, and additional fluids in maternal tissue, ten pounds of an average thirty-pound pregnancy weight gain is composed of liquids. It is needed for building the fetus's body cells, for the developing circulatory system, for the delivery of nutrients, and for the excretion of wastes. Your body needs extra fluids during pregnancy, too, to help combat constipa-

nancy, too, to help combat constipation, prevent dry skin, regulate body temperature, and to reduce the risk of urinary tract infection. Drinking enough water can also keep you from retaining too much fluid (a.k.a. swelling) by helping your body flush out waste products. Hot weather and physical activity can increase your fluid needs greatly, and so can early pregnancy vomiting or diarrhea anytime; not replacing that lost fluid can lead to dehydration. You can be sure you're taking in enough fluid when enough is coming out; you should be urinating pale or colorless urine frequently.

When tallying your fluid intake, remember to also count fluids that don't come from the tap (or your water bottle). Milk (which is two-thirds water) taken in liquid or frozen form (such as frozen yogurt), and soups and broths should figure in. Fruits and vegetables count, too—five typical servings equal about two fluid servings—as do decaffeinated coffee or tea, sparkling water, and juices.

Particularly in early and late pregnancy, your frequent trips to the bathroom may tempt you into cutting back on fluids. Don't. The excreted urine is carrying out a vital task: removal of waste products from your system and your baby's.

Prenatal vitamin supplements: a pregnancy formula taken daily. When it comes to your nutritional needs during pregnancy, nothing can

wisdom of the ages?

Pregnancy superstitions run the gamut from possibly plausible to downright peculiar. Definitely falling into the latter category is this one: Pregnant women centuries ago were told that if they didn't drink enough water, their babies would be born dirty. (Care for some soap with that glass of water, ma'am?) While there's obviously no truth to the actual superstition (and besides, all babies get dirty quickly enough—especially in the diaper area), there is some wisdom behind the advice. Getting enough water during pregnancy is extremely important.

compete with a well-balanced diet. The vitamins, minerals, and nutrients that come from a variety of wholesome foods are better than anything science can manufacture. And beyond the many already documented, there are likely many more properties in natural foods important for good health that have yet to be discovered or are impossible to recreate in a laboratory. But sometimes, despite your best intentions and your best efforts (after all, you *did* try to eat that bowl of cereal between trips to the bathroom to throw up), your diet may one day be lacking in a vitamin, another day—a mineral or two.

Enter the prenatal vitamin supplement. The point of taking vitamin supplements during pregnancy (or at any other time) isn't so you can let your diet slide, but to provide insurance in case it should slide inadvertently. It's also to keep you from

LOSE THE GUILT

▼ ▼ ▼

Maybe you really tried to eat well today. Or, maybe you didn't try as hard as you could have, or as hard as you tried yesterday. Maybe you tried, but a tough day at the office or a particularly harsh bout of nausea stood in the way of your efforts. As you tally up your Daily Dozen, you realize just how far short you came, and that familiar feeling starts swelling in the pit of your stomach. No, not bloating. Guilt.

Throw it away—before it has a chance to rise up and make you miserable. Guilt has no place in any eating plan—and, in fact, it's the reason most eating plans fail. (Eating ice cream makes you feel guilty; feeling guilty sends you once again to the freezer for more ice cream; run out to the corner market for another half-gallon, and repeat.) For an eating plan to be successful anytime, but especially during pregnancy, it has to provide feelings of pleasure, not remorse.

Here's some straight talk about a pregnancy diet. There are more than a Daily Dozen reasons why eating an excellent diet is good for you and good for your baby. (Just skim through the last few chapters, if you're not convinced.) And striving

for excellence in eating is well worth your while. But the bottom line is, if you maintain a healthy lifestyle (avoid drugs, tobacco, alcohol; exercise and get good prenatal care) and eat an overall well-balanced diet (one that consists of a nice mix of fruits, vegetables, whole grains, and proteins, without an excess of junk foods), you and your baby are in great shape—literally. If you miss your recommended intake of vitamin C one day because you were nowhere near a fruit or vegetable, don't beat yourself up—just blend yourself up a smoothie tomorrow for breakfast. If your cravings send you diving spoon-first into a big bowl of sugar-frosted cereal two days in a row, don't despair; just dive into a big salad for dinner. If you spend an entire week in your second month eating nothing but dry crackers (the dry, refined type) and ginger ale (the sugary kind), don't worry—you've got weeks ahead to make up for it. In the meantime, neither you nor your baby will suffer.

So do your best to eat right, and when your best isn't all that good, lose the guilt—and try to do better next time. Pregnancy should be filled not only with good food, but good feelings, as well.

being shortchanged should storage, cooking, or exposure to air rob foods of the vitamins and minerals you're counting on. In the case of nutrients that are difficult to obtain in adequate quantities from diet alone, such as iron and folic acid (and, for strict vegans, calcium, vitamin D, vitamin B_{12}), a supplement makes the task easier. And studies show that women who take prenatal vitamins before and during pregnancy dramatically lower the risks of having babies with spina bifida and cleft palate (due, most probably, to the folic acid content of the supplements) and also may be less likely to give birth prematurely. But remember that prenatal vitamins don't supply protein, fiber, certain important minerals, and energy (calories) necessary for a healthy pregnancy. Vitamins are considered supplements, not substitutes for a balanced diet.

The formula you take should be especially designed for pregnancy. Ask your practitioner to prescribe or suggest one, or select one yourself that contains the vitamins and minerals in approximately the same dosages as the following formula:

▲ No more than 4,000 IU (800 ug) of vitamin A. Many manufacturers have reduced the amount of vitamin A in their vitamin supplements or have replaced it with beta-carotene, a much safer source of vitamin A.

▲ At least 400 to 600 mcg of folic acid (folate).

▲ 250 mcg of calcium. If you're not getting enough calcium in your diet, you will need additional supplementation to reach the 1,200 mg needed during pregnancy. Do not take more than 250 mg of calcium (or more than 25 mg of magnesium) *along with* supplementary iron, since these minerals interfere with iron absorption. Take any larger doses at least two hours before or after your iron supplement.

▲ 30 mg of iron

▲ 50 to 80 mg of vitamin C

▲ 15 mg of zinc

▲ 2 mg of copper

▲ 2 mg of vitamin B_6

▲ Not more than 500 ug of vitamin D

▲ Approximately the DRI for vitamin E (15 mg), thiamin (1.4 mg), riboflavin (1.4 mg), niacin (18 mg), and vitamin B_{12} (2.6 mcg). Most prenatal supplements contain two to three times the DRI of these. There are no known harmful effects from such doses.

▲ Some preparations may also contain magnesium, fluoride, biotin, phosphorous, pantothenic acid, or a combination of these.

Do not take any other nutritional supplements without your doctor's approval. When taken in supplement form (not in food), some nutrients (such as vitamins A and D) are toxic in large doses (doses higher than those found in prenatal vitamins). In addition, some supplements may contain herbs that are not safe to take during pregnancy.

▲ ▲ ▲

Q *"My midwife prescribed some prenatal vitamins for me. But they make me extremely nauseated. How can I get the benefits of a supplement if I can't keep it down?"*

IDEAL . . . GET REAL

▼ ▼ ▼

Now that you have The Pregnancy Diet—a well-balanced eating plan that provides you with all the important nutrients you need for a healthy pregnancy and your baby needs for a healthy start in life—all you have to do is follow it.

And chances are, you'll be able to. Much of the time. Or, at least, some of the time. On those days when you manage to actually sit down for breakfast. And when lunch isn't something you grab off a catering tray in the conference room. And when dinner is something you actually get home in time to cook.

But let's face it. Not every pregnant woman—probably not even those with the will power of a triathlete and a genuine fondness for broccoli—will be able to score a perfect twelve on the Daily Dozen, or live and breathe those Nine Basic Principles every single day of their nine months.

And that's okay. The Pregnancy Diet represents the ideal—the best of all possible nutritional worlds. Something to shoot for, absolutely. But nothing to shoot yourself over if you sometimes (or even often) fall short. So if you find you can't reach the ideal every day—or even once a week, or even once during your entire pregnancy—don't stress. Don't be hard on yourself. And certainly, don't give up. But do realize that there are many ways to come close—ways that are probably pretty attainable for you—and to reap as many baby-friendly benefits as possible. And who knows—you might actually be coming closer to that ideal than you think.

THE PREGNANCY DIET IDEAL	GET REAL
VITAMIN C: 3 servings daily	Pour a tall glass of orange juice before you dash out the door in the morning to do carpool for your toddler. Good job—you've bought yourself two servings of vitamin C.
CALCIUM: 4 servings daily	Back home, a bowl of Wheaties, banana, and milk starts your day; later you finish your toddler's half-eaten grilled cheese at lunch; a scoop of frozen yogurt tides you over until dinner—and don't forget that OJ you had for breakfast was calcium fortified. 3 servings of calcium—not bad.
GREEN LEAFY AND YELLOW VEGETABLES AND YELLOW FRUITS: 3 to 4 servings	Your dinnertime salad counts as one serving. And weren't there some shredded carrots hidden among the lettuce leaves and tomatoes? That's two. (Hey—those tomatoes give you another vitamin C serving. See, you've made it to three in that department.) Don't forget that handful of dried apricots you munched while you were waiting at the bank. Guess what? You're already there.

THE PREGNANCY DIET IDEAL	GET REAL
OTHER FRUITS AND VEGETABLES: 1 to 2 servings	That blueberry pie you ate for dessert—count it toward one (while trying not to think about the extra calories). And didn't you slice half a banana into your cereal bowl this morning? You're on a roll— 1½ servings!
WHOLE GRAINS AND LEGUMES: 6 or more servings	That half-eaten cheese sandwich was on whole wheat bread— right? That's one serving. The Wheaties count for another. The half-bagel you wolfed down midmorning is another. Your side at dinner was long-grain and wild rice. There's another one. Can't forget those crackers you ate before you got out of bed to keep the queasies away. And you have to count that crust from the blueberry pie (well, at least this one time). You've gotten your six servings already. Great job.
PROTEIN: 3 servings	This is a no-brainer. There's that milk from the cereal, the cheese from the sandwich, the frozen yogurt, and the grilled chicken you had for dinner—plus the protein from all those grains. That was easy.
IRON-RICH FOODS	There's some iron in those peas and dried apricots you ate today. Way to go.
FATS: 4 servings	This is easy. Make that too easy. You probably made it at least halfway with the blueberry pie. And don't forget the dressing on that salad, or the light cream cheese on the bagel.
CALORIES	Your day's diet totals approximately 1,900 calories. Assuming your prepregnancy weight was 125 pounds, you're right on target— plus you have almost 100 calories to spare. (Scratch that—you already spent it on the granola bar you found under the car seat. The good news—that realization just brought your grain total up to seven.)

LAUNCH A SNACK ATTACK

▼ ▼ ▼

Poking around the fridge for some good healthy snacks to round out your day and your Daily Dozen? Give these a try:

- 1 hard-cooked egg* (deviled, if you're feeling ambitious), and a glass of V-8

- Cooked soybeans (edamame)

- Apple slices with peanut butter (if you don't have allergies; see page 136)

- Soy chips or crisps (they're high in protein, low in fat, crunchy and yummy); Pirate's Booty or Veggie Booty

- Whole wheat crackers with low-fat cheese slices

- Low-fat yogurt with granola sprinkled on top

- A mozzarella stick and some frozen grapes

- Fruit smoothie

- Multigrain waffle

- Air-popped popcorn, sprinkled with parmesan cheese and chili powder

- A small potato, microwaved and sprinkled with cheddar cheese

- A handful of almonds or walnuts and raisins

- Dried apricots, apples, pears, figs, or cranberries and a wedge of cheese

- Half a whole wheat flour tortilla, rolled up with shredded cheese and tomato

- Carrot and celery sticks with hummus spread

- A cup of tomato soup (choose a low-sodium brand or use the recipe on page 285), topped with a small scoop of cottage cheese

- A carrot muffin and milk or cheese

- A small box of dry cereal

- Soy nuts and raisins

---

*Keep a supply of hard-cooked eggs, preferably omega-3-rich ones, in your refrigerator for a quick protein fix.

A Don't give up—switch around. The pharmacy shelves are lined with prenatal supplements, and one is bound to sit better with your stomach. Your practitioner can recommend some good options such as a coated one, or one that has a slow release formula, or one that has a greater amount of vitamin B6 (which combats nausea). You can also try taking your supplement with a meal or taking it with a pre-bed snack so you can sleep through the queasiness it causes. Also, check out the tips on page 17 for taking vitamins while combating morning sickness.

Q *"I'm using an over-the-counter store brand of prenatal vitamin instead of the brand my obstetrician prescribed. Is that okay?"*

A Don't dismiss over-the-counter prenatal vitamins just because they're not technically what the doctor ordered. Most of them contain the same formula as the prescription prenatal vitamins and can cost much less. To be sure, check the labels and compare—or ask your OB.

Q *"I usually am very diligent about taking my prenatal vitamins very day. But yesterday I completely forgot to take one. Should I take an extra one today?"*

A Remember that your prenatal vitamins should never be used in place of a healthy diet. So assuming you're being pretty good about

following The Pregnancy Diet, if you miss a day or two of taking the vitamin supplements (or if queasiness leads you to throw them up or skip them once in a while)—you've lost nothing except a little insurance. Don't double up on your supplement today if you missed it yesterday.

Q *"When is the best time of the day to take my vitamins?"*

A If you're suffering from nausea, any time of the day that you're best able to keep the prenatal down is the best time to take it. If queasiness isn't an issue, try to take it down during a meal that includes a little fat to help you absorb those fat-soluble vitamins (A, D, E, and K). And make sure you chase it with plenty of fluids to help it dissolve well. If it's an iron supplement you're taking, avoid eating or drinking something high in calcium (as calcium impedes iron absorption) or fiber (ditto) along with it; instead, accompany your iron with food or drink high in vitamin C (which will aid in iron absorption).

▼ ▼ ▼

The Expectant Gourmet

IF YOU'RE LIKE MOST PREGNANT WOMEN, it's not making the decision to eat well that's challenging (everyone wants what's best for their baby), it's actually changing the way you eat to make sure you *are* eating well.

For some, it might be as easy as adding an extra fruit or two to their day, or drinking another glass of milk. (In fact, you may already be a whole lot closer to putting away those Daily Dozen than you think; check out the quiz on the next page.) For others, it might take a little more effort—remembering to ask for the whole wheat bagel at the deli instead of the plain; opting for the side salad or fruit cup instead of the fries with that sandwich; switching from ice cream to frozen yogurt.

For card-carrying junk-food fans who still cling to the possibility that ketchup can be counted as a vegetable and a chocolate bar with nuts as a good source of protein, the changes—and the effort required to effect them—will be substantial. But so will the benefits, for their health and their baby's.

Whether your diet just needs a little fine-tuning or a major overhaul, you'll find the tools you'll need to make those changes in this chapter.

Evaluating Your Eating Habits

YOU PROBABLY ALREADY HAVE A good idea of how well you're eating, but taking this quiz will help you confirm what you already know:

1. My typical breakfast consists of:
   a. Bacon and eggs, "wheat" toast with margarine, and calcium-fortified orange juice
   b. A bowl of Cheerios with sliced strawberries and skim milk, grapefruit sections on the side
   c. A bowl of hot pink, neon blue, bright green, and canary yellow sugar-frosted cereal loops, no milk (it makes them soggy)

2. My typical lunch consists of:
   a. Tuna salad on an onion bagel, bag of potato chips
   b. Grilled chicken with arugula, roasted red pepper, mozzarella cheese, and portobello mushroom on multigrain bread
   c. Who has time for lunch? I just grab a chocolate bar from the vending machine.

3. My typical dinner consists of:
   a. Canned vegetable soup, two slices of frozen pizza, frozen yogurt
   b. Grilled fish, broccoli and cheddar on a baked potato with skin, red leaf lettuce salad, fresh fruit

   c. Fast-food burger, fries, apple pie, coffee with creamer

4. You have an early-morning meeting at the office and have no time for breakfast. What do you grab to eat on the way?
   a. Corn muffin and a decaf latte
   b. Yellow peach and a carton of yogurt
   c. A prenatal vitamin and a can of diet soda

5. A typical snack during the day is:
   a. Packaged crackers and cheese spread
   b. Dried apricots and walnuts
   c. Potato chips and onion dip

6. Your favorite fruit is:
   a. Raisins
   b. Cantaloupe
   c. Fruit roll-up

7. How many fruits do you eat daily?
   a. 1 to 2
   b. 3 to 4
   c. Does a fruit roll-up count?

8. How do you get your vitamin C?
   a. A glass of orange juice
   b. A fresh orange
   c. Prenatal vitamin

9. Your total calcium intake for a typical day includes:

a. Calcium-fortified orange juice, cheese on pizza, frozen yogurt

b. Skim milk in cereal, fruit and yogurt smoothie, cheese sandwich, steamed broccoli

c. The yellow square they put on burgers . . . and how about that creamer?

10. The color of your bread is:
a. White
b. Brown
c. I gave up bread because it's a carbohydrate.

11. What types of drinks do you have in your refrigerator?
a. 2 percent milk, apple juice
b. Skim milk, calcium-fortified orange juice, sparkling water
c. Diet soda

12. What's in your freezer?
a. Frozen pizza, frozen chicken nuggets, frozen yogurt
b. Frozen vegetables, frozen veggie burgers, frozen blueberries
c. Frozen Snickers bars

13. Your salad is made out of:
a. Ready-made iceberg mix (with shriveled carrots and cabbage), cucumbers
b. Romaine lettuce, red peppers, tomato, sunflower seeds
c. What's a salad?

14. Your favorite grain is:
a. Quick-cook brown rice in a bag
b. Bulgur wheat or quinoa
c. White rice (and refried beans)

15. What's in your pantry?
a. Canned fruit in syrup
b. Canned fruit in juice
c. Candy

16. How many glasses of fluids do you drink a day?
a. About 6
b. At least 8
c. Coffee counts, right?

17. Your favorite dessert is:
a. Fresh peach pie
b. Fresh peaches
c. Death by Chocolate

18. When you want something to munch on during the game, what do you reach for?
a. Salted pretzels
b. Raw vegetables and fresh tomato salsa
c. Chocolate chip cookies

19. What's your oil of choice?
a. Vegetable oil
b. Olive or canola oil
c. Margarine, melted

20. Where do you keep the fruit in your house?
a. In a fruit bowl on the dining room table
b. In the center of my refrigerator
c. What fruit?

Now it's time to add up your score. For every question you answered *a*, give yourself one point. For every *b*, give yourself two points. For every *c*, give yourself zero points. Final score: _____

So how did you do? If you scored:

31 to 40: Great job! You're already eating well.

16 to 30: Not bad at all. You're doing pretty well already—and with a few tweaks, you'll be right on track.

0 to 15: Get ready. Your diet needs a major overhaul.

A more precise way to evaluate your diet is to keep a food diary (see diary, page 112). Over the course of five days, write down everything you eat and drink (including the amount). At the bottom of each column, tick off the number of portions you consume in each category. Remember, this is not a test (there's no "passing grade," no reason to cheat); just an evaluation. Be specific, accurate, and honest when you fill it out so that you get the clearest idea of your eating habits; no one will be seeing your lists besides yourself.

Once your chart is completed, you'll be able to get an honest picture of your eating habits. Have you met or exceeded The Pregnancy Diet recommendations for healthy eating? Come close? Are there many Daily Dozen categories that you need to improve on, or just one or two? Is there any category that needs major overhauling (such as junk food or caffeinated beverages)? Are you eating too many proteins and not enough calcium foods? Or are you heavy on the fruit but light on the green leafies?

Keep in mind that variety is important for good overall nutrition, too. So consider: Are you eating the same thing for lunch pretty much every day? (Even if that lunch is healthy, you'd probably be better off mixing it up a bit to ensure you're getting the right combination of vitamins and minerals daily—a grilled chicken salad one day, an egg salad wrap the next.) Are bananas always your fruit of choice? If so, you're getting a great source of potassium, but very little in the way of vitamin C, so consider slicing your banana up with kiwi. Widening your diet to include a diversity of foods is as important as making sure those foods are nutritious on their own.

DEAR FOOD DIARY

▼ ▼ ▼

DAY 1	DAY 2
BREAKFAST	BREAKFAST
LUNCH	LUNCH
DINNER	DINNER
SNACKS	SNACKS

DAY 1	DAY 2
PROTEIN FOODS _____	PROTEIN FOODS _____
CALCIUM FOODS _____	CALCIUM FOODS _____
VEGETABLES _____	VEGETABLES _____
FRUITS _____	FRUITS _____
WHOLE GRAINS _____	WHOLE GRAINS _____
REFINED GRAINS _____	REFINED GRAINS _____
IRON-RICH FOODS _____	IRON-RICH FOODS _____
HIGH-FAT FOODS _____	HIGH-FAT FOODS _____
JUNK FOODS _____	JUNK FOODS _____
CAFFEINATED BEVERAGES _____	CAFFEINATED BEVERAGES _____
WATER & OTHER FLUIDS _____	WATER & OTHER FLUIDS _____

DAY 3	DAY 4	DAY 5
BREAKFAST	BREAKFAST	BREAKFAST
LUNCH	LUNCH	LUNCH
DINNER	DINNER	DINNER
SNACKS	SNACKS	SNACKS

PROTEIN FOODS _____	PROTEIN FOODS _____	PROTEIN FOODS _____
CALCIUM FOODS _____	CALCIUM FOODS _____	CALCIUM FOODS _____
VEGETABLES _____	VEGETABLES _____	VEGETABLES _____
FRUITS _____	FRUITS _____	FRUITS _____
WHOLE GRAINS _____	WHOLE GRAINS _____	WHOLE GRAINS _____
REFINED GRAINS _____	REFINED GRAINS _____	REFINED GRAINS _____
IRON-RICH FOODS_____	IRON-RICH FOODS _____	IRON-RICH FOODS _____
HIGH-FAT FOODS_____	HIGH-FAT FOODS _____	HIGH-FAT FOODS _____
JUNK FOODS _____	JUNK FOODS _____	JUNK FOODS _____
CAFFEINATED BEVERAGES____	CAFFEINATED BEVERAGES ____	CAFFEINATED BEVERAGES ____
WATER & OTHER FLUIDS _____	WATER & OTHER FLUIDS_____	WATER & OTHER FLUIDS_____

Making a Change for the Better

WHETHER YOUR EATING HABITS are almost there or have a long way to go, following these steps will make that change for the better easier to make:

Change your mind. Don't confuse healthy eating with dieting, a word that has understandably left a bitter taste in most women's mouths. Healthy eating, unlike dieting, isn't synonymous with deprivation. Instead of thinking of the changes you'll be making in terms of what you'll be denying yourself, think of them as the good ways you'll be feeding yourself and your baby. Focus on the foods you'll be adding to help provide your baby with all the nutrients he or she needs.

Change slowly. Changing too quickly to new eating or lifestyle habits usually backfires. Instead of making sweeping, sudden changes (such as going cold turkey off all refined grains), take baby steps toward your goal. For example, switch from corn flakes to a whole-grain cereal the first few days. Start ordering your sandwich on whole wheat bread a couple of days later. Drop that midmorning cinnamon roll the following week, adding a whole-grain muffin in its place. Before you know it, most of the grains you eat will be whole.

Not only will the slow approach to change make it easier to handle, but it'll probably make it last longer, too. And studies show that the longer you remain on a healthy diet, the greater the chance of changing your habits for good.

Take it one day at a time. It's definitely daunting to think about changing your diet completely for nine months—so don't think that way. Instead, take your dietary changes one day at a time. Focus on each day, and do the best you can on that day. But if you don't do so well one day (or even a few days in a row), don't look back, don't get discouraged, and don't give up. Just tackle the next day as a brand-new one (the first day of the rest of your Pregnancy Diet), with new opportunities for eating better.

Reinvent food. Even if you hated spinach when your mother forced you to eat it, you might actually enjoy it as an adult. Take a fresh look at foods you never liked before; with a new perspective and new preparations, you may find they're actually pretty good. Instead of serving spinach up in the form of your childhood nightmares, eat it raw in a Spinach Strawberry Salad (see page 314), lightly steamed as a bed for grilled salmon, or stuffed with cheese inside rolled chicken breasts.

Put fruits and vegetables front and center. Bury the fruits and vegetables you bring home from the supermarket in the bottom of the produce drawers, and you'll forget about them. By the time you remember, you'll be greeted by soft peaches, moldy grapes, wilted lettuce, and shriveled carrots. Place the fruit that doesn't need refrigeration in a bowl on the kitchen table (bananas, for instance) and the others in the front of the middle shelf in the fridge.

Plan, plan, plan. The reality of life is that it gets in the way a lot. You meant to get up early to brown-bag a healthy lunch, but you overslept—and ended up grabbing a package of cheese crackers from the vending machine instead. You had every intention of stirring up a healthy chicken stir-fry for dinner but realized when you got home from the market that you'd forgotten to buy the chicken—so you end up dining on peanut butter and jelly. The way around these sorry (but probably all-too-real) scenarios is to plan ahead. See page 116 for tips.

Keep your lifestyle in mind. Here's another dose of reality: If you have to undergo major life changes in order to change the way you eat, your new habits won't stand a chance. If mornings have you running to catch an early commuter train, a full sit-down breakfast probably isn't in the cards. Instead, blend your breakfast in a Breakfast Booster Shake (see page 427), to be slipped into a thermos and sipped on the train along with a bag of crunchy dry cereal and freeze-dried fruit. Or pack a healthy brown-bag breakfast-to-go the night before (Triple Blueberry Muffins, page 256 which you've cleverly baked ahead and stashed in the freezer, yogurt, a peach, and a single-serving bottle of calcium-fortified orange juice). If business sends you to restaurants most nights, scout for healthy choices on the menu (see page 184 for tips on eating well while eating out). If your budget's tighter than your jeans are getting, you'll probably balk at shelling out big bucks on field greens and fresh raspberries—no matter how nutritious they are. Instead, opt for more ordinary—but still nutritious—produce, and save yourself a bundle while eating healthier than ever (see page 195 for tips on eating well on a budget).

Don't succumb to peer pressure. A colleague brings in a box of French pastries to celebrate a new deal, and everyone dives in headfirst. Don't make your office workers' bad habits your own, especially if you've already changed for the better. Have a bite or two if you can't resist, and then turn your attention back to the healthy snack you brought from home.

PLANNING AHEAD

▼ ▼ ▼

The very definition of a habit is that it's something you do all the time, without thinking. Which is why habits can be tough to change. When it comes to eating habits, the best way to overcome that challenge is to start thinking—and planning—ahead of time about what you're going to eat, rather than leaving it up to chance. Advance preparation allows you to throw out the old I-can't-eat-healthy-because-I-have-nothing-healthy-to-eat excuse—and help make a habit out of eating well. Here are some realistic plan-ahead tips:

■ **Plan for between-meal hunger.** If healthy snacks are always within arm's reach, you'll never have to make a trip to the vending machine (for that chocolate bar) or to the corner grocery store (for a bag of chips) when hunger strikes. Bag some crunchy freeze-dried peaches and toasted almonds to tote in your briefcase, stash some soy chips in your desk drawer and some granola bars in your car, and keep the fridge filled with ready-to-munch hard-cooked eggs, cheese sticks or individual wedges, cut-up raw vegetables, and fresh fruit.

■ **Plan for shopping.** Don't just dash to the supermarket with some vague idea of what you'll be eating. (That's how you forgot the chicken for the stir-fry.) Take a few minutes to draw up a weekly (or daily, if you market that often) menu and arm yourself with a shopping list that covers it all. If that's too much prep work for the spontaneous you, at least make sure your cupboards, fridge, and freezer are filled with healthy choices you can make meals out of (see page 119).

■ **Plan for what you can realistically do.** Don't plan for meals you don't have time to

Don't eat your words. If you're really serious about changing your eating habits, get serious about changing them. Don't vow one day that the bag of potato chips you're munching from is your last, only to buy another one three days later. Make a plan and stick to it. You'll feel better reaching a goal you set.

Think before you don't eat. If your biggest eating challenge is not eating at all (you're a breakfast or lunch skipper from way back), you'll need to make a concerted effort to make sure you're eating three to six times a day, regularly. Not enough time in the morning to sit down at the breakfast table? Try setting the alarm to go off earlier. Or take breakfast to work: a container of cereal and banana, with an individual serving of milk; instant oatmeal, dried apricots and blueberries mixed with nonfat dry milk (add hot water to finish it off); a container of yogurt topped

make. The Veal Stew with Wild Mushrooms (30 minutes prep time; 1½ hours to braise) sounded fabulous in the cooking magazine, but if you're likely to get home from work at 8 P.M. to an empty pot and an empty stomach, it wasn't a wise choice for dinner. Fantasy dinners like that typically end up staying just that—a fantasy—with reality taking the form of frozen dinners . . . or a bag of chips.

■ **Plan on produce.** When formulating your dinner menu, get into the habit of using a vegetable as your starting point—instead of thinking of meat as the "main." For example, instead of deciding on a steak for dinner (with a small salad on the side), plan to prepare a large salad of baby greens, roasted peppers, and mushrooms, and laying the sliced steak on top (and maybe some thinly sliced Parmesan cheese; see Steak Salad, page 328). Instead of featuring grilled chicken (with a cameo by coleslaw), make the star of your dinner show grilled asparagus and shiitake mushrooms (cast on a lovely bed of greens); the chicken will appear (and taste) delicious on top.

■ **Plan for tomorrow tonight.** If mornings are rushed for you, there's a good chance you'll dash out the door before you can fix yourself a good breakfast. And as for packing a brown bag when you're late for the train? Forget about it; it'll never happen. So instead of leaving tomorrow's meals up to chance—and up to real life—spend a few minutes before you turn in at night preparing breakfast (put the fruit and the yogurt in the blender jar, and refrigerate it for smoothie-ing in the morning; prepare a bowl of cold cereal and dry fruit ready to be covered with milk; heap some cottage cheese in a cantaloupe half and leave it in the refrigerator covered in plastic wrap overnight (add a defrosted muffin in the morning); or prepare cheese and fresh spinach on a whole wheat tortilla ready to microwave). And while you're at it, pack a lunch, too. (Bag the turkey, cheese, lettuce, and tomato separately from the bread so mushiness won't set in by morning.)

with fresh or frozen (thawed) strawberries; or Swiss and tomato in a pita.

If eating a big lunch fills you up (too much), don't forget about the meal altogether; split it. Have a salad early on, then snack on half a whole wheat bagel with vegetable cream cheese later.

If breakfast or lunch just aren't something you can get excited about, make them more exciting—or at least, more appealing. Eat something you love, even if it's not traditional breakfast fare. After all, there's no rule that says breakfast has to be a bowl of cereal or eggs (and besides, rules about eating are made to be broken); breakfast can be anything that appeals in the morning—whether that's a slice of pizza, a Breakfast Burrito (page 244), even cold leftovers from last night's chicken and rice stew. Make lunch more inviting by sharing it with a friend, your spouse, or a good book, or, pack a picnic lunch to eat in the park in nice weather. Don't feel like preparing lunch for just one? Make a little extra at dinner and eat leftovers for lunch the next day.

Don't be a martyr. No matter what impression you got from your own mom, you don't have to be a martyr to be a mother (or mother-to-be). Besides, martyrs don't last long on special diets. Feeling like you're depriving yourself all the time will only make you feel grumpy—and hungry. Find ways to substitute like for like (see page 21 for some suggestions). Or find ways to make a less-wholesome food a little healthier instead of forcing yourself to eat something healthy that you're so not in the mood for. For instance, your sweet tooth's aching for an apple—in pie form. Instead of trying to talk it into a plain apple, compromise with a baked apple—stuffed with cinnamon and raisins, microwaved, and sprinkled with toasted walnuts. Once in a while, skip the substitutions and treat yourself to the actual food you're craving—even if it's oozing with caramel and fudge. Just don't start treating yourself that generously on a daily basis—keep in mind why you were changing your old habits in the first place.

Avoid tempting places. You're less likely to stray if you stay away from the places that have become guilty by association with your bad food habits. If you can't resist the fried chicken and biscuits at a favorite restaurant, resist the restaurant for a while. If passing a pair of golden arches makes your mouth water for a quarter-pound burger and fries, save yourself the drool, and take alternative routes when you're hungry. If late-night movies in the den have always been accompanied by late-night raids on the refrigerator, watch your movies in the bedroom.

Think positive. If you say at the outset, "I'll never be able to eat well for nine months," you probably won't. Walk into a restaurant exclaiming, "I can never resist the pecan pie here," and you're pretty sure to order it. Insist that you can't make it through the morning without three large coffees, and you'll talk yourself into a ten-o'clock sag the first day you try. Instead, boost your spirits and your willpower with a positive outlook. Walk into that restaurant and tell yourself that not only will you be able to pass up the pecan pie (though you might very well take a few bites from the slice next to you), but you'll really savor those fresh strawberries (especially with some whipped cream). Order your second coffee decaf, and linger over the fact that it's warm and satisfying instead of the fact that it's caffeine-free. Get your mind to work for you instead of against you. Be your own best spin doctor. Tell yourself (and it's true!) that you can break your bad habits and take on better ones. You've never had a better reason.

Taking Stock of Your Kitchen

REFURBISHING YOUR EATING HABITS will probably call for some kitchen renovations as well (thankfully, not the kind you need a contractor for).

First, take a good look at your pantry. What are the shelves filled with? Are there chips and neon cheese balls as far as the eye can see? A collection of sugar-frosted cereals? A parade of processed foods—fruits in syrup, packaged macaroni and cheese, cans of high-sodium soup? Are your eyes blinded by the white rice and pasta? Next, survey your fridge. Is that a sugary fruit drink where the juice should be? A year's supply of diet soda? Is that whole milk next to it? Bologna in the cheese compartment? Chocolate éclairs from the bakery in the produce drawer (they stay fresher that way) but no actual produce?

If you answered yes to many of these questions, you'll probably agree it's time for a change. Unless your willpower is a match for the kind of temptation that comes with frosting or that leaves your fingers a cheesy orange, your best bet—if you're really committed to eating your best—will be to cleanse your cupboards and start fresh. Out of sight is out of mind, or at least, out of reach. So keep any wholesome foods you managed to find (the low-fat cottage cheese you normally buy anyway, the can of peaches in juice that you bought by mistake), eighty-six the rest (or donate them to a junk-food-loving neighbor or the local food bank), and start restocking with The Pregnancy Diet in mind.

On to the supermarket.

Shopping for a Healthy Kitchen

AS YOU WALK THE SUPERMARKET aisles, think about this: Just about every edible item you drop into your cart will end up in your stomach—and eventually in baby. The trick will be to fill that cart the way you'd like to see yourself filled and the way you'd like to see baby filled. Fortunately, that's not as difficult as it sounds.

The following tips can help you end up at the checkout line with a cart you can be proud of:

▲ Be organized. Consider writing your menus down for the week (you can use your own recipes or the ones starting on page 238) and creating a shopping list or lists from those menus. This will prevent you from getting stuck in the shopper's twilight zone—wandering the aisles looking for inspiration and finding it in a half-gallon of fudge brownie swirl. And it will save time—especially if you don't have to shop as often. Write your grocery list by food group (or aisle location in the store) so you don't end up visiting the produce section two or three times in one shopping trip.

▲ Don't let your diet get clipped by coupons. Coupons can provide terrific savings, but they can also convince you to select foods that weren't on your list (and probably shouldn't be on it). If you're a coupon clipper, concentrate on ones for household products and (eventually) baby items, like diapers.

▲ Plan around the seasons. Although most fruits and vegetables are available year-round, produce will be more flavorful, fresher, and more nutritious in season. (And it'll cost less, too.)

▲ Don't shop when you're about to drop. If you start the marketing expedition when you're on your last legs of the day, your chances of finishing it successfully are slim.

▲ Eat something before you go. A growling stomach will lead you astray—and down the aisle of temptation—every time. Have a snack before heading off.

▲ Leave the kids at home (if you can). Not only are children a distraction while you shop (and you'll need to be focused if you're going to get this job done), but their pleas for cookie-crunchy cereal may send your resolve crumbling. Hire a sitter for an hour or two or leave them home with dad or a willing friend.

▲ If it's not on the list (and doesn't belong on it), don't buy it. Beware of marketing ploys—and compelling packaging—that may tempt you to buy beyond your shopping list. Picking up a healthy food that didn't make the list but has caught your eye is fine, though.

▲ Banish boredom. Look for something new, exciting, and healthy each time you market. A baby vegetable you've never seen before, an exotic tropical fruit, an intriguing grain to add to your pilaf. Your taste buds will be grateful for the variety.

▲ Be fresh. Usually, you'll get more vitamins, minerals, and fiber and less fat, sugar, salt, and calories from fresh foods than from processed. When you can't find fresh or time is tight, opt for canned and frozen vegetables and fruits without added salt or sugar. They can be nutritionally equivalent or even superior to fresh, particularly when the fresh is out of season or hasn't been stored properly.

Cruising the Food Aisles

Y OU'VE GOT A SHOPPING LIST IN hand, and you're ready to roll. But before you and your cart take on the supermarket, it helps to have the floor plan in mind. Here's a run-down of the aisles you'll be cruising, and what you should be looking for in each area:

Produce aisle. Green means go. And in the produce aisle, so does red, yellow, blue, orange, and pur-ple. Stock your wagon high with fresh fruits and vegetables, picking the ripest, richly colored (see page 140), and fragrant fruits and veg-etables. (For fruits especially, a sniff test will usually be very telling.) Look here, too, for fresh herbs to stir up intriguing flavor in whatever

you're cooking. See page 126 for tips on selecting salad greens. When practical, opt for organic produce, which is grown without pesticides (see page 124).

Dairy aisle. Look for skim milk, non-fat or low-fat yogurt, cottage cheese, hard cheese, and eggs (choose the omega-3 eggs for a healthful dose of this brain-boosting fatty acid) in this aisle. And don't forget the orange juice and other fresh natural fruit juices you'll find here (opt for the calcium-fortified). Remember to check expi-ration dates (see page 154 for more).

Bakery aisle. You don't have to avoid this aisle when you're shopping (unless you can't resist the bins of doughnuts

A GOOD EGG

▼ ▼ ▼

S almon and other fatty fish are a great source of the baby-brain-nourishing omega-3 fatty acids, but did you know that eggs can be, too? DHA eggs, now widely available, come courtesy of chick-ens fed a diet containing sources of omega-3 fatty acids, often flaxseed or marine algae. The eggs taste just like reg-ular eggs (nothing fishy going on here). Researchers have found that eating DHA eggs not only nourishes your baby's brain but can also help prevent preterm labor (women at risk of preterm delivery who eat DHA eggs have an average gesta-tional period that is six days longer than that of women who eat regular eggs). So boost your intake of these essential fatty acids every time you whip up an omelet by cracking open these especially good eggs.

and sweet rolls); just be selective. In most markets you'll encounter a good selection of whole wheat and whole-grain breads, tortillas, wraps—and even some baked goods that qualify as healthy food. Also look for packaged whole wheat bread, pita, and rolls, but read the ingredients to make sure they're "whole" and not just "wheat." (Some fresh wraps and tortillas may be found in the refrigerated dairy case.)

Meat aisle. Choose only extra-lean cuts of beef, chicken, pork, turkey, veal, or lamb. Don't drop into your cart any packages that smell even vaguely funky, are leaking, or have old "sell by" dates—even if they're a bargain. See page 158 for more on safe meat handling.

Seafood aisle. Your eyes and nose will serve you well here. Fresh fish should *look* fresh, with moist gills, shiny skin, and clear bright eyes. Fillets should also be shiny, not dull. The flesh should spring back without leaving an indentation when you press it lightly with your finger, and should have no smell or a mild smell (like an ocean breeze, not like a bait box). If something smells fishy in this department, you might want to recast your dinner menu back in the meat aisle. When you're shopping for seafood, also remember to bring along the fish safety guidelines for pregnant women (see page 169).

Canned-goods aisles. You'll need to study this aisle carefully, choosing only foods that have come through their canning process with their nutrition intact. Look for low-sodium vegetables, vegetable soups, and tomato sauce, canned salmon and sardines, nonfat evaporated milk, fruit packed in juice (not syrup). Don't pick up any dented, swollen, or rusted cans.

Dry-goods aisles. Color is key here, too, since your goal will be to avoid the whites of this aisle. And you may find there's a whole new world of eating waiting for you when you make the move from refined products to whole grain. Read labels carefully, and stock up on dried beans, whole-grain and soy pastas, brown and wild rice, whole-grain flour, and assorted other whole grains. See page 130 for more on choosing grains.

Cereal aisle. Unlike the produce aisle, where vibrant hues indicate wholesome freshness and nutrition, bright colors here are never a good sign. Brown (in its various shades, but chocolate doesn't count) is a better bet, though you'll want to read the labels thoroughly, too, to make sure the box you're dropping into your cart is filled with whole grains (such as whole wheat or oats). A piece of helpful supermarket trivia: The middle shelves (which are located at eye level) are generally devoted to the less healthy cereal choices that are often impulse buys. So keep your eyes up or down and reach for the lower or upper shelves to pull out a whole-grain cereal worthy of your cart. In addition to ready-to-eat whole grains, stock up on oatmeal (rolled oats are best; quick cook better than instant; unflavored instant better than fla-vored), whole wheat farina (most are refined; check the label), Wheatena, and wheat germ (which can be added to just about any cereal to pack in a little extra nutrition).

Frozen food aisle. Don't hang out too long in this aisle—though in your overheated pregnant state, that might be tempting. Also tempting will be the impulse to grab an armful of frozen entrées and desserts that don't mesh with your nutritional mission. Instead, read labels to locate entrées that are high in nutrients and lowish in sodium (for those nights when cooking's just not an option, many markets now carry brands formerly carried only in health-food stores), vegetarian sausages and veggie burg-ers, all-natural frozen fruit-juice con-centrates, whole-grain waffles, frozen vegetables and fruits (without added salt or sugar), low-fat or fat-free frozen yogurt (scan nutrition labels to find ones with plenty of calcium) or fruit-only Popsicles.

Other aisles. Don't forget to pick up some dried and crunchy freeze-dried fruits, nuts (see page 136), all-

fruit jam, dried herbs and spices, lemon juice, olive oil, canola oil, and safflower oil (see page 143 for more on choosing oils).

▲ ▲ ▲

Q *"My friend shops at a health-food store. Is there any reason to go to one?"*

A These days, you don't have to shop at a health-food store to eat healthy. While you'll probably be able to find a wider selection and assortment of healthy foods (includ-ing grains, fruit-juice sweetened baked goods and cereals, organic produce, more wholesome frozen dinners, soy and other vegetarian products) at stores that specialize in them, more and more local super-markets are also stocking them—not only in the "health food" section, but in just about every aisle. Realize, too, that not everything in a health-food store (or in a health-food aisle) is healthy. You'll need to look beyond buzzwords like "organic," or "all nat-ural," which sometimes merely pro-vide cover for foods that are high in calories or saturated fat. So be as thorough in your label-checking when you're scanning health food as you are with any other packaged food. One department of the health-food store that may be particularly unhealthy for pregnant women is the supplement section; steer clear of all supplements and herbal preparations that are not specifically prescribed by your practitioner.

Q *"I'm interested in eating as healthy as I can during my pregnancy. Should I only buy organic produce?"*

A It's unclear whether organic produce is more nutritious than conventional produce, though it is likely to be as close to pesticide-free as possible—a definite plus, since the pesticides you consume through your diet are shared with your baby both in utero and through breast milk. But whether there are dietary benefits beyond that pesticide-free plus (there certainly are environmental benefits to produce being grown without chemicals) is up in the air. So far, the small body of reliable studies that have been done are contradictory. Some don't show any significant nutritional difference between organic and conventional foods, while others show that organics do boast more nutrients. And while the jury is still out on taste (most people say that organic doesn't have much of a taste edge), fruits and vegetables that are grown without pesticides are usually fresher when they hit the market. That's because they're more perishable and must be rushed to the market within days. (Much of the conventional produce can tough it out during long stays in refrigerated warehouses.)

Keep in mind that organic does not necessarily mean "safe," either. Though it won't be contaminated with pesticides, it could—like any produce—be contaminated with bacteria, which is why washing is a step you shouldn't skip just because you've bought organic. In other words, no nibbling on those farmer's market blueberries before they've been brought home for a thorough rinse. (Scrubbing conventional produce with water and produce wash, or peeling it, can eliminate or greatly decrease pesticide residue.)

Since 2002, the U.S. Department of Agriculture has in place a set of national standards that food labeled "organic" must meet, whether it is grown in the United States or imported from other countries. The USDA merely regulates the labeling of organic products, making no claims that organically produced food is safer or more nutritious than conventionally produced food, only that organic food differs from conventionally produced food in the way it is grown, handled, and processed (without pesticides, chemical fertilizers, weed-killers, genetic modification, germ-killing radiation, hormones, or antibiotics). According to the USDA Organic Seal guidelines, foods labeled "100 percent organic" must contain only organically produced raw or processed products. Foods labeled as "organic" must have at least

95 percent organically produced ingredients (excluding water and salt). Foods that contain 70 percent organic ingredients can use the phrase "made with organic ingredients." Foods that contain less than 50 percent organic ingredients cannot use the word "organic" on the main label, only on a side label that lists all ingredients.

Not confused enough? For more information on the USDA's organic products regulations, go to their website: www.ams.usda.gov.

▼ ▼ ▼

Foods That Make the Grade

IN CASE YOU HAVEN'T NOTICED, supermarkets are getting bigger and bigger—and the selection offered in them is becoming more and more dizzying. The mom-and-pop stores of yesterday (complete with their modest assortment of products: the four brands of cereal, the three kinds of soup, the two varieties of bread)—could now be housed in a single aisle of the typical mega-superstore, with room to spare.

Which leaves you with a much tougher job than yesterday's shoppers —of sifting through the staggering array of items, and deciding which to pass by, which to drop into your cart. The downside of these supermarkets-on-steroids—this could take a while. The upside—there are more wholesome choices than ever before.

Where to begin choosing? First, you'll need to check out the following directory of healthy foods—what to look for in everything from soup (beans) to nuts. Think of it as your yellow pages guide to nutritious eating (except you'll need to do the walking through the supermarket aisles, so bring your comfortable shoes). Next, you'll have to open your mind. After all, it's a lot easier to reach reflexively for the iceberg lettuce and corn flakes than it is to change the way you shop and eat. Resist the urge to stick with the familiar (and less than healthful) foods and broaden your culinary and nutritional horizons. This primer should help:

Salad greens. A salad is a salad, no matter what type of leaf you put in your bowl, right? Well, yes. But while any salad is better than no salad, there's a wide range of nutritional value in the wide range of salad greens on most market shelves. So it's smart to become salad savvy before heading to the produce section. You should know, for instance, that most (but not all) greens are good sources of folic acid; some supply a huge amount of

DRESSING FOR SUCCESS

▼ ▼ ▼

Want the skinny on salads? Dressing can fatten them up a lot more than you think. Just 2 tablespoons of the typical salad dressing (and keep in mind that most people dress for excess, often using 4 or more tablespoons to top their bowl) contains 12 to 16 grams of fat and 150 calories. Here are some ways to dress down your salad, while dressing up its taste.

■ Make your own. A simple vinaigrette prepared at home is at least as delicious as a store-bought dressing and a lot more healthy. (Many packaged brands contain a paragraph or two of artificial ingredients and whopping amounts of sodium and sugar.) Using more vinegar and less oil (2 to 1 ratio) than most recipes call for won't compromise taste but will trim excess fat. If that's too tangy for your taste buds, try half vinegar to half oil. (If you like things really tangy, you can cut down even more on the oil, but don't cut it out entirely because you won't absorb as many of the salad's nutrients without it; see page 97). Use a tastier, milder vinegar, such as balsamic or rice (or try substituting citrus juice, such as

lemon or orange, for some or all of the vinegar), add plenty of fresh or dried herbs, and maybe some grated Parmesan cheese, and you may not miss the extra oil at all. Opt for olive oil instead of vegetable (see page 143 for the reason why). For low-fat dressing ideas, see the recipes starting on page 314.

■ Make creamy healthy. Instead of using mayonnaise or sour cream in your home-made creamy dressings, substitute yogurt or buttermilk (see Creamy Caesar Dressing, page 332). If that's too tart for your tastes, compromise: Mix these low-fat (and high-calcium) ingredients with the traditional high-fat ones. Using whole-milk yogurt will increase the calories somewhat, but will result in a much creamier dressing that's still far lower in fat (and higher in calcium) than a mayo-based one.

■ Toss it. When you ladle dressing on top of a salad, you're liable to use a lot more than you would if you just added enough to coat the leaves lightly and evenly. So try tossing when you can. When you can't toss, use a smaller spoon to dish out the dressing.

---

vitamin A, while others are richer in calcium and iron. As is so often the case with produce, color is key; and in the case of greens, the greener the better. Dark-leafed romaine has seven times as much beta-carotene, two times the calcium, and twice the potassium of iceberg, which pales in comparison both in hue and nutri-

tion. But even within the same head of romaine, there's a difference—the darker, outer leaves offer more vitamins than the blanched inner leaves. Red is also a good color for greens; those with a red-pigment offer up more vitamin C.

In an iceberg rut? Break out and become a salad explorer:

▲ *Arugula* has a subtle peppery yet sweet-tangy flavor. High in omega-3 fatty acids (see page 98 for why this is so important), calcium, and vitamin K, it's great for salads (such as Crunchy Pear Salad, page 315) and in sandwiches (such as Market Chicken Pita, page 269) and wraps. You can also wilt it slightly by serving with a warm dressing, or placing under warm fish or chicken.

▲ *Boston (or Bibb) lettuce* has a buttery feel and a subtly sweet taste that almost melts in your mouth. A head of Boston lettuce resembles a flowering rose and its tender leaves make a perfect salad needing only a light dressing, preferably a vinaigrette. Boston teams well with tomatoes. It contains a nice amount of vitamin A and folic acid.

▲ *Dandelion greens.* Sure, it's a weed, but when young, the green jagged leaves of the yellow flower you hate on your lawn you may love on your salad. These greens are tangy and somewhat bitter, and they mix well in a salad of milder greens. They're overachievers in the nutrition department, scoring high in vitamins A, E, C, and K, as well as calcium. Just don't eat the ones on your lawn.

▲ *Curly endive and escarole.* Curly endive has lacy dark green leaves and creamy inner leaves. Escarole has broad, coarse, crumpled leaves with light inner leaves. Both add crunch to a salad and both contain a good amount of vitamin A and folic acid.

▲ *Iceberg lettuce* is the familiar mild-flavored pale salad green favored by many, and of salad bar fame. It comes as a head of tightly packed leaves (or, more often these days, in ready-to-eat shredded form). While it adds a crispy texture to salads and sandwiches, it has a humble share of nutrients. Still, two cups of iceberg lettuce provide a good amount of folic acid. And tossed with some shredded carrots, tomato wedges, and purple cabbage, you've got yourself a respectable bowl of nutrients and fiber. And if you're a confirmed iceberg fan, you're definitely better off composing a salad out of ingredients you like than giving up on salads altogether because you don't like dark green lettuce.

▲ *Leaf lettuces* have large, loosely packed leaves that do not form a heart. The most common types are green leaf or red leaf (with leaves

wisdom of ☀ the ages?

Here's an ancient custom that has modern applications, particularly for pregnant women: It was customary for the Romans to precede their banquets with refreshing salads, which they believed enhanced the appetite. Here's one that may not: In Elizabethan times, dried lettuce juice was used to aid sleep.

KEEPING THOSE VITAMINS IN

▼ ▼ ▼

Buying fresh produce is one way to ensure you're getting great nutrition. But keeping those nutrients in the produce once you've brought it home is another. Bear these tips in mind:

■ Use ripe produce as soon as possible after purchasing, or refrigerate quickly. Fresh fruit makes a pretty centerpiece, but being on display for days robs those pears, grapes, and apples of their natural nutrients. (You can ripen fruit on your table, though.) Keep an eye on your crisper drawer so you won't lose track of produce before it loses many of its vitamins and minerals.

■ When you're prewashing and cutting up fruit and veggies for easy snacking, refrigerate them as soon as possible to reduce the subtraction of nutrients and the multi-plication of germs. And don't store in water (the water will end up with all the vitamins). See facing page for lettuce storing tips.

■ Keep beverage containers closed. Orange juice loses vitamin C when exposed to air. Milk loses nutrients when exposed to light.

■ When cooking vegetables, remember that less is more. That means less water (opt for steaming or over boiling, and avoid doing cold-water plunges) and less cooking time. (stop when they're crisp-tender). Vegetables that have lost their color (as when a green bean or carrot goes from bright to dull) have probably also parted with many of their vitamins. And stop in the name of nutrients before you dump that cooking water; instead, refrigerate to use it in broths, soups, or sauces.

that are shaded to deep red at the edges). Leaf lettuces contain vitamin A, folic acid, potassium, and even some calcium. Their degree of crispness is midway between romaine and Boston; their taste is mild and delicate; they are also good candidates for a light vinaigrette.

▲ *Mesclun greens* are a mixture of many different salad greens, usually tender baby ones, including arugula, dandelion, frisée, mizuma, oak leaf, mâche, radicchio, and sorrel. All these greens are rich in nutrients, especially vitamins A and K. Try them in Mucho Mango Salad, page 319, or Pomegranate Salad, page 316.

▲ *Mustard greens* are dark green leaves with a peppery pungent flavor. They are best for soups and stews, or sautéed like spinach, but they can always be eaten raw in a salad. They are high in vitamins E and C, folic acid, and calcium. They're delicious in Spicy Greens with Ginger Dressing, page 404.

▲ *Romaine lettuce,* best known as Caesar salad's lettuce of choice, has long leaves with light green hearts and darker green tips. It has a crisp texture and an assertive, but not bitter, taste that can hold up well to just about any dressing. Romaine lettuce is high in vitamin C, vitamin A, calcium, and folic acid. Great romaine salads here include It's Mediterranean to Me Salad, page 323, Shrimp Caesar Salad, page 330, and Taco in a Salad, page 327.

▲ *Radicchio* is a red-and-white cabbage-shaped head of lettuce that can grow to orange or grapefruit size. The leaves are slightly bitter yet slightly sweet (much like endive). Because it's one of the more expensive types of salad greens, it's often used as a color and flavor accent in a salad rather than as one of the main ingredients. It's also delicious brushed lightly with olive oil and grilled. Radicchio contains a nice amount of vitamin E and potassium.

▲ *Spinach.* The dark green leaves can be small and smooth (baby spinach) or large and wrinkled. Baby spinach is much milder tasting, but also usually more expensive. Packed with nutrients, including folic acid, vitamins C and K, and iron, spinach can be eaten raw in salads or cooked in soups and pasta dishes, sautéed on its own (with some garlic or shallots) or as a bed for fish (as in Ginger Steamed Halibut, page 369) or poultry.

▲ *Watercress* is sold in bunches of small dark leaves that have a slight peppery mustard-like taste. High in vitamins C and K, watercress is a popular garnish, or can be used as a spirited sandwich or salad ingredient, or as a wilted bed for fish (Sautéed Halibut with Watercress, Mango, and Avocado, page 368) or poultry.

Choose lettuces that are free of blemishes and that look lively. Avoid any greens with brown spots, those with a sour or rotten smell, or those that have limp, withered leaves that have brown or yellow edges. You can buy most greens prewashed in packages or in bulk, which saves time, but definitely not money.

If you're buying greens the old-fashioned way, you'll need to wash and dry them before using. Separate the leaves from their base (by tearing the leaves, not cutting them), plunge them into a bowl filled with cold water (you can add to the water a little produce wash—a liquid soap designed for rinsing off pesticide residue—found in produce departments). Gently swish them around with your hands. Be sure all the sand, dirt, and bugs are washed away. Rinse thoroughly (especially if you've used a produce wash). Then dry them in a salad spinner or lay them on paper towels or a clean kitchen towel and blot dry. Be sure your greens are completely dry before you

MICROWAVE SMARTS

▼ ▼ ▼

It cooks, reheats, defrosts—and saves time. That is, if you know how to use it. Armed with the following tips, you might really be able to turn your microwave into the little engine that could:

■ Start with micro-safe containers. Check to make sure the containers you're zapping your dinner in are safe for use in a microwave. (Not all plastic containers are.) High temperatures can cause some non-microwaveable materials to release unwanted chemicals into your meal. For the same reason, use microwave plastic wrap only—and don't let the wrap touch the food. Better still, use a paper towel or paper plate to cover your food before you zap it.

■ To maximize the retention of nutrients when cooking vegetables in the microwave, add only a few drops of water. Too much water, and the nutrients will be washed away. Even better, keep your vegetables on top of the water (with a microwave-safe rack) so you're steaming, rather than boiling. Be sure, too, to keep your microwaving time to a minimum, so that your broccoli ends up crisp and green, not soggy and gray. Three minutes (for 2 cups) should be the ticket to crisp-tender.

■ Use your microwave for all it's worth. Sure, it's great for reheating those leftovers from last night. But there are plenty of other ways to work microwave magic. Here are a few:

■ Before squeezing an orange, lemon, or lime for its juice, microwave the fruit on high for 20 seconds. You'll get more juice flowing.

■ Toast nuts in a flash by spreading them out on a plate and heating them on high for 2 to 3 minutes, stirring every minute.

■ Make your own bread crumbs by cutting a slice of bread into cubes, and microwaving on high for 1 to 2 minutes, stirring once. Then crumb in a blender, and toast as per nuts.

■ Thaw a 6-ounce can of frozen juice concentrate by removing any metal lid and microwaving on high for 30 seconds.

■ For tear-free onions, trim the ends off a whole onion and heat on high for 30 seconds.

make your salad. If you're not going to use them right away, store washed greens by loosely wrapping them in paper towels and then sealing them in plastic bags or a large plastic container. They will stay fresh for up to

a week in your refrigerator (the sooner they're used after washing, the more nutrients they'll retain).

Grains. First, a quick botany lesson: Grains are the seed-bearing parts of grasses. An inedible husk (chaff) is the outermost layer of the grain. The next layer is a protective coating called the bran, which is rich in fiber. Inside the bran is the endosperm (the starchy part of a grain) and the germ, the part of the grain that is highest in nutrients. When the husk is removed, the resulting product is called groat or berry. When the bran is removed, the product is called pearled or polished. When grains are refined, the husk, bran, and germ are removed, leaving only that starchy, nutritionally modest endosperm.

As a result of being stripped down to the endosperm, refined grains suffer a dramatic loss of such vital nutrients as folic acid, vitamin B_6, iron, and zinc. They also have nothing left in the way of the trace minerals—selenium, magnesium, zinc and copper—that most people don't get enough of. Most of the fiber's gone, too.

Just how much difference does a whole grain make? Compare whole wheat flour to white flour: whole wheat flour contains four times more fiber, two times more copper, six times more magnesium, three times more potassium, two times more selenium, four times more zinc, and twenty times more vitamin E than white flour. That's a pretty convincing profile.

That's not to say that refined grains should never touch your lips. First of all, avoiding them altogether, while possible (especially if you don't eat out a lot) isn't always practical; there are sometimes when whole wheat's just not an option (like when you're lunching at the average pizza place). And to those used to the white stuff, it isn't always preferable; to some, the taste of refined is a favorite. Since most are enriched with vitamins and minerals, opting for a serving of refined is fine—as long as you're not often making them your carb of choice. Instead, aim to make whole grains the mainstay of your diet. And though whole wheat's the most obvious—and the most widely available—way to accomplish that, there are many other great grain options, yours for the picking off your supermarket shelves:

▲ *Amaranth* is a grain that has a nutty flavor and sticky texture and is rich in protein, iron, calcium, B vitamins, and fiber. It can be used as a substitute for wheat and other grains in breads, pastas, pancakes, and cereals; it can be added to soups and stews as a thickening agent; it can be popped like popcorn.

▲ *Barley* contains phytochemicals, thiamin, niacin, vitamin E, and important minerals. The best type to eat is hulled barley because it's in its whole-grain form. Barley can be served as a side dish (instead of rice or salads in pilafs, see Barley Risotto with Wild Mushrooms, page 415, and

Pomegranate Pilaf, page 416) or in a soup or stew (see Beef and Barley Soup, page 297). Barley flour can be substituted for all-purpose flour in most recipes.

▲ *Buckwheat*, also called kasha, has a strong, grainy flavor. Buckwheat can be cooked as a substitute for rice or mixed with other grains (as in Three-in-One Pilaf, page 419), and buckwheat flour can be used to make pancakes and other baked goods. Rich in vitamin E, buckwheat also contains fiber, B vitamins, potassium, some iron, calcium, manganese, and phosphorus.

▲ *Bulgur*, used often in Mediterranean cooking, has a chewy tender texture. Bulgur is cracked whole wheat that has been lightly cooked and parched. It contains niacin, vitamin B_6, folic acid, pantothenic acid, and other minerals. Best known as an ingredient in Middle Eastern tabouli salad, bulgur can be used instead of rice or couscous in stews, salads, pilafs, soups, casseroles, or stuffing. And it also makes a yummy hot cereal.

▲ *Corn* is the only cereal grain native to the Americas. Whole-grain yellow corn is a fairly good source of vitamin A and contains smaller amounts of vitamin C, folic acid, and other B vitamins. It is also rich in potassium, magnesium, iron, zinc, and selenium. Blue corn contains the amino

acid lysine, making it a richer protein. Corn that hasn't been stripped of its whole goodness is called non-degerminated (as opposed to the refined, which is called degerminated). Use whole grain cornmeal for baking, breading (as in Pan-Fried Trout with Tomatoes and Watercress, page 383), and for making polenta. Use fresh or frozen corn in cooking (see Turkey Breast with Corn and Edamame Salsa, page 365).

▲ *Millet* is a mild-tasting crunchy grain that's a good substitute for rice in stews, soups, or casseroles. Millet flour can be used in bread or stuffing (try it in grain form in Red Peppers, Stuffed with Millet Pilaf, page 420). Rich in protein, iron, magnesium, potassium, and fiber, millet also contains good amounts of niacin, thiamine, and riboflavin, vitamin B_6, folic acid, and a little vitamin E.

▲ *Oats* are traditionally used as a breakfast cereal (oatmeal, granola, muesli). They're a soft grain that is less affected by the refining process than are other types of grains—though you should opt for rolled oats when you can (especially in baking), using instant when you're on the run. Oats contain protein, fiber, folic acid, niacin, pyridoxine, pantothenic acid, iron, magnesium, zinc, potassium, manganese, calcium, and copper. Try oats in Tomato-Layered Mini Meat Loaves (page 343), Power Breakfast

THE WHOLE TRUTH ABOUT WHOLE WHEAT

▼ ▼ ▼

Finding whole grain in the bakery department is as easy as scanning the shelf for bread and rolls that are labeled "wheat," right? Not exactly. Wheat (or oat, or corn) specifies only the type of grain, not whether it's whole or not. Nor does reaching for brown baked goods mean you'll be bringing home whole-grain goodness. A little caramel color can lend less nutritious loaves the wholesome hue that whole grains come by naturally.

To ensure you're dropping the whole grains and nothing but the whole grains into your cart, you'll need to be a little more thorough in your background check. First, check out the big print—a loaf of whole wheat bread will proudly wear the banner "100 percent whole wheat." Then, look to the fine print. Since ingredients are listed in descending order of weight (see page 146 for more on deciphering food labels), a loaf of whole wheat bread will list "whole wheat flour" as its first ingredient. Other words that will top the list of a whole grain product: "whole wheat," "whole-grain wheat," "whole-oat flour," "whole-grain oats"—you get the picture. Beware of tags like "multigrain," "seven-grain," and "nutri-grain"—again, this only lets you know that the product contains multiple grains, not necessarily whole grains. You'll have to investigate further to be sure that those seven grains are mostly or wholly whole.

The same rules apply to cereals and other grain products as well. Read up on your favorite cereals to be sure that the "oat" cereal you're buying is made from "whole-grain oat flour," not just "oat flour."

The following glossary should help you in the screening process:

■ "Wheat flour" means the flour is made by grinding wheat and typically does not contain the bran or germ.

■ "Enriched flour (wheat)" is wheat flour (no bran or germ) that has been enriched with nutrients that are lost during the refining process.

■ "Enriched flour (flour)" can be any type of grain flour (rye, oats, barley, or soybeans, for instance) that has been enriched with nutrients.

■ "Stone-ground wheat flour" describes merely how the wheat grain (without the bran or germ) was milled. Whether it was ground by stones or machines, it's still refined if it doesn't specify "whole."

■ "Whole wheat flour" is wheat flour that includes the bran and germ. And that's the ticket to a wholesome product.

Bars (page 254), Raisin Bran Muffins (page 263), and Fruit-and-Oat Meal (page 248).

▲ *Quinoa (KEEN-wah),* with its unique fluffy texture and delicate taste, is both hardy and nutritious.

Quinoa is a quick-cooking whole grain that is extremely high in protein, iron, potassium, riboflavin, calcium, magnesium, and B vitamins. It can be substituted for almost any grain in almost any recipe, from soup to salad to pilaf (as in Three in One Pilaf, page 419).

▲ *Rice* comes in many forms. White rice has been stripped; brown rice, with its tan color and chewy nutty flavor, has the greatest amount of fiber and nutrients. It comes in short or long grains. Wild rice (really a grass) has a chewy texture and strong nutty flavor and is high in protein. When preparing rice, don't rinse it before cooking, because that washes away nutrients. Enjoy wild rice in Pomegranate Pilaf, page 416, or brown rice in Stove-Top Brown Rice Pilaf, page 414.

▲ *Spelt* has been popular in Europe for centuries but is gaining a following in this country, as well. Spelt has a nutty taste and chewy texture and is an attractive alternative to the common varieties of wheat. Spelt flour can be substituted for wheat flour in breads, pastas, cookies, crackers, cakes, muffins, pancakes—you name it. It's a good source of protein, thiamin, riboflavin, copper, iron, magnesium, and zinc.

▲ W*heat berries* are a hard, red winter wheat with short rounded kernels. They have a nutty flavor and firm chewy texture. High in protein, wheat berries can be added to cooked cereal, pilafs, soups, stews, stuffing, breads, muffins, and other baked goods. Try them in Wheatberry Salad with Red Pepper, Carrots, and Red Onion (page 421).

When purchasing grain in its natural state, look for the best quality (whole pieces with few broken, scratched, or deteriorated grains). Keep grains in an airtight container and store in a cool, dry place.

Beans. When you were a kid, the rhyme "beans, beans, they're good for your heart . . ." was a surefire way to get the giggles going. As an adult, this song still rings true (though hopefully, you're over the giggles). Beans *are* truly good for your heart (and your blood sugar, and your blood pressure). They're high in protein, low in fat, and are a valuable source of fiber. Beans also contain thiamin, folic acid, copper, iron, magnesium, manganese, phosphorus, potassium, zinc, selenium, pantothenic acid, calcium, riboflavin, and niacin. There are many types of beans available on supermarket shelves. Experiment with them all:

▲ *Black beans* are medium black-skinned beans with tan insides. They have an earthy, sweet flavor and are indispensable in Mexican cooking. Try them in Purée of Black Bean

BEANS AND GAS

▼ ▼ ▼

Sure, beans are good for you, but they might not make you feel so good—or so sociable. The quality that makes them good fodder for playground ditties makes many who eat them live to regret it. Worse for you, the gas and bloating that are often served up after a bean dish can be particularly pronounced and uncomfortable when you're pregnant.

But there is hope for bean lovers (and those who love them). Soaking beans before cooking starts can dissolve the gaseous starches that can cause discomfort. Here's a good way to soak your beans: In a large pot, place 1 pound of dried beans in 10 or more cups of water. Boil for 2 to 3 minutes, then cover, and set aside overnight. By morning, nearly 90 percent of the indigestible sugars will have dissolved into the soaking water. Drain, then rinse the beans thoroughly before cooking them.

You might also ask your practitioner about whether you should try a product called Beano, which has food enzymes that break down the complex sugars in beans, making them more digestible. While no studies have been done on pregnant women, Beano is probably safe to use during pregnancy or during breastfeeding.

Soup, page 290, or Black Bean Quesadillas, page 275.

▲ *Black-eyed peas,* a Southern delight, are tan with a small black eye-shaped spot.

▲ *Chickpeas,* also called garbanzo beans, are round and firm with a nutty flavor. A favorite in salads (toss Crunchy Chickpeas, page 331, into your next bowlful).

▲ *Great Northern beans* are white beans with a delicate flavor. They're terrific in soups and with braised meat, or with fish (Seared Scallops on White Beans and Kale, page 388, and Roasted Mediterranean Sea Bass with Red Pepper and White Beans, page 375).

▲ *Kidney beans* are dark red outside, tan inside, and kidney-shaped. A standard in chili (Turkey Chili, page 291), they also toss well in a salad (Taco in a Salad, page 327).

▲ *Lentils,* actually legumes, come small red, brown, black, or green with a mild, earthy, yet elegant flavor. They can be served in salads or soups (like Red Lentil and Tomato Soup, page 286).

▲ *Navy beans* are small and white with a mild flavor and powdery texture. They are excellent in soups, chowders, and stews.

▲ *Pinto beans* are reddish beans streaked with pink or have a mottled beige and brown color. Their earthy flavor and powdery texture make them a favorite for chili, refried beans, and other Mexican dishes.

Nuts. In a nutshell, you don't have to be a health nut to enjoy the healthy benefits of these tasty, crunchy morsels. Nuts are loaded with cop-

per, manganese, magnesium, selenium, zinc, potassium, as well as vitamin E—all important for your developing baby. And while it's true that nuts are high in fat, it's mainly the good-for-you kind. (Of course, don't confuse good-for-you with all-you-can-eat; overdoing the nuts will pile on the pounds.) Plus, they're versatile. While many prefer to snack on them right out of the jar, nuts can also be tossed into salads, pasta, meat, or fish dishes, as well as in baked goods. In other words, whatever you're cooking—go nuts!

When choosing nuts, look for raw (you can toast them lightly yourself, if you like) or dry roasted (preferably unsalted). Oil-roasted varieties, obviously, contain added oils—which means more calories (and if the fats used to roast are saturated or trans-fats, more unhealthful calories). They're also more likely to be high in sodium. Check out these nuts:

▲ *Almonds* are delicious on their own, but their delicate flavor blends well with just about any kind of cuisine. Use them chopped in baking (they're yummy in Heavenly Chocolate Cake, page 434, or Cherry Cobbler, page 446), sliced in meat, poultry, fish, or grain dishes, toasted and slivered with vegetables and salads (like Spinach Strawberry Salad, page 314). Almonds are a good source of calcium, riboflavin, niacin, and vitamin E.

PASS ON THE PEANUTS?

▼ ▼ ▼

A peanut butter and jelly sandwich is as American as apple pie—probably more so. But there's sad news for some of those who crave this lunch-box staple. Researchers have found that expectant mothers who have (or have had) food allergies of any kind or a history of eczema and who eat highly allergenic foods (such as peanuts) during pregnancy and lactation may be more likely to pass on allergies to those foods to their offspring. The American Academy of Pediatrics recommends that women with a family history of allergies, especially nut allergies, should consider skipping peanut products during pregnancy and while breastfeeding. If you or your baby's father has such a history, discuss with your practitioner about whether you should pass on the peanuts, nuts, or other allergenic foods.

SOWING THE SEEDS

▼ ▼ ▼

Though they're really a category of their own, seeds are often lumped together with nuts because they share that nutty taste as well as many of the same vital nutrients. Try these—sprinkled on salads, in your cooking, or just plain:

■ *Flaxseed* is an oil seed that was popular in ancient times and is now experiencing a well-deserved comeback. Also known as linseed, it has a nutty flavor, lots of fiber, and high levels of omega-3 fatty acids. Don't pop flaxseeds in your mouth— instead, grind them (or buy them ground) and use in cereal, breading, and baking (see page 435 for more facts on flax).

■ *Pumpkin seeds* are usually roasted, then eaten by the handful, tossed in salads, or mixed with grains. They can also stand in for walnuts or pine nuts in pesto. They're a good source of dietary fiber, protein, vitamin E, zinc, copper, iron, magnesium, calcium, potassium, and phosphorus, as well as a rich source of mono- and polyunsaturated fat.

■ *Sesame seeds* are rich in oil and flavor, especially when they're toasted. They find themselves in some of the world's finest cuisine, from Asian (the seeds and oil made from them is often used in stir-fries) to Middle Eastern (in tahini and hummus). They also top some of the best baked goods. Sesame seeds contain protein, vitamins A and E, zinc, calcium, copper, iron, magnesium, phosphorus, and potassium. Try sesame seeds in Asian Slaw, page 324.

■ *Soy nuts,* also legumes, are the crunchy roasted version of soybeans. Soy nuts are high in folic acid and protein, and make for tasty and nutritious snacking. Toss them into trail mix, too.

■ *Sunflower seeds* are the hulled seeds of the sunflower plant. Packed with vitamin B_6 and folic acid, sunflower seeds are also rich in vitamin E, iron, thiamin, manganese, copper, zinc, and potassium. They are great tossed in trail mix, salads, pesto, or baked goods.

▲ *Brazil nuts,* actually large seeds of giant trees that grow in the Amazon, are sweet and creamy, with a coconut-like taste. They are chock-full of protein, fiber, selenium, magnesium, phosphorus, and thiamin—and are rich sources of linolenic acid, which converts to omega-3 fatty acid in the body. They're best for snacking, though they're delicious baked into Tropical Bar Nones, page 433.

▲ *Hazelnuts,* also called filberts, have a sweet, rich flavor, great for baking. Their bitter brown skin is usually removed before eating. (Toasting them first makes this easy to rub off.) Hazelnuts contain vitamins E and B_6, biotin, and folic acid. Try them in Pan-Fried Trout with Tomatoes and Watercress, page 383.

▲ *Macadamia nuts* are brown in color with an extremely hard shell. The nut is small, round, and creamy white with a very creamy texture. Macadamia nuts contain protein and a lot of fat (though 80 percent of that fat is monounsaturated fat, which helps lower artery-clogging LDL cholesterol in the blood). They are also high in calcium, magnesium, phosphorus, and potassium—as well as high in price compared to other nuts. Feeling flush? Toss them into your next batch of cookies, or into Mucho Mango Salad, page 319.

▲ *Peanuts,* America's favorite nut, aren't really nuts at all—they're legumes. Peanuts are a good source of protein, niacin, phosphorus, magnesium, folic acid, and vitamin E, and have dozens of uses beyond peanut butter. (If you have a history of allergies, see page 136 and consult with your practitioner before opening that jar of peanuts or peanut butter.)

▲ *Pecans* are a good source of baby-friendly protein, iron, calcium, vitamins A, B, and C, potassium, and phosphorous. Think outside the pie, here, and add them to pilaf (like Pomegranate Pilaf, page 416), stuffing, quick breads, and vegetable dishes, or try them in Apple Cranberry Crisp, page 444, or

I Can't See the Black Forest for the Cherries Cake, page 436.

▲ *Pistachio,* that greenish-yellow cocktail party favorite, is an excellent source of protein. It's low in saturated fat and the nut family's richest source of potassium. (Two ounces of pistachios contain more potassium than one medium banana.) It's also a good source of vitamns C, A, and B_6, as well as magnesium, folic acid, iron, and calcium. Toss pistachios into your mouth, as well as into your salads, desserts, or your vegetables. (They're tasty tossed over Broccoli Vinaigrette, page 392.)

▲ *Walnuts* are a tasty source of protein, fiber, and those all-important omega-3 fatty acids. Add them toasted or un- to your trail mix, to your cereal (as in Fruit-and-Oat Meal, page 248), your salads, stuffings, pilafs and pasta dishes (Alotta Broccoli with Chicken and Penne, page 302), and baked goods (Pumpkin Pie Muffins, page 262, or Carrot Pineapple Cake, page 437).

Because they're full of oil, nuts go rancid easily. It's best to store them in your refrigerator or freezer. You can tell if nuts are rancid when they have a faint fishy odor; when in doubt, always toss them out.

Herbs and spices. Culinary herbs are a wonderful addition to just about anything you're cooking up. They're one of the best ways to stir in fat-free flavor naturally—allowing you to kick up the taste in a recipe without kicking in too much salt. You may already be using some dried and fresh herbs in your cooking, but maybe there are some you haven't explored yet. Fresh provide a much richer taste and headier aroma than jarred varieties, but there's a place for both in your kitchen. You'll need to use at least three times the amount of fresh when substituting fresh for dried in a recipe (depending on the strength of the herb). Try these at home:

▲ *Basil* lends robust flavor to pasta, meats, vegetables, salads, and tomato dishes. There are many varieties of basil, including lemon, purple, licorice, lettuce-leaf, Thai, and the most common, sweet basil. It's most commonly found in Italian cuisine, although it also appears in Asian foods. Try it in Salmon with Basil and Tomatoes, page 380; or Tomato and Roasted Red Pepper Frittata, page 243.

▲ *Chives* are excellent snipped into soups, salads, and potato, egg, and cheese dishes, usually just before serving. The long stems have a sweet mild oniony flavor and the blossoms are edible as well, adding intriguing flavor and color to salads. Toss them into Chicken Pot Shepherd's Pie, page 362.

HERB HAZARDS

▼ ▼ ▼

There's a difference between culinary herbs (such as the ones listed on this page) and the medicinal herbs that have been gaining popularity in alternative medicine circles. And that difference is particularly important when it comes to pregnancy. Medicinal herbs are drugs and, like all drugs, they should be avoided during pregnancy (unless prescribed by a doctor who knows you are pregnant). Even seemingly benign herbs (such as those in some teas) are capable of inducing diarrhea, vomiting, and even heart palpitations. Remember, too, that herbal preparations are not tested, approved, or regulated by the FDA, so their safety has not been clinically established. Take care when choosing your culinary herbs; make sure you don't confuse them with medicinal herbs.

▲ *Cilantro,* which is actually the leaves of the coriander plant, looks a lot like parsley, but tastes and smells a lot different. Its distinctively pungent flavor (it's definitely not subtle) is used abundantly in Mexican and Asian cuisines. Let it assert itself in a Breakfast Burrito, page 244, Salmon Poached in Thai Carrot Broth, page 381, and Curried Broccoli and Tofu, page 394.

THE PROOF IS IN THE PIGMENT

▼ ▼ ▼

The best way to make sure you're getting the most out of your diet is to follow the rainbow—at least, the one in your produce aisle. If your food palate is mostly brown and beige (as in burgers and fries, not as in whole bread), it's time to add some color to your life—and to your dinner plate. It's best to choose the most vibrantly colored fruits and vegetables available because the pigments that make such produce so visually appealing (a class of phytochemicals called carotenoids) are packed with powerful disease-fighting antioxidants. The fruits that sport them are also high in the nutrients most valued in baby-making. Check out these hot hues:

RED. Red is the color of lycopene, one of nature's superstar phytochemicals. Tomatoes, both raw and cooked (though when cooked they offer more), are a great source. So, too, are ruby red (or pink) grapefruit, watermelon, persimmon, and guava. Other reasons to see (and eat) red because of their high antioxidant content: strawberries, cranberries, cherries, and pomegranates.

ORANGE AND YELLOW. Fruits and vegetables that are orange or yellow are usually rich in baby-friendly beta-carotene. Color your world with winter squash (from butternut to kabocha to delicata), carrots, sweet potatoes, apricots, yellow peaches, cantaloupes, mangoes, papayas, pumpkins, and yellow and orange peppers. Other yellows and oranges, such as oranges, tangerines, lemons, and pineapples, are also high in Vitamin C.

GREEN. Some dark green vegetables are an excellent source of two carotenoids (lutein and zeaxanthin) that help preserve eyesight; others contain indoles (which may reduce the risk of breast cancer). Some are also a great source of baby-friendly folate (folic acid). Besides lettuces (see page 126), stock up on broccoli, articokes, green peas, green

---

▲ *Dill* leaves are fine, feathery, flavorful, and aromatic and are used for seasoning potatoes, meats, fish, salads, breads, and soups. Dill also adds its distinctive taste to pickles and vinegars. Enjoy dill in Salmon Hash Patties, page 253, or Seared Scallops on Succatash, page 387.

▲ *Marjoram* is very close in flavor to oregano, though milder, sweeter, and more citrusy. Pair marjoram's small gray-green leaves with meat and fish dishes, as well as stuffings.

▲ *Mint,* with its sharp, pointed, toothed leaves is popular in many cuisines. For culinary purposes, tangy, sweet spearmint is the mint of choice. Add it to your egg recipes, salads, steamed vegetables, fruit desserts and beverages, such as Minty

beans, avocados, honeydew, spinach, kale, swiss chard, brussels sprouts, green grapes, okra, green peppers, zucchini, kiwi, and parsley.

BLUE. The antioxidant anthocyanin makes the blueberry blue and is a powerful cancer fighter. You won't, however, find it in those boxes of Fruit Loops; that blue (and pink, and yellow, and green) comes by its color an entirely different way.

PURPLE. Purple (or red) grapes contain lutein and zeaxanthin; plums, prunes, blackberries, and purple cabbage are also rich in antioxidants. Beets are rich in the antioxidant betacyanin.

WHITE. While not really a color, don't overlook the white of paler fruits and vegetables. Garlic, onions, shallots, scallions, and leeks contain compounds that protect DNA and may block carcinogens. And endive, mushrooms (particularly wild varieties), celery, and pears are rich in flavonoids (another phytochemical), that protect cell membranes.

▲ *Parsley,* which is grown either as a flat leaf (Italian) or curly leaf, is a natural breath freshener that also adds zest to vegetables, fish, chicken, stews, salads, and soups. Parsley is filled with vitamins and minerals, so use it liberally—not just as the traditional garnish. Add to Here's the Beef Stew, page 336, and Sauteed Shrimp and Linguine, page 305.

▲ *Rosemary* is a fragrant, needle-shaped herb that lends unmistakable flavor and aroma to anything roasted, braised, stewed, or grilled—including chicken, pork, beef, lamb, fish, vegetables, and potato dishes. Just the right touch in Braised Roast Beef in Tomato Sauce, page 337, and Rosemary Lemon Chicken, page 350.

▲ *Sage* adds a unique taste to meats, fish, egg, stuffing, and cheese dishes. Its long oval, slightly fuzzy leaves contain beneficial phytochemicals. It will add a robust flavor to Pan-Roasted Vegetables, page 411.

Medley, page 400; Any Day Breakfast Parfait, page 247; Melon Cooler, page 453; and Iced Watermelon Water, page 424. It also makes a lovely garnish.

▲ *Oregano* is a small, strongly flavored leaf that lends distinctive taste to Greek, Mexican, Spanish, and Italian dishes. It's delicious in Shrimp with Feta, page 385.

wisdom of ☼ the ages?

Here's another old wives' tale to help you figure out if you're carrying a boy or a girl: Eat a clove of raw garlic. If the smell of garlic seeps out of your pores, it's a boy. If no garlic smell is detected at all, it's a girl. But here's a better suggestion: If you really want to find out if it's a boy or a girl (and you don't want to have bad breath or heartburn), ask at the ultrasound.

THE JOY OF SOY

▼ ▼ ▼

Asian cultures have long known the joy of soy—and its many health benefits. Admittedly, the spread of soy has been slower going in the States. For years, only vegetarians and health-food fans toyed with soy. These days, however, the soy invasion is in full deployment; you can find soy in its many nutritious forms in supermarkets and specialty markets the country over—and even served up at coffee bars. Don't pass soy by when you spy it on the shelf. Not only is it rich in protein, calcium, fiber, some vitamins, and phytochemicals, but it offers a host of health incentives for those who partake, from reducing the risk of certain cancers, to lowering LDL cholesterol, to possibly minimizing calcium loss from bones. And its chameleon-like properties make it one of the most versatile ingredients (it blends in and adapts well no matter what you're cooking, from a latte to a stew) you'll find anywhere in the market. So look up some recipes that call for soy (or try Curried Broccoli and Tofu, page 394 or Grilled Tofu, page 413) and start experimenting with soy in one or all of these forms:

■ *Soybeans* can be used instead of pintos for refried beans. Or added cooked and chilled to salads, or tossed into a bean soup. Japanese cuisine features green soybeans as a snack (edamame)—more and more Americans are enjoying these tasty pods (steamed and lightly salted) between meals, too. Look for them in the frozen foods section, or sometimes in produce, and try them in Vegetable and Edamame Soup, page 289, and Kale and Shiitake Mushroom Salad, page 405.

■ *Tempeh* is made from fermented soybeans (it tastes much better than it sounds) and shaped into a firm cake. It can be sliced and cooked like meat, poultry, or fish; a good source of vegetarian protein—plus something to turn to when you have an early pregnancy aversion to the real thing. Try it in stir fries, in casseroles, steamed, baked, or grilled.

■ *TVP* (textured vegetable protein) is a defatted dehydrated soy protein in a flaked form that wouldn't fool a meat lover, but does, again, taste better than it sounds. It makes a satisfactory substitute for ground beef, especially if you'll be cooking it in a highly flavored sauce, as in chili.

■ *Tofu* (also called bean curd) is made from soy milk that has been allowed to coagulate into cheeselike cakes (yet again, a lot better than it sounds). It's white in color, comes in

▲ *Savory,* a member of the mint family, has a peppery flavor with a hint of mint and thyme. Use its slender green leaves in fish, vegetables, cheese and eggs, soups, beans, and tomato dishes.

▲ *Thyme* also contains phytochemicals and adds a savory taste and distinctive aroma to meats, poultry, fish, vegetables, stuffing, and much more. Enjoy thyme in Diner Eggs, page 241; Flounder with Carrots,

various textures (smooth and creamy to extra firm), and can be used like tempeh. Although tofu evokes the "yuck" factor for many people, it really has little taste on its own (much like a plain yogurt, but with less tang) and can take on the flavoring of whatever you cook it with. Use firm or extra-firm varieties when you're baking, grilling, or stir-frying; soft when you're pureeing it (Soft tofu makes a great high-protein thickening agent in soups, sauces, and smoothies).

■ Soy milk can be used as an occasional substitute for cow's milk or when you're looking for a change of pace with your cereal. Choose soy milk that's fortified with calcium and vitamin D if you're using it instead of cow's milk (if you're a vegan or you're lactose intolerant). Make sure you choose a soy milk that's not loaded with sugar or other ingredients you don't want. Soy cheese is a good nondairy alternative to regular cheese.

■ Miso is a fermented paste of soybean combined with a grain (rice, wheat, or barley). This salty paste is used to make miso soup or as a flavoring for many other foods.

In making your discoveries about the joy of soy, keep in mind that as versatile and nutritious as it is, it shouldn't be the only source of protein in your diet. As with all good things, enjoy soy in moderation.

Fennel, and Leek, page 371; and Fettuccine with Turkey and Wild Mushrooms, page 299.

Oils and other fats. What oil do you reach for when you're dressing your salad or stir-frying your chicken? What fat do you use in your baking, spread on your bread, or sprinkle on your vegetables? Think one's as good as another? Not so. Some are healthier for the heart, while others are healthiest for your developing baby—and some really aren't healthy at all. All contain about the same number of calories (and those calories can add up quickly if there's a lot of hidden—or not so hidden—fat in your diet). Keep in mind, too, that while pregnant women are well protected against the effects of cholesterol, others in their families over the age of two aren't. Here are the fat facts:

▲ Olive oil, a mainstay of that healthy Mediterranean diet, is widely considered the heart healthiest type of oil. That's because it's high in monounsaturated fat, known to reduce bad cholesterol (LDL) without decreasing the good cholesterol (HDL). It also protects cells through antioxidant activity. And it tastes great (though it can be an acquired taste) in salads and in savory cooking (not sweet baking). Olive oil, however, is low in other essential fatty acids, so it shouldn't be the only type of oil in your diet.

▲ Canola oil and the fatty acids found in fish are extremely important for their DHA (omega-3 fatty acid) content, crucial during the third trimester for your baby's optimum brain growth and development (see page 98). Researchers are also discovering that canola oil contains important phytochemicals. Because it has such a mild flavor, it's very versatile. Use it in cooking or baking of any kind, and in salad dressings.

▲ *Vegetable oils* (such as safflower oil) are high in linoleic acid, a polyunsaturated fat essential for you and your baby. There have been reports that linoleic acid benefits your baby's immune system, and because it works like another fatty acid (DHA), it helps in the proper development of the fetus's brain. It also possibly reduces the risk of preeclampsia in the mother. Polyunsaturated fats are beneficial in preventing coronary heart disease and diabetes, but while they reduce bad cholesterol (LDL), they also decrease good cholesterol

(HDL). Use as you would canola oil. Peanut (unless you or the baby's father has a history of allergies; see box page 136) and corn oil are also good choices. They are higher in monounsaturated fat than safflower oil (which is a good thing), but lower in polyunsaturated fat than safflower oil (not a good thing).

▲ *Saturated fats,* found in animal products, dairy products, and many processed foods like bakery products and snack foods, should be kept to a minimum because they raise cholesterol levels. With the exception of palm oil and coconut oil, they are solid at room temperature, and melt in cooking. Butter is loaded with saturated fat, so limit your intake of butter (but choose butter over margarines that contain trans-fats; see below).

▲ *Trans-fatty acids* or trans-fats take the cake when it comes to heart

FAST FAT FACTS

▼ ▼ ▼

So where's the beef—or rather, the best cut of beef or other meat? If you're looking for less fat, choose beef, pork, or lamb that have *loin* or *round* in their names. Be picky, selecting cuts that look leanest (with little marbling). Trim any extra fat before cooking. For ground beef, choose lean or extra lean. (It's more expensive, but it'll cook down less, leaving you with more cooked weight.) When eating poultry, favor the breast, and be sure not to eat the skin (which is 85 percent fat). Cook without the skin when you can; when you can't, remove it before eating.

HOME, HOME (AND HEALTHIER) ON THE RANGE

▼ ▼ ▼

Wondering why grass-fed beef has been capturing so many headlines these days, while also scoring a spot in more and more meat cases? Because cows (like people) are what they eat. And while you might think "grazing" when you think cattle, most American cows are actually fed grain or other high-calorie feed, to fatten them up quickly. Keeping them pent up also keeps them fatter.

Grass-fed beef eat the old-fashioned way, by grazing on the range. Not only is their feed vegetarian, but they have to work for it, resulting in much leaner, lower-calorie meat. What's more, grass-fed beef is as much as six times higher in omega-3 fatty acids than grain-fed, plus much higher in vitamin E and beta-carotene. Try it in steaks, as well as ground for hamburgers, stews, and casseroles. All these health advantages come at a price; grass-fed beef is generally more expensive. Keep in mind, too, that grass-fed beef isn't necessarily organic; for beef to be both grass-fed and organic, the label must say so. For another extra-healthy, extra-lean, and extra-tasty red meat, try buffalo, too.

disease—they're even more heart unhealthy than saturated fats. They raise LDL blood cholesterol levels (the bad kind) and reduce HDL (the good cholesterol)—and if that's not reason enough to steer clear of them, they also increase triglycerides and insulin resistance (which means that they pave the way for type II diabetes). Plus, trans-fats are just plain gross. They're not naturally occurring fats—they're by-products of a chemical process in which liquid vegetable oils are hardened to produce solid fats like margarine or shortening. Trans-fats are found mostly in processed foods, especially baked goods (such as snack crackers and pastries). The FDA is now requiring manufacturers to list the amount of trans-fats on the nutrition label, so it's easier than ever to keep them out of your shopping cart. Even better, more and more manufacturers are voluntarily reformulating their products to cut down on or cut out trans-fats. When buying margarines, look for ones made mainly with monounsaturated fats, canola, or olive oil, or those with zero trans-fats.

Playing Label Detective

JUST BECAUSE FOODS ARE LABELED, it doesn't necessarily make shopping easy (just a little easier). Manufacturers, for the most part, design their labels to entice and sell, not to inform. Their goal is to convince the consumer that their product is worthy of your shopping cart—and they do this by putting the stuff they want you to read (the hype: "Great taste!" "Natural ingredients!" "Wholesome!") in big type, and the stuff they're hoping you won't notice (such as the ingredients list and the nutritional information) in smaller print. So figuring out which foods should make it into your cart and which are better left on the shelf takes a sharp eye (and maybe a magnifying glass), as well as the knowledge you need to sort the fact of the small type from the fancy of the large. Here are some clues to keep in mind when you're playing label detective:

Ingredients list. You'll find out a lot about a product just by skimming this list—and you may often be surprised at what you find. All ingredients in a product must be listed on the package in order of predominance, with the first ingredient the most plentiful and the last the least. So a fruit and grain bar that lists its first four filling ingredients as: "sugar, high fructose corn syrup, corn syrup, mixed berry puree" clearly has a lot

more sugar than it does fruit or grain. A "whole-grain" bread that lists "wheat flour" and "sugar" before "whole wheat flour" has little in the way of whole wheat and a lot in the way of refined flour and sugar. A meat and tomato pasta sauce that buries "meat" at the bottom of the list after salt and modified food starch—or worse, lists only "meat flavor"—won't be giving you much in the way of protein.

A good way to look at ingredient lists is to remember that the first five ingredients make up the bulk of the food. If there's little nutrition in those first five, there's little nutrition in that food, even if there's fruit listed seventh or whole grain listed ninth. You should also scan the small print of the list for ingredients the manufacturer is not likely to brag about elsewhere on the label, such as hydrogenated or partially hydrogenated vegetable fats, lard or other animal fats, starchy fillers, and artificial preservatives, colorings, and flavorings.

Nutrition information. Want just the facts, ma'am? Don't look for them on the front of the box, where manufacturers aren't compelled to share them. (Have you ever seen a label that boasts "loaded with saturated fats" or "now with lots more sugar"?)

THE BIG-TYPE HYPE

▼ ▼ ▼

The FDA's reins on label libel are tighter than they've ever been before. There are regulations that specify uniform definitions for terms that describe a food's nutrient content (such as "light," "low-fat," and "high-fiber," see box on page 148) to ensure that manufacturers mean what they say when they use them on a product. There are also rules controlling claims about the relationship between a food and a disease (such as calcium and osteoporosis, and fat and cancer). But even within the parameters set by the FDA, the consumer can get fooled. Many terms are still unregulated (meaning that they can mean anything or nothing at all), including "natural," "wholesome," and "smart." "Healthy" isn't always healthy, either; a cereal labeled as such can be loaded with sugar, refined grains—even artificial colors and flavors. Here are some other tricks of the label trade:

■ "Fortified with 6 vitamins and iron" looks impressive, especially in that extra-large print. And for the most part, fortification with vitamins and minerals is a good thing. But fortification alone does not make a food healthy—especially if it's just tossing some vitamins and minerals into a food that's nutritionally weak. Just about all junk food, after all, is fortified.

■ That macaroni and cheese dinner you bought looks healthy at first glance because that banner across the front announces "Cheddar and Other Natural Flavors." But it's anybody's guess what the "natural flavors" are. And it's likely that the six chemicals listed in small print on the side of the box went unread while your attention was diverted to the big-type hype. And just how far down the list is that cheddar, anyway?

■ There's nothing like pancakes in the morning—especially when the mix you've bought proudly claims "no preservatives" on its front label. Look a little closer, though, and you'll see what the manufacturer probably isn't as proud of: the artificial colors and other chemical additives listed in the ingredients. So don't be fooled by declarations about what isn't in a product; read on about what is.

■ The label calls the box of baked goods in your shopping cart "bran muffins." Good choice, right? Not necessarily. For a bran muffin to earn its name, no more than a pinch of the rough stuff needs to be added to the recipe. Search for *bran* in the ingredients list to see if these bran muffins really are. Does it come second, after whole wheat flour? Or fifth, after white flour, sugar, corn syrup, and enriched flour? Remember, manufacturers like to highlight ingredients they think will sell best. (Who's going to buy a box of "white-flour muffins"?)

LABELS DEFINED

▼ ▼ ▼

Some words you'll find on a label mean very little. Some mean nothing at all. But there are a number of terms currently regulated by the FDA that must fit specific guidelines. Look for these words on the products you're buying, and you'll know exactly what you're looking at:

FREE: The product contains no amount of (or only a trivial amount of) fat, saturated fat, cholesterol, sodium, sugars, or calories—depending on what goes before the word *free*. For example, "calorie-free" means fewer than 5 calories per serving, and "sugar-free" and "fat-free" both mean less than 1/2 gram (g) per serving

LOW-FAT: Contains 3 g or less of fat per serving

LOW-SATURATED FAT: Contains 1 g or less of saturated fat per serving

LOW-SODIUM: Contains 140 milligrams (mg) or less of sodium per serving

VERY LOW SODIUM: Contains 35 mg or less of sodium per serving

LOW-CHOLESTEROL: Contains 20 mg or less of cholesterol and 2 g or less of saturated fat per serving

LOW-CALORIE: Contains 40 calories or less per serving

LEAN: Meat, poultry, seafood, and game meats that contain less than 10 g of fat, 4 1/2 g or less of saturated fat, and less than 95 mg of cholesterol per serving and per 100 g

EXTRA LEAN: Meat, poultry, seafood, and game meats that contain less than 5 g of fat, less than 2 g of saturated fat, and less than 95 mg of cholesterol per serving and per 100 g

HIGH: Contains 20 percent or more of the daily value (DV) for a particular nutrient in a serving

GOOD SOURCE: Contains 10 to 19 percent of the DV for a particular nutrient per serving

Instead, turn to the back or the side for the evidence you're searching for. "Nutrition Facts" gives an excellent nutritional profile of the product you're thinking about buying. It tells you how many calories, grams of fiber, sugar, sodium, fat, protein, vitamins, minerals, cholesterol, carbohydrates, and trans-fat each serving of the food contains in grams or milligrams. It also tells you the percentage of the DV (daily values) of these nutrients there is in a serving for the average person consuming 2,000 calories a day.

Now, this may seem like a lot more than you need to know about a product—and probably a lot more than you know what to do with. But the point of reading nutrition labels isn't so that you can calculate grams or add up percentages. (After all, The Pregnancy Diet Daily Dozen already ensures that you're getting

REDUCED: Contains at least 25 percent less of a nutrient or of calories than the regular product

LESS (or FEWER): Contains 25 percent less of a nutrient or of calories than a reference food. For example, pretzels that have 25 percent less fat than potato chips could carry a "less" or "fewer" claim.

LIGHT: Contains one-third fewer calories or half the fat of the reference food *or* the sodium content of a low-calorie, low-fat food has been reduced by 50 percent. (Beware: "Light" can also be used to describe texture and color, as long as the label explains the intent, for instance, "light brown sugar.")

MORE: Contains 10 percent of the DV more than a reference food

For more information on food labels and definitions, call the FDA's Food Safety Hotline at 888-723-3366 or go to www.fda .gov/Food/LabelingNutrition/default.htm.

▲ An item is low in a nutrient if it contains 5 percent or less of the DV.

▲ Foods containing 20 percent or more of the DV for a nutrient are considered a good source of that nutrient.

▲ Foods containing 5 percent or less of the DV for fat are low in fat (though they still might not be healthy; remember to read the rest of the nutritional facts as well to see if the food passes the nutrition test with the rest of its ingredients). You should try not to exceed 20 percent DV for fat in a main-course dish and 10 percent DV for fat in a side dish, snack, or beverage.

Serving size. What's in a serving? The nutrition information provided on a food label is based on the serving size listed. But get that product home, and the size of the serving can vary a whole lot, depending on who's

the amounts of nutrients you need, without doing the math; besides, the DV for pregnancy is often different from that listed on the label.) It's to figure out whether the product you're picking up is worth dropping into your cart. Some good rules of thumb to keep in mind:

▲ Try to select foods that contain no more than 3 grams of fat for every 100 calories.

PREPARING IT ALL

▼ ▼ ▼

Once you're home from your food-shopping expedition you'll need to make sure you're up on the ABC's of storing and preparing your bounty safely and healthily. See Chapter Seven for tips.

dishing it out and who's eating it. So if the label says that a serving is half a cup and it's likely you'll eat a cup and a half, remember that all the numbers will triple (including the calories and grams of fat). And if the serving size is for a cup and you'll be eating only half a cup, you'll have to halve the nutrient numbers promised on the label.

BAR NONE?

▼ ▼ ▼

They fit neatly in a purse, glove compartment, desk drawer, even your pocket. They're loaded with vitamins and minerals—and they're filling enough to keep you going when you're on the run. But do nutrition bars have what it takes to take the place of a meal when you're expecting? If only healthy eating were that easy and convenient.

While most bars offer plenty of vitamins and minerals, they come by their nutrients through fortification, not because they're real food. (Besides, if you're taking a prenatal supplement and eating a healthy diet, you don't need those extra vitamins and minerals.) And though they're usually high in protein, they're often just as high in sugar (or sugar substitutes) and fat. Bottom line on bars: Snacking on them occasionally is fine; counting on them regularly to stand in for meals isn't.

Eating Safely When You're Expecting

EATING IN THE TWENTY-FIRST CENTURY is pretty safe business, even for the pregnant consumer. Gone are the days when the dinner table often offered up a bounty of bacteria along with otherwise wholesome foods—when the roast was accompanied by a side of *Clostridium botulinum,* the milk served with a helping of shigella, the water with a host of cholera. Modern food preparation, packaging, and storage techniques now team up to ensure that most of what you pull off your supermarket shelf can be popped into your mouth without a second thought about safety. Still, eating well when you're expecting—even in this era of refrigeration, shrink-wrapping, and vacuum-sealing—takes a little extra prudence, as well as a few more second thoughts about safety. There are some edibles (and drinkables) you'll need to avoid altogether while you're eating for two, others that you'll need to limit, and still others that you'll be able to indulge in freely with a few preparation precautions.

Keeping Your Kitchen Safe

THINK THAT YOU HAVE MONTHS before you'll have to worry about making your kitchen safe for baby? While it's true that you can hold off on installing child-proof latches on the cabinets and knob covers on the stovetop, there are many other precautions you should be taking around your kitchen right now to protect your growing fetus—not from pinched fingers or accidental burns, but from food-borne bacteria and other toxins that can make both of you sick. So before donning your extra-large apron in the kitchen, remember to:

Wash your hands. Mom (and the Health Department) does know best when it comes to this first rule of safe cooking and eating. Washing your hands in hot soapy water before preparing food is your best line of defense against the spread of bacteria in the kitchen. Break out the soap, too, after you've handled raw meat, poultry, fish, or eggs—all of which can harbor dangerous bacteria. Rewash, also, after blowing your nose, going to the bathroom, changing a diaper, or attending to another germ-charged activity.

Wash your rags. That dish towel you just dried your hands with looks pretty clean, doesn't it? Take a closer look (like under a microscope) and you might change your mind—as well as your towel. Kitchen rags, sponges, and towels provide a perfect breeding ground for bacteria, which thrive in moist environments. To avoid drying your hands, wiping your counter, and

HOME IS WHERE THE HEALTH IS . . . OR IS IT?

▼ ▼ ▼

MYTH: Food prepared at home is much safer than restaurant food. Most food-borne illnesses are contracted from food at restaurants.

FACT: Actually, you're more likely to pick up a bug at home than at your favorite restaurant. That's because most (though certainly not all) professional food handlers have been trained in safety techniques and are more likely careful about how food in restaurant kitchens is prepared, cooked, and stored. Think about this, too: Most home kitchens probably wouldn't pass inspection by the Health Department. Would yours?

cleaning your dishes with a veritable petri dish of microorganisms, wash rags and towels often in hot soapy water or in the washing machine (with a little bleach if possible). Replace sponges at least once a month, and wash them thoroughly with soap and water or in the dishwasher at the end of the day. You can also microwave the cellulose types (when wet) for two minutes on high to wipe out harmful bacteria. To avoid spreading germs around your kitchen, use paper towels for kitchen cleanup.

Mind your surfaces. Bacteria multiply far faster than rabbits, especially when left to their own devices on kitchen surfaces. To thwart their reproductive efforts, clean counter tops and sinks with soapy water or cleansers often. Don't put defrosting meats and poultry (even those that are wrapped in plastic or paper) directly on the refrigerator shelf; place paper towels and a dish under defrosting meats and poultry to catch the juices. Use a different cutting board for produce than you use for meat, poultry, and fish, and wash them in the dishwasher after each use. (Or if they're too large to fit, with hot, soapy water.) When boards get scarred from too much use, discard them. (Bacteria like to hide—and multiply—in pitted surfaces.)

Keep utensils separate. One knife that gets around—from the raw

chicken breasts to the cheese to the tomatoes—can spread a whole lot of bacteria around your kitchen. If you're using one knife for several food-prep steps, wash between uses with hot soapy water. Better still, keep different knives for different purposes (one for raw meat and poultry, another for produce).

TAKING OUT TONIGHT?

▼ ▼ ▼

Have so little energy left after your long day that you've decided to blow off cooking altogether and stop for takeout? Here's how to make sure you're not bringing home bacteria along with your ready-made meal:

■ **Check out the display.** Avoid buying cooked foods that may have mingled with raw meats, fish, or poultry in the store display case (or may have been dished out with utensils that have touched them), or that haven't been refrigerated.

■ **Screen the salad bar.** Does it have a "sneeze guard?" Is it well refrigerated? Does it look clean? Are there separate utensils for all items?

■ **Screen the food.** If a take-out food looks wilted, withered, or off color, or if it has a funny odor, don't purchase it. If it's too late for that, don't eat it.

Keeping Your Foods Safe

YOU'VE SHOPPED FOR THE MOST nutritious ingredients, and you're ready to turn them into a delicious meal. To ensure that what goes into you (and your baby) is as safe as it is nourishing, keep these general recommendations in mind when preparing, serving, and storing foods:

▲ Keep cold foods cold (at or below 40°F). Don't keep perishables (meats, fish, poultry, cut raw or cooked produce, dairy products) at temperatures above 40°F for more than two hours. Refrigerate foods that won't be served or cooked immediately. Store highly perishable foods (milk, fish) in the

THE DATING GAME

▼ ▼ ▼

How can you tell if a food you're about to purchase or that's been sitting in your refrigerator for a while is too old to eat? Play the dating game by checking out the label.

■ Labels on products such as flour and grains, baked goods, cereals, and some canned goods, generally read: "Best if used before" or "Best if used by" or "Best before." These foods generally won't be dangerous after the date stated, but they may very well begin to taste stale. Best to toss them.

■ On perishable products that require refrigeration and have a shorter shelf life—such as cheese, yogurt, or eggs—the labeling usually reads: "Expiration date," "Use by," or "Use before." In most cases, it means the food should no longer be consumed after that date passes. In the case of yeast, it means it will have lost its rising power.

■ On milk, which is highly perishable, there is a "sell by" date—and though the milk should be pulled from the grocer's shelves after that date, it will usually be safe to use for another week if it's refrigerated at home.

■ Meats are safe for only three to five days (two days for ground meat) after that "sell by" or "pull" date, unless you bring them home frozen (they can last six months in the freezer). Poultry and seafood should be consumed within two days of the "sell-by" date.

Another trick of the dating game? To bring home foods with the latest dates possible, check the back of the supermarket shelf. Grocers usually put the older items up front (to get rid of them before they expire).

back of the refrigerator. (The storage areas on the door don't stay as cold.)

▲ Keep hot foods hot (at or above 140°F) until serving. Reheat leftovers thoroughly until hot and steaming; bring gravies and soups to a rolling boil before you ladle them up.

▲ Here's bad news for the buffet table: Do not leave food at room temperature for more than two hours (one hour on a hot day, so be especially careful during those summer barbecues). Refrigerate or freeze leftovers as soon as possible. (That after-dinner coffee and conversation can wait until after cleanup.)

▲ Keep raw and cooked foods separate.

▲ Do not refreeze foods that have been thawed at room temperature, or have been brought to room temperature after thawing, or have been kept more than a day or two after thawing, even in the refrigerator.

▲ Pay attention to "sell by" and "use by" labels on foods (see previous page). When in doubt, throw it out—even if there are no obvious signs of spoilage. Definitely throw out any food that has an off color or odor.

▲ Don't double dip (dip a carrot into salsa, take a bite, and then dip the same carrot again) or eat straight from a container with the same spoon. Bacteria from your mouth can contaminate the food—even if it's refrigerated afterward.

▲ Wash the lids of canned foods before opening to keep dirt and bacteria from getting into the food. Also, clean the blade of the can opener after each use. Drop it in the dishwasher afterward.

wisdom of ☼ the ages?

Not surprisingly, old wives have spent a lot of time in the kitchen over the ages—and have spun more than a few tales around the stovetop. Among them— you shouldn't put hot food in the refrigerator because it will spoil. In fact, the old wives are way off base on this one. The longer a food (hot or cold) sits out at room temperature, the greater the chances bacteria will multiply—and the faster it will spoil. A good mantra to remember when cooking foods that won't be eaten right away: Cool slightly; then don't hesitate, refrigerate.

Safe Produce

NOTHING IS MORE WHOLESOME THAN fresh fruits and vegetables from the supermarket produce section—right? For the most part, yes. Unless the fresh peach or apple you're about to bite into is sporting a layer of pesticides or is covered in unwholesome bacteria it picked up from a picker who didn't wash his hands.

Luckily, there are many ways to make sure the produce that's supposed to keep you healthy is healthy:

▲ Go for locally grown produce (when possible). For one thing, it's usually fresher than imports (which means it's likely to retain more nutrients). For another, it doesn't require post-harvest pesticides to preserve it during a long cross-country (or even international) journey. Try to buy fruits and vegetables in season (for the same reasons). Keep in mind that imported produce may contain both more bacteria and more pesticide residue (unless it's certified organic), since regulations on both sanitation and chemical use are more lax in some foreign countries.

▲ Go organic. Whenever it's available and affordable and looks good, opt for organic. It isn't less likely to contain bacteria, but at least it won't be covered with pesticides.

▲ Switch off. Choosing a variety of fruits and vegetables doesn't only

PRODUCE-PHOBIC?

▼ ▼ ▼ ▼

Is a fear of chemical residue keeping you and produce apart? Don't let it. As long as you follow the basic principles of fruit and vegetable safety (always wash fruits and vegetables; choose organic when you can; vary the produce you eat; and, when in doubt, peel), you won't have to pay the price in pesticides. In fact, many types of fruits and vegetables actually contain natural substances that protect you (and your baby) against the effects of chemical contamination (not only from the produce you eat, but also from other sources in your environment). So fear not your produce! For more information on chemical residue and pesticides on produce, contact the EPA National Pesticide Information Center at (800) 858-PEST (7378) or http://npic.orst.edu.

PASTEURIZED, PLEASE

▼ ▼ ▼

Pasteurization may be the best thing that ever happened to a glass of milk (or a wedge of cheese), but it shouldn't stop at dairy products. To protect yourself and your unborn baby from harmful bacteria, such as listeria or *E. coli,* make sure that the juice you drink is also pasteurized (not "raw")—even if it means bypassing your favorite cider mill.

guarantee better nutrition, but safer eating as well. That's because different chemicals are used on different types of produce; vary your produce, and you won't ingest too much of any. (Of course, if you choose organic, you won't ingest any at all.)

▲ Be picky when it comes to fruits and vegetables; toss those that look moldy or smell funny. (It's okay to eat produce that's bruised, though.)

▲ Don't forget to date your produce, too. Don't buy (or use) prepackaged produce that is close to its expiration date—or that doesn't look fresh or isn't refrigerated.

▲ Wash the surfaces of all fruits and vegetables, even those you plan to peel (including melons)—otherwise

the knife or peeler you're using can pick up surface germs and transmit them to the part of the produce you'll be eating. (Keep in mind that organic produce is just as likely to carry bacteria as the conventional variety.) Don't soak produce (you'll end up throwing out many of the vitamins with the soaking water), and don't use soap (a produce wash is best). If necessary, use a small scrub brush to remove dirt. Wash the brush frequently in the dishwasher.

▲ Double-check before you don't wash. Most prepackaged letuce is already washed—usually triple-washed. But some isn't.

NO SPROUTS FOR YOUR LITTLE SPROUT

▼ ▼ ▼

Raw sprouts (alfalfa sprouts or bean sprouts, for instance) may look pretty (and pretty healthy) on top of your salad or stuffed into your sandwich, but what's not pretty is the bacteria they may harbor. Sprouts have been linked sometimes to outbreaks of *E. coli,* and salmonella and, unfortunately, should be avoided when you're pregnant or breastfeeding.

Safe Meat, Poultry, and Fish

BUILDING A BABY? THERE'S NO MORE efficient source of baby-building protein than lean meat, poultry, and fish. To cash in on the protein without tapping into any bacteria that may have come along for the ride:

▲ If freezing store-bought meat, poultry, or fish, unwrap them from the plastic or paper wrapping they came in and seal in aluminum foil or specially designed freezer bags to prevent freezer burn. (Don't forget to label them so you won't be left with unidentified frozen objects).

▲ Defrost meats, poultry, or fish in the refrigerator, in cold water (changing the water every 30 minutes), or in a microwave oven, rather than at

room temperature. Food defrosted in the microwave should be cooked immediately.

▲ Marinate meat, poultry, or fish in the refrigerator. Don't reuse marinade that has touched raw meat or poultry. (Set some aside before marinating).

▲ Cook all meat, poultry, and fish thoroughly (see box on page 161 for appropriate temperatures).

▲ Keep hot meats hot and cold meats cold. If you're bringing chicken salad to a picnic, be sure it's transported on ice. Don't let cooked hot meats stay out at room temperature for more than two hours (one on a hot day).

A MEAT MYTH THAT'S ALL WET

▼ ▼ ▼

MYTH: Raw meat and poultry should always be rinsed before cooking to wash away the bacteria on the surface.

FACT: Cooking meats and poultry to the right internal temperature (see box, page 161) will almost always kill all the bacteria lurking on the surface—and inside. Rinsing doesn't wash enough bacteria

away; it does, however, splash germs and bacteria into the sink (and, if you're not careful, onto countertops), so if you insist on rinsing (even though you now know that it's pointless and risky) you'll need to clean up thoroughly afterwards. (Fish, on the other hand, will stay fresher if it is rinsed and patted dry before freezing or when brought home from the store.)

WHAT DID YOUR DINNER HAVE FOR DINNER?

▼ ▼ ▼

Wondering whether the chicken you're having for dinner may have ingested a few too many chemicals before ending up on your plate? Here's some reassuring news: You don't have to pass on the protein to keep your unborn baby safe. As with produce, there are plenty of ways to minimize the exposure you (and your baby) will have to unwanted chemicals when meat (or poultry) is on the menu:

■ Be partial to certain parts. Most chemicals ingested by an animal tend to congregate in its fat and fatty organs. To avoid their entry into your system (and baby's), stick to lean cuts of meat (steaks, for instance, that have less marbling; extra-lean ground beef) and the white meat of poultry. Though organ meats (liver, kidneys, brains, sweetbreads) offer plenty of vitamins, the trade-off (plenty of chemicals) isn't worth it; eat these infrequently.

■ Skin and trim. For the same reasons, take the skin off your poultry before cooking when it's possible; when it's not possible, remove the skin before eating.

Trim meat of all visible fat. When sautéing ground beef, drain well before continuing with the recipe; always discard fat that has accumulated during cooking (instead of reusing for sauces). Skin fish, too, and trim dark meat off fish steaks and fillets.

■ Vary the meat you eat. Try not to play meat favorites (steak for dinner every night—unless, of course, early pregnancy queasiness dictates main course monotony). Including a variety of meat and poultry in your diet will help ensure that you're not taking in too much of any kind of chemical.

■ Spring for organic. If it's available in your market and isn't too pricey, opt for meat and poultry that is raised without hormones or antibiotics—and preferably, on an organic diet.

■ Consider grass-fed. Grazing cows are healthier cows; see page 145.

For more on meat and poultry safety, call the USDA meat and poultry hotline at (888) 674-6854. See page 169 for more on minimizing the risks of contaminated fish.

▲ Don't stuff meat or poultry until it is ready to go into the oven. Stuff lightly (about ¾ pound of stuffing per pound of turkey), keep it moist, and cook until the center of the stuffing reaches at least 165°F on a meat thermometer. After cooking, store the stuffing and meat separately. Safer still, don't stuff at all; bake the stuffing in a separate pan, basting occasionally with broth to keep it from drying out (a bonus: the stuffing will develop a crusty top; if you prefer soft stuffing, bake it covered with foil).

NOW YOU TELL ME?

▼ ▼ ▼

Does this chapter have you worried about all the things you'd have done differently if only you'd known? Like sucking down that sake (and that huge plate of sashimi) two days before the pregnancy test came back positive? Eating a salami sandwich before reading the section on luncheon-meat risks? Ordering your hamburger rare twelve times before finding out that you shouldn't "have it your way" (unless your way is "well done") when you're expecting?

Relax. Most women have at least a few expectant encounters with food or drink that aren't considered fit for pregnant consumption (especially before they find out they're expecting)—some have many. In the vast majority of cases, there's no harm done. (For instance, sushi and salami only rarely contain organisms that cause illness.) So use this chapter as a guide to making your pregnancy diet as safe as you can make it from now on—but don't use it to drive yourself crazy about what's already behind you.

▲ Cook meat until brown in the middle, never pink or red. (Be aware, though, that this so-called "color test" can be misleading because cooked color varies considerably. For example, freezing and thawing may influence a meat's tendency to brown prematurely, even if it's not yet cooked through.) Using a meat thermometer will give you a better reading of meat safety (see box, facing page). Order meat "medium well" or "well" in restaurants (even at the risk of offending the chef), just to be on the safe side.

▲ Cook chicken and other poultry until the juices run clear and it reaches the appropriate temperature (see box, facing page). Traces of pink near the bones do not mean the poultry is not well cooked; the color leaches out from the bones. Sadly, you'll also have to order duck (which is often served up rare, especially the breast, and is definitely juicier and tastier that way) well done.

▲ *Do not* eat raw meats or poultry, because they can harbor microorganisms.

▲ *Do not* eat raw or rare fish or seafood. See the box on page 169 for more on fish safety and types of fish that are safe to eat during pregnancy and the box on page 163 for information about the safety of smoked seafood.

▲ Heat ready-to-eat hot dogs and sausages (whenever possible choose those that are low in fat and nitrate-free; see page 171) and meat or poultry leftovers until steaming hot all the way through. Luncheon meats should be eaten sparingly—

first, because they often contain nitrates (check out the health-food market for those that don't), and second, because they may be contaminated with listeria (see box, page 163). Heating luncheon meats until steaming will eliminate the listeria risk, but will also make the meats less appealing (steamed salami, anyone?). Better yet, wait until your pregnancy is over to bite into that bologna sandwich.

IS IT DONE YET?

▼ ▼ ▼

How do you make sure that your dinner isn't half-baked—and thus, potentially harboring germs that could make you sick? By taking your dinner's temperature (a high enough temperature means you won't be serving bacteria along with that roast or that fish). Don't rely on the pop-up thermometers that come with some poultry; invest in a good-quality instant-read meat thermometer, and use it faithfully (wash it after each use with hot soapy water). Of course, you'll also need to know where to stick it—as well as what temperature to look for once you have. Here's a guide:

FOR ROASTS, STEAKS, OR CHOPS MADE FROM BEEF, VEAL, PORK, OR LAMB: Insert the thermometer in the center or the thickest part of the meat, away from any bone, fat, or gristle.

FOR GROUND MEAT OR POULTRY, CUTLETS, FISH, AND CASSEROLES: Insert the thermometer in the thickest part of the food. For burgers, insert sideways.

FOR CHICKEN, TURKEY, DUCK, OR GOOSE: Insert the thermometer in the inner thigh area, where the leg meets the body of the bird (but be sure it isn't touching the bone).

The following foods can be considered safely cooked when they reach these temperatures:

BEEF, VEAL, LAMB, OR PORK ROASTS, CHOPS, OR STEAKS: medium—160°F; well done—170°F

GROUND BEEF, VEAL, LAMB, PORK: 160°F

PRECOOKED HAM: 140°F

WHOLE CHICKEN OR TURKEY: 165°F

GROUND CHICKEN OR TURKEY: 165°F

CHICKEN BREASTS: 165°F

STUFFING: cooked in bird or alone—165°F

FISH: 145°F

EGG CASSEROLES: 160°F

MOLD AND MOMS-TO-BE

▼ ▼ ▼

You had good intentions of filling your fridge (and your tummy) with Daily Dozen goodies when you bought that extra container of cottage cheese and pint of strawberries. But somehow you never got around to eating them, and when you finally dug them out for a healthy breakfast, a blue fuzz has started multiplying across the top of the cottage cheese, and a green one is sprouting on the strawberries. Do you scrape and eat them or dump them? Here are some guidelines about mold for the mom-to-be:

■ If small fruits (grapes, berries, strawberries) become moldy, throw them out. If a few berries at the top of a box are moldy, it's okay to eat the rest as long as you've screened them carefully.

■ If a hard fruit or vegetable (apple, potato, broccoli, onion, for instance) or hard cheese has a small area of mold, it's safe to cut the mold away (plus a half-inch margin of safety) and eat the rest. Moldy soft fruits (peaches, plums, melons, tomatoes) should be tossed.

■ Soft dairy products (cottage cheese, yogurt, sour cream, butter) that are sprouting mold should be discarded—even if the mold is only on top. Ditto moldy meat and leftovers.

■ Moldy bread, grains, peanut butter, nuts, sauces, and jams should be thrown away (even if the mold is only in one area). And always remember—when in doubt, throw it out.

Safe Dairy

THERE'S NO QUICKER WAY TO FILL your calcium requirement (and to pick up a good bonus of protein) than by stopping at your market's dairy case. And most dairy products are as safe as they are nutritious. To ensure safe dairy eating:

▲ Never use raw (unpasteurized) milk or cheeses. This is one case where processed (or at least, pasteurized) is better.

▲ Store all dairy products in the refrigerator (even pasteurized products can become contaminated after pasteurization), and do not use them after the expiration date or if they smell or look suspicious.

LISTERIA ALERT

▼ ▼ ▼

Food contaminated with the harmful bacteria listeria can cause an illness called listeriosis. This serious illness is particularly dangerous for pregnant women (who are at increased risk of contracting listeriosis because of their suppressed immune system): It can lead to premature delivery, miscarriage, or serious illness in the fetus. And, unlike other bacteria, listeria enters the bloodstream directly and can get to the baby quickly. Take these steps to reduce your risk of getting listeriosis:

■ Steer clear of smoked fish. Refrigerated smoked seafood—such as salmon, trout, whitefish, cod, tuna, or mackerel—most often labeled as "nova-style," "lox," "kippered," "smoked," or "jerky," should not be eaten by pregnant women unless it is cooked (as in a casserole) or is shelf stable smoked fish.

■ Heat deli meat. See page 160 for more.

■ Stay away from unpasteurized soft cheeses. Soft cheese such as feta, goat cheese, blue cheeses (Roquefort for instance), Brie, Camembert, and soft Mexican-style cheese or any cheese that is made from raw (unpasteurized) milk can be contaminated with listeria. If you're not sure whether a soft cheese is pasteurized, don't eat it unless it's cooked until bubbling. Pasteurized dairy products are safe to eat, so a ricotta, or fresh mozzarella, feta, blue, or Brie cheese labeled "pasteurized" is safe for the pregnant. Hard cheeses, processed cheeses, cream cheese, cottage cheese, and yogurt are also safe bets.

For more information, contact the FDA Center for Food Safety and Applied Nutrition at 888-723-3366; visit www .foodsafety.gov; or contact the Centers for Disease Control and Prevention at www.cdc.gov/foodsafety.

Safe Eggs

THOUGH THE CHOLESTEROL IN EGGS isn't a problem during pregnancy, contamination with salmonella could be. Washing eggs before using them doesn't guarantee safety, since most eggs are contaminated before the shells form. However, there are steps you can take to make sure all the eggs that end up on your table are good eggs:

▲ Only buy eggs that have been kept refrigerated. Once you've brought them home, store them in the fridge;

MILK SENSE

▼ ▼ ▼

Not surprisingly, what goes into a cow (including the chemicals in her diet) can end up in her milk. To keep it from ending up in your milk (and cheese, and yogurt):

■ **Forgo the fat.** Whole-milk dairy products (whole milk, whole-milk cheese, cream cheese, and cottage cheese, whole-milk yogurt) may have more flavor, but they also have considerably more fat. Which doesn't just translate to more calories, but potentially more chemicals (as is the case with meat and poultry, fat is the storehouse for chemicals that end up in a cow's milk). So make skim or low-fat dairy products the mainstay of your diet (using whole-milk yogurt to make a creamier slaw or salad dressing is fine, though).

■ **Reach for organic.** When it's available and affordable, consider buying organic—especially when you're getting a whole-milk dairy product, butter, or cream. But be sure that they're organic *and* pasteurized.

they can stay fresh for three weeks (assuming the expiration date hasn't passed). And because even hard-cooked eggs can become contaminated, don't leave these out at room temperature longer than two hours.

▲ Cook eggs until the whites are set and the yolks have begun to thicken (they shouldn't be runny). Hard-cooked eggs can stay fresh in the fridge for one week.

▲ Do not use raw eggs in salad dressings (try one of the Caesar salad recipes starting on page 330 instead of a traditional one), sauces (hollandaise), or whipped up in desserts that won't be cooked (mousse).

Don't eat homemade foods that contain raw eggs, including ice cream, mayonnaise, eggnog, cookie dough, and cake batter (even if it's finger-licking good); the commercial counterparts of these foods are safe to eat, since they're made with pasteurized eggs (a heating process that kills bacteria without harming or cooking the egg). Pasteurized eggs (and egg whites) can also be bought for home use, and are safe to use raw in prepared foods or to serve undercooked.

▲ Don't use an egg that is cracked when you buy it or cracks on the way home—disease-causing organisms can get in too easily.

▲ Choose eggs from cage-free chickens, when possible. Cooped-up hens may be more likely to produce contaminated eggs. (Precautions should still be taken with cage-free eggs, though, since the possibility of cont-amination—though smaller—does exist.) You might also want to look for organic eggs, which come from chickens not treated with antibiotics or growth hormones.

Off the Menu

THOUGH MOST FOODS ARE SAFE FOR pregnant consumption, there are a few that should stay off the menu entirely until after delivery.

Alcohol. Wine with dinner? Cocktail before? Not when you're expecting. As you probably already know, total tee-totaling during pregnancy is recommended not only by doctors and midwives, but also by the United States Surgeon General (in the form of labels plastered on all bottles of wine, beer, and other alcoholic beverages). And for good reason. Alcohol crosses the placenta in concentrations almost identical to those in the mother's blood (which means each drink is shared equally with the unborn baby); studies link regular drinking during pregnancy (even regular moderate drinking) to a variety of very serious birth defects and complications, including low I.Q. Researchers have also found that children heavily exposed to alcohol in the womb are at higher risk for developing drinking problems and even psychotic symp-toms in young adulthood. Since no "safe" upper limit of alcohol consumption has been determined—and even occasional light drinking hasn't been completely cleared—on the wagon is by far the safest place for you to stay during your nine months.

Which doesn't mean that you should worry about the wine, beer, or cocktails you drank before you found out you were expecting. What it does mean is that you should give up alcohol the moment you know you're pregnant (in the best of all pos-

DON'T MIX THIS

▼ ▼ ▼

Recreational drugs, cigarette smoking, and pregnancy don't mix—in fact, they can lead to numerous long-term problems for your fetus. So play it safe. Stay away from both tobacco and drugs during pregnancy and lactation. See *What to Expect When You're Expecting* for reasons why and tips on how to quit.

WINE IN DINNER?

▼ ▼ ▼

Hungry for some coq au vin or beer-braised short ribs, but not sure whether pregnancy alcohol prohibitions carry over to the stove? Feast away, within reason. In general, the longer the stints on the range or in the oven, the less alcohol remains. And although alcohol does not cook out completely when you add it to a stew or baked dish (the amount of alcohol that actually cooks off varies on how long the food has been cooked; see below), the

alcohol that remains will not add up to much, especially in the context of a single serving. So unless you're planning on drinking three cups of sauced sauce, you've got nothing to worry about. To be extra safe, stick to recipes that require cooking times of at least half an hour, avoiding those that expose the alcohol to only passing heat (such as flambéed cherries), or choose alcohol substitutions in your recipes instead (see box, facing page).

IF YOU BAKE OR SIMMER FOR:

THE AMOUNT OF ALCOHOL REMAINING IS:

15 minutes	40 percent
30 minutes	35 percent
1 hour	25 percent
1½ hours	20 percent
2 hours	10 percent
2½ hours	5 percent

sible pregnancy scenarios, you'd give it up when you first start trying to conceive). If you decide to take a very occasional celebratory sip or two, do so with food, which slows the absorption of alcohol into the system. For tips on giving up alcohol, see *What to Expect When You're Expecting.*

Raw fish and seafood. It's sad news for those who like to eat it raw—

pregnancy isn't the time to do that. Preparing fish and other seafood properly is as important as choosing the right varieties (see box, page 169). Shellfish, including clams, mussels, oysters, and scallops should always be thoroughly cooked, since they can carry the bacteria or viruses that can cause hepatitis or food poisoning. Same for fish, which can carry any number of potentially harmful

STANDING IN FOR THE SAUCE

▼ ▼ ▼

Is your kitchen an alcohol-free zone since you've been expecting? Here are some ways to stir comparable flavor into your favorite recipes, without the sauce:

INSTEAD OF	TRY
Amaretto (2 tbsp)	Almond extract ($^1/_2$ tsp)
Beer	Ginger ale or chicken broth
Brandy	Apple cider, apricot juice
Calvados	Apple juice concentrate
Champagne	Ginger ale or sparkling white grape juice
Cognac	Peach, apricot, or pear juice
Dry red wine	Grape or cranberry juice (cut the sweetness with red wine vinegar), or beef broth
Framboise	Raspberry juice
Cassis	Cherry, blueberry, or pomegranate juice
Frangelico	Hazelnut or almond extract
Grand Marnier	Orange juice concentrate
Kirsch	Juice from raspberries, currants, or cider
Port wine (or sweet sherry)	Grape or pomegranate juice
Rum	White grape juice or pineapple juice
Sake	Rice vinegar
Sherry or bourbon	Orange or pineapple juice
Vermouth (sweet)	Apple or grape juice
Vermouth (dry)	White grape juice mixed with white wine vinegar
White wine	Chicken broth, diluted cider vinegar, or white wine vinegar

organisms that cooking kills. Fish should be cooked until it easily flakes with a fork and reaches the appropriate temperature (see box, page 161); seafood until it's firm. Marinating raw fish in lime juice or anything else (as in ceviche) or dipping in a hot sauce does *not* kill microorganisms and is an unsafe way of preparing seafood in pregnancy. Off the menu during pregnancy: All raw seafood and fish (including sashimi and sushi rolls that contain raw fish), as well as seafood or fish that's served "seared," rare, or in tartares or carpaccios. Refrigerated smoked seafood (such as lox or smoked salmon) is also off the menu because of the risk of listeria (see box, page 163).

Undercooked or raw meat and poultry. See page 158 and box, page 161, for safe meat and poultry tips.

Unpasteurized soft cheeses. See box, page 163, for the list of soft cheeses that are off the pregnancy menu.

Raw eggs. See page 163 for more.

TRY THESE INSTEAD

▼ ▼ ▼

What happens if your pregnancy cravings get in the way of sensible and safe eating? Not to worry. There are many ways to safely satisfy those yearnings— even when they're for foods you're supposed to be steering clear of. Try these sensible substitutions:

INSTEAD OF	TRY
Sushi with raw fish	Rolls made with cooked fish or vegetables
Raw shellfish	Steamed or boiled shellfish
Swordfish	Roasted or grilled halibut
Rare hamburger	Well-done hamburger (add more toppings to compensate for loss of flavor)
Salami	Hot open brisket sandwich; grilled slice of turkey breast
Caesar salad dressing made with raw eggs	Creamy Caesar Dressing (see page 332)
Raw sprouts	Cooked sprouts
Store-bought fresh-squeezed juice (unpasteurized)	Juice squeezed at home

JUST FOR THE HALIBUT

▼ ▼ ▼

Despite the fact that they can't breathe, fish (at least those that swim or spawn in inland waters that have been used as receptacles for chemical wastes) have not escaped the scourge of industrial society: pollution. Certain fish contain high levels of polychlorinated biphenyls (PCBs) or mercury. And because of the potential risk to the unborn (and to the already born, through contaminated breast milk), it's recommended that pregnant and breast-feeding women be more cautious in their seafood consumption than the general population and stick to fish that are con-

sidered safe. You can also play it safer by trimming dark flesh off fish, by skinning fish before cooking, and by cooking fish well. (Remember that, as with most environmental risks, occasional exposure is unlikely to be hazardous to your fetus. So don't lose any sleep over the mahi mahi or swordfish dinners you tucked away early in your pregnancy; just refrain from ordering those from now on.)

According to Environmental Protection Agency (EPA) guidelines, during pregnancy and lactation, you should:

AVOID	LIMIT TO 6-OZ/WEEK	LIMIT TO 12-OZ/WEEK	
Shark*	Freshwater fish caught by family and friends	Shellfish	Tilapia
Swordfish*		Salmon	Ocean perch
King Mackerel*	Canned albacore tuna	(Caught wild or organic	Sea bass***
	Fresh tuna (contains more mercury than canned, so eat infrequently)	farm-raised is better then conventional farm-raised)	Halibut***
Tilefish*			Cod
Mahi mahi**			Farm-raised trout
Grouper**		Flounder	Store-bought freshwater fish
Amberjack**		Sole	
Fish from contaminated waters		Snapper	Canned light tuna
		Pollack	Catfish
		Haddock	Sardine

For the latest information on fish safety call the FDA at (800) 332-4010, or contact the EPA at (800) 490-9198 or their website: www.epa.gov/waterscience/fish.

*These fish contain high levels of a form of mercury called methyl mercury that may harm the fetus's developing nervous system. (This is true of regular consumption; don't worry if you've already eaten some of these fish.)

**These fish sometimes contain toxins.

***Smaller fish are better than larger ones.

Use with Care

THESE ARE THE "YELLOW LIGHTS" OF pregnancy eating—foods that aren't strictly off the menu, but that should be served up only with a side of caution. Proceed prudently with the following:

MSG. Monosodium glutamate is used as a flavor enhancer of protein foods in many Asian dishes, canned or packaged broths, and processed foods. Though MSG is considered safe to use during pregnancy, some people have bad reactions to it, including pressure in the temples, headaches, and upset stomach. MSG has not been shown to cause problems for the fetus, yet it might be wise to limit your consumption of MSG during pregnancy, especially if you do have a sensitivity to it. Limit the amount of (or preferably, leave out) flavor enhancers containing MSG in your cooking, ask that it be omitted from your meals at Asian eateries, and avoid processed foods that list it as an ingredient.

Processed foods. Do you usually run for cover (or, at least, for the nearest health-food market) at the mention of the word *chemical*? If so, you might want to sit back down and continue reading. Not every food that lists chemicals among its ingredient list is necessarily bad (or

dangerous) for you, just as every food that doesn't list any is automatically safe and healthy.

All foods, from garden-variety tomatoes to laboratory-variety tomato-flavored sauces, are made of chemicals. A just-picked, organically grown strawberry, for instance, is composed of acetone, acetaldehyde, methyl butrate, ethyl caproate, hexyl acetate, methanol, acrolein, and crotmaldehyde. How's that for a chemical profile?

Chemical additives found in processed foods are synthesized in the lab from a wide variety of organic and inorganic materials, or extracted from completely natural sources (sodium caseinate from milk, lecithin from soybeans). Some are suspected of being harmful (those that are indisputably proved to be harmful are taken off the market). But the good news is that more are believed to be harmless (and some even beneficial—such as the chemical ascorbic acid, otherwise known as vitamin C). From what is know right now, the danger to a developing fetus from chemical additives in food is extremely remote.

Still, many processed foods are far from nutritious (especially if they're made from refined grains and saturated fats)—and typically, the greater the number of unpronounceable additives a product contains, the less wholesome it is. Keep

THE BIOTECH BOOM

▼ ▼ ▼

GMO's, or genetically modified foods (in which a gene from one organism is introduced into a species to produce a more desirable crop), may be coming to a dinner plate near you—and sooner than you think. Almost half of all the corn grown in this country is genetically modified; more than three-quarters of all U.S. soybeans have also been genetically reprogrammed, with probably many more such foods on the way. Is the biotech boom a boon or a bane? Supporters say that biotechnological advances are not only safe, but can make food more nutritious, and crops more resistant to insects (reducing the need for pesticides). Critics of these crops say there are too many unanswered questions about how these changes in our food supply will ultimately affect our health. And consumer groups are responding to those unanswered questions by calling for greater oversight of biotech foods by the government, including better labeling. In the meantime, if you'd like to avoid bringing biotech home, bring home organic; organic foods aren't allowed to contain GMO's.

---

that in mind when making processed food selections.

Nitrates. Good news for those pregnant (or not): In recent years, the levels of nitrates in processed foods has come down and now present much less of a risk than in the past. Nitrates are used as a preservative in processed meats (actually keeping the amount of bacteria down). But they can be converted in your stomach to nitrites or nitrosamines, powerful carcinogens (something you don't want at anytime during your life, and especially not when you're pregnant*). Smoked and cured meats such as bacon, ham, cured pork, sausage, dried beef, luncheon meats, salami, and frankfurters often contain nitrates— though varieties sold in health-food markets may be smoked naturally, without nitrates. The same goes for smoked fish.

Even though the risk from nitrates is not as great as it once was, there are other reasons to cut back on the amount of smoked and cured meats and fish you eat while you're expecting. For one thing, all are very high in sodium and some also in fat. For another, some are linked to listeria (see page 163).

So what to do? Look for smoked meats that do not contain nitrates (or sodium nitrites, as they are sometimes called), and eat those that do only rarely or not at all during pregnancy

---

*It has not yet been determined whether or not nitrosamines are harmful to a fetus.

HOW SWEET IT IS

▼ ▼ ▼

Not so sweet on the empty calories sugar offers, especially now that you're trying to eat efficiently for two? Thinking of turning to a low-calorie substitute to satisfy your sweet tooth instead? Sugar substitutes are a mixed bag for pregnant women; some are almost certainly safe, others possibly unsafe, still others questionable. Here's what's known about the most popular sweeteners, so far:

SUCRALOSE (SPLENDA). Made from sugar, but chemically converted to a form that's not absorbable by the body, sucralose appears to be the best bet safetywise for pregnant women seeking sweetness with no calories and little aftertaste. Feel free to sweeten with sucralose (unlike other sugar substitutes, it retains its sweetness when cooked), or to use products (drinks, baked goods, and ice cream) that have been sweetened with it, as long as they're otherwise healthful. Keep in mind that moderation's probably smart even with sucralose.

ASPARTAME (EQUAL, NUTRASWEET). The research jury's still out on this widely used sugar substitute. Many practitioners consider it harmless, and will okay light or moderate use in pregnancy. Some experts, on the other hand, are less convinced of the sweetener's safety (in pregnancy and out) and recommend that expectant moms be especially cautious in their use of aspartame until more results are in. (Women with PKU—phenylketonuria—must limit their intake of phenylalanine and are generally advised not to use aspartame.) In the meantime, it's probably wise to keep your use to a minimum. Adding a packet to your midmorning tea or enjoying a container of aspartame-sweetened yogurt is probably fine. Regularly filling up on aspartame-sweetened diet soft drinks or desserts probably isn't.

SACCHARIN. No problems in expectant humans have been linked to saccharin use, though studies show an increased cancer risk in the offspring of pregnant animals who ingest the chemical. Still, since saccharin hasn't been proved safe for use in pregnancy—and since it does cross the placenta, and is eliminated very slowly from fetal tissues—it makes sense to avoid saccharin while preparing for pregnancy, around the time of conception, and during

and while you're breastfeeding. When you opt for nitrate-containing meats, avoid cooking them at very high temperatures (fried ham and bacon, for instance); nitrites are most dangerous when they form under these conditions. (But do heat until steaming those that pose a listeria risk; see page 163.) And since eating a vitamin C–rich food with nitrate-containing foods will help prevent the formation of nitrosamines, serve up your smoked meat with a side of tomato or a glass of O.J. (Food manufacturers often add vitamin C derivatives, listed as sodium erythrobate or ascorbate, to counter-

pregnancy itself. Don't worry, however, about saccharin you had before finding out that you're pregnant, since the risks, if any, are certainly extremely slight.

ACESULFAME-K (SUNETTE). This sweetener, 200 times sweeter than sugar, is approved for use in baked goods, gelatin desserts, chewing gum, and soft drinks. At this point there is little research proving its safety during pregnancy, but no research showing it's unsafe—so if you choose to sweeten with Sunette, do so in moderation.

SORBITOL. This relative of sugar is found naturally in many fruits and berries. With half the sweetness of sugar (but more calories than most sugar substitutes), it is used in a wide range of foods and beverages and is safe for use in pregnancy in moderate amounts. But it does present a problem in large doses: too much can cause diarrhea.

MANNITOL. Less sweet than sugar, mannitol is poorly absorbed by the body and thus provides fewer calories than sugar (but, again, more than most sugar substitutes). Like sorbitol, it is safe in modest amounts, but large quantities can cause diarrhea.

STEVIA (TRUVIA). This zero-calorie sweetener is made from erythritol (a fermented

sugar alcohol that's found in grapes and pears) and the leaf of the stevia plant. There's no clear research on its safety during pregnancy, so until more is known, it makes sense to avoid it during pregnancy.

LACTOSE. This milk sugar is one-sixth as sweet as table sugar and adds light sweetening to foods. For the lactose intolerant (see page 208), it can cause uncomfortable symptoms; otherwise it's safe.

HONEY. There's been lots of buzz about honey these days. Scientists say that honey may be a healthy sugar alternative, due to its high levels of antioxidants. Darker varieties of honey (such as buckwheat honey) are the richest in antioxidants, and that's sweet news. But here's the sticky part: honey is definitely not low-cal. It has 64 calories per tablespoon—even more than sugar's 45.

FRUIT JUICE CONCENTRATES. Safe and nutritious, fruit juice concentrates are smart (if not low-cal) sweeteners to rely on during pregnancy. You can substitute them for the sugar and liquid in many recipes; they can be found in a wide variety of commercial products. Plus, they're more likely to be made with other nutritious ingredients, such as whole-grain flour, than are products sweetened with sugar or other sugar substitutes.

balance the nitrates in a processed food.)

Tap water. Most water in this country is perfectly safe for pregnant—and nonpregnant—guzzling, right out of the tap. Still, water safety varies from community to community. To find if

you should be drinking the water that flows from your tap, check with your local water supplier or health department, the Environmental Protection Agency (EPA)*, or a consumer

*EPA Safe Drinking Water Hotline: 800-426-4791; Environmental Defense Fund: www.edf.org, www.scorecard.org, or 800-684-3322.

BREWING UP TROUBLE?

▼ ▼ ▼

Had a hard day? Feel like curling up on the sofa with a good book and a steaming cup of herbal tea? Before you reach for those leaves, make sure you're not brewing up trouble with your tea. The effects of herbs in pregnancy have not been well researched and until more is known, the FDA advises that pregnant (and breastfeeding) women use herbal teas with caution.

If you enjoy herbal-type teas, read labels carefully. Some brews that seem to be fruit based also contain a variety of herbs. Stick to green or black tea that comes already flavored or make your own using juices, orange or lemon rinds, fruit slices, cinnamon, cloves, ginger, or other familiar ingredients and decaffeinated tea. And never brew a homemade tea from a plant growing in your backyard unless you are absolutely certain what it is and that it's safe for use during pregnancy.

advocacy group. You might also want to find out:

▲ Is the water chlorinated or filtered? (Filtering water is the safest way to purify; chlorinating risks the possibility of overly high levels of chemicals, though in most cities that chlorinate, levels are below the danger point.)

▲ Is there runoff from farms or industries, or possible seepage from underground gas storage tanks, into reservoirs or other water sources? (These can raise the level of hazardous chemicals in the water.)

▲ Is there leaching of lead or other metals from pipes in the water supply? (This may be the case in your own home if lead has been used to solder the plumbing pipes.) Lead exposure can lead to serious problems for a pregnant woman and her unborn child.

If your tap water fails the safety test, invest in a filter for your kitchen sink (what kind depends on what turns up in your water). The filter will last longer if it is used only for cooking and drinking and not for the dishwasher or other purposes. Or use bottled water for drinking and cooking. (Be aware, however, that bottled waters are not automatically free of impurities. To check the purity of a particular brand, contact the National Sanitation Foundation, 800-673-8010 or www.nsf.org.) Avoid distilled waters (from which beneficial minerals, such as fluorides, have been removed).

If you suspect lead in your water, or if testing reveals high levels, changing the plumbing is the ideal solution, but it isn't always feasible. To reduce the levels of lead in the water you drink, use only cold water for drinking and cooking (hot leaches more lead from the pipes), and run the cold-water tap for about five minutes in the morning (as well as any time the water has been off for six hours or more) before using it. You can tell that lead-free fresh water from the street pipes has reached your faucet when the water has gone from cold to warmer to cold again.

If your water smells and/or tastes like chlorine, boiling it or letting it stand, uncovered, for twenty-four hours will evaporate much of the chemical.

▲ ▲ ▲

Q *"I can't get through the day without drinking coffee. Do I have to give up caffeine completely now that I'm pregnant?"*

A Java lovers rejoice—in moderation. Most evidence seems to suggest that light coffee drinking (about two cups a day) doesn't pose a problem during pregnancy. Choose to drink more, however, and there's less cause for celebration. Heavy caffeine intake (more than five cups of coffee a day) has been linked to low birth weight and miscarriage, and the research on a three- to four-cup-a-day habit has

ENERGY IN A CAN?

▼ ▼ ▼

Looking for a pick-me-up now that pregnancy fatigue's got you down? Wondering whether a jolt from one of the many energy drinks lining supermarket shelves these days may be just the ticket? Well, think (and read the labels) before you drink. Those drinks may provide an energy boost, but they provide it primarily courtesy of the large amounts of caffeine and sugar they contain. And though they're packed with vitamins and minerals (which you're getting plenty of from your diet and your prenatal supplement), they also boast a number of questionable ingredients for the pregnant set, including some herbs. So pass on the cans, and seek your energy boost the natural way instead (see page 34).

been inconclusive. (Some studies have found it harmless in pregnancy; others have not.)

Bottom line—as long as you can stick to one or two cups a day, you and Joe won't have to part company while you're expecting. (Keep in mind that espresso-based coffee drinks contain far more caffeine than regular brews.)

Q *"I've lost a taste for coffee early in my pregnancy, but I'm craving chocolate. Do I still have to worry about my caffeine intake?"*

A You'd be surprised at how quickly the caffeine adds up even when coffee's not on the menu. Caffeine hides not only in coffee, but also in soft drinks, coffee-flavored yogurt, tea, and chocolate, not to mention some over-the-counter drugs such as headache and cold remedies. However, you have nothing to fear caffeine-wise if an occasional (or even daily chocolate bar) is your only source of caffeine; an average one contains only 30 mg, as opposed to 137 mg in a cup of coffee.

Q *"I drink only two or three cups of coffee a day, but my midwife suggested that I cut down to one. If there's no harm to light caffeine intake, why is she advising that I limit caffeine?"*

A She may have a number of reasons up her white-coated sleeve—all of them pretty good. For one, coffee and tea have a diuretic effect. Not only does that effect draw fluid and calcium—both vital to your health and your fetus's—from the body, but it also steps up those already too frequent trips you make to the bathroom. For another, coffee and tea, especially when taken with cream and sugar, are filling and satisfying without being nutritious—and can easily spoil your appetite for the nutritious food you need. (The same is true of caffeinated soft drinks.) Another black mark for coffee (even

when it's taken "light"): Caffeine can exacerbate your normal pregnancy mood swings (who needs that?) and prevent you from getting the rest you need (especially when you drink it after noon). Finally, caffeine interferes with your body's ability to absorb iron that both you and your baby need.

Of course, cutting back is easier said (by your midwife) than done (by you)—particularly if you're a longtime coffee drinker. See the next question for some advice.

Q *"I'm a coffee and soda junkie, but I'd like to give it up now that I'm pregnant. How can I break—or at least cut back on—the caffeine habit?"*

A Since light caffeine drinking is safe during pregnancy—and breaking a heavy caffeine habit cold turkey can be painful, literally—you'd probably be smart to take a gradual approach to your caffeine withdrawal. Cut back first to a safe level of caffeine consumption (no more than two cups a day), and get used to that before slashing your intake any further. Substituting decaf for some of each cup you normally drink (again, as long as your caffeine total doesn't exceed two cups) will allow you to wean yourself off both the taste and the kick of the real stuff more easily. Keep reducing the amount of regular and increasing the amount of decaf until your cups are completely caffeine-free.

Another way to cut back on the caffeine in your cup—make it a latte. Cut the coffee back to half a cup, and fill it to the brim with hot skim or low-fat milk.

Afraid you'll miss the lift you get from your morning caffeine fix? You'll get a longer-lasting boost from exercise, as well as from regularly eating foods rich in complex carbohydrates and protein. Though you'll doubtless sag for a few days while your body adjusts, you'll soon feel better than ever. (Of course, you'll still experience the normal fatigue of pregnancy.)

If you drink cola for the taste, you can substitute caffeine-free soft drinks occasionally, but soft drinks shouldn't be a staple of the pregnancy diet. Instead, quench your thirst with flavored sparkling waters served up straight or mixed spritzer-style with unsweetened fruit juices.

▼ ▼ ▼

Eating Well Whenever, Wherever

YOU CAN RECITE the Daily Dozen in your sleep (and often do, according to your spouse). You've become a connoisseur of nutritious foods and an expert in preparing them safely. You're completely committed to eating well while you're expecting. And then, real life threatens to get in the way. Business lunches (and breakfasts, and dinners) challenge your resolve—and your ability to simultaneously feed your clients and your baby what they're hungry for (client: sushi and sake; baby: poached salmon and steamed broccoli). The airline you've chosen for a three-hour flight tosses a bag of snack mix your way and calls it lunch. The destination you've chosen for a before-baby getaway is known less for its green leafies and more for its white gravy. The buffet tables at the holiday parties you're waddling to and from are veritable land mines (from the raw oysters to the possibly unpasteurized Brie to the eggnog). Or money and time are as tight as your clothes, and you're not sure you have enough of either to eat the way you should. Fortunately, you can feed your baby well no matter what circumstances real life throws at you.

On the Job

MIXING BUSINESS WITH BABY-growing is always challenging (what you really need is an afternoon nap, what you really have is an after-noon presentation), but never more so than at meal and snack times. You packed a well-balanced brown bag (good for you!), but left it at your front door. (Oh, well—there's always the coffee wagon!) Your morning meeting puts you face-to-frosting with a pile of Danishes. Your stom-ach's been growling since 11, but you're not on break until 2. Here's how to make sure that your 9-to-5 job doesn't conflict with your 24/7 job of feeding baby right:

Stock up on supplies. Though tra-ditional office supplies (computer, files, notepads, pens) are essential for the working woman, a very different set of supplies is essential for the preg-nant working woman. Fill your desk drawer, your locker, your briefcase, and your purse with a selection of healthy snacks and quick bites to ward off hunger pangs between meals. A convenient fridge makes snack-stashing easier, but isn't a necessity. For great snack ideas, see page 106.

Brown-bag it. Leaving your next meal up to chance is never a good idea when you're trying to eat well, but it's

WHAT'S FOR LUNCH?

▼ ▼ ▼

Here are some lunch-in-a-bag sug-gestions:

■ Any of the sandwiches starting on page 266

■ A thermos of hot or cold soup (see recipes starting on page 281), a wedge of cheese, a roll

■ Leftovers from last night's dinner

■ Baked potato stuffed with leftover steamed broccoli and cheese (heat it up in the office microwave)

■ Cottage cheese, cut-up fruit, and whole wheat bagel

■ Low-fat yogurt, a handful of nuts, a gra-nola bar, a ripe peach

■ A hearty salad (see recipes starting on page 326), whole wheat roll

■ A turkey-and-cheese wrap in a whole wheat tortilla

■ Turkey Chili or Vegetarian Chili (pages 291 and 293) topped with cheese and chopped tomato, side salad

wisdom of ☀ the ages?

In the Chinese culture, a pregnant woman is expected and encouraged to continue working throughout her pregnancy because it's believed that pregnancy "labor" eases delivery. And if you have to work anyway—wouldn't that be nice to believe?

an especially bad idea when you're trying to eat well on the job. So unless you know where your lunch will be coming from (and no fair having it come from the vending machine), don't leave home empty-handed. Pack up a healthy lunch (and a healthy breakfast, too, if you don't have time to eat before you run; see the recipes starting on page 240). See the box on page 279 for some lunch suggestions in a bag; also see page 279 for sandwich ideas.

Serve it hot. Cold sandwiches for lunch every day starting to leave you cold? Think hot instead. Bring a thermos of hot Broccoli and Cheese Soup, page 281, or Hearty Fish and Potato Chowder, page 296. Use the office microwave to warm up some chicken breasts and pasta, brown rice and steamed vegetables, or tuna melt on seven-grain bread.

Keep it cold. Take advantage of the office refrigerator (if there is one) and put any perishable foods you've brought from home in it. Or, pack your lunch in an insulated soft-sided bag with an ice pack to keep it cold.

If you're using paper lunch bags, create layers by double-bagging to help insulate the food.

Think drink. Getting enough to drink is important for all pregnant women, especially those who spend all day in offices with dry circulating air. Stay hydrated by keeping a tall glass or bottle of water at your desk and refilling it often (giving you the chance to both stretch your legs and catch up on water cooler gossip). For those times when you'd rather have a little flavor (or nutrition) in your fluids, bring a thermos of milk or a half-pint of juice. And though it's hard not to think coffee when you're thinking drink on the job, it's smart to limit your caffeine consumption. (See page 175 for reasons why.)

Stick to a schedule. Never find time for meals when you're at work? Start thinking of baby's next meal as a deadline you must meet. (Even if you're not hungry, baby is.) So plan for a lunch break at the same time each day, and follow through as though your job (of baby-growing) depended on it. If your work takes you out to late lunches or dinners, have a healthy snack at your regular lunch or dinner hour to tide you (and baby) over until you and the clients can stop talking turkey and start eating it.

Make it easy. Feeding baby on the job doesn't have to be complicated,

stressful, or time consuming. Whenever possible, take the easy way out.
Cook dinners with brown-baggable
lunches in mind (like Rosemary
Lemon Chicken, page 350, or
Tomato-Layered Mini Meat Loaves,
page 343). Toss juice or milk boxes
(the kind that don't need refrigeration)
into your purse so you won't have to
run for the nearest deli for a drink. Let
someone else do the peeling and chopping; visit a nearby salad bar for lunch
and pile your plastic container high
with fresh fruits and vegetables.

While Traveling

NEVER AGAIN WILL IT BE SO EASY
to travel with baby on board.
(No diapers! No car seats! No child-
proofing hotel rooms!) Still, whether
you're flying from Phoenix to Fargo,
driving from Detroit to Denver, or
visiting Vancouver or Venezuela,
being pregnant and peripatetic poses
certain challenges—especially when
it comes time to feed your hungry
load. After all, it's easy for your diet
to wander when you're roaming.

How, for instance, can you eat
regular meals when you're on an
irregular schedule? (You just lost four
hours to a time change, or two hours
sitting on a tarmac.) How can you
handle hunger that strikes midair,
between train stations, or miles from
the nearest highway rest stop? And
what do you do when you can't drink
the water or eat the local produce?

You won't have to stick close to
home to stick close to your pregnancy diet. What you will have to
do is include baby's nutritional
needs in your travel plans:

On a Plane

▲ Plan ahead. Call the airline to find
out what food, if any, will be served
on your flight. Flying during a mealtime doesn't guarantee you'll get a
meal or even a snack. Many airlines
serve a meal only on longer flights in
coach (though some have a decent
selection of meals and snacks available for purchase); some limit service—no matter how far you're
flying—to pretzels and soft drinks.
(Of course, even if a meal is provided, it doesn't mean it will be edible or filling, so see below.)

▲ Pack a snack (or a meal). Even if
you'll be served a meal or will be able
to buy one, and even if you planned
ahead and ordered a special one,
chances are that what you'll find on
your tray won't fill your tummy—or
your Daily Dozen. Not by a long
shot. Besides, you never know when
that meal or snack will be coming. (A
delay on the ground could postpone it

for hours.) Instead of leaving your hunger in the hands of the flight attendants and air traffic control, always pack a healthy meal or a substantial snack, as well as a few light snacks in case the flight stretches on, in your carry-on bag. Consider a cold sandwich or salad, a cheese stick and crackers, some grapes or other fresh fruit, a granola bar, a bag of trail mix. Check out www.tsa.gov to find out what you can bring along from home and what you'll have to purchase once you've passed through security (like drinks and yogurt).

▲ Keep the fluids flowing. Flying can be dehydrating because of the low humidity in aircraft cabins, so be sure to drink a lot before and during the flight. Besides keeping yourself from dehydrating, increasing your fluids will also send you to the bathroom often—a great way to stretch your legs and prevent circu-

lation problems. But plan on picking up your own bottle of water before you board. First, because beverage service can take forever on a jumbo jet, and those tiny plastic tumblers may not satisfy your thirst. Second, because the tank water on many planes does not meet federal safety standards, and water on the cart may come from the tap. (Of course, canned and individual bottled beverages are always safe bets.)

In a Car

▲ Plan ahead. If your car trip will be a long one, find out (by checking travel guides, automobile associations, websites) if there are frequent rest stops on the highway, and if possible, what types of restaurants are available on the road. (Keep the eating-out tips on page 184 in mind when making those pit stops.)

▲ Pack a bag. Whether you're venturing fifty miles for a quick visit or meeting, or crossing country on your road trip, don't leave home without a snack bag. Include beverages, fresh whole fruits, cut-up vegetables, sandwiches (pitas and wraps make for neater eating), and other healthy snacks to munch on. (Use a cooler to keep perishables fresh and drinks cold.) If you're in it for the long haul, you can always pull off the interstate and restock your snack supply at a local supermarket.

FILL 'ER UP

▼ ▼ ▼

When you stop to fill up your car with gas, don't fill yourself up with junk food from the convenience store. Most gas station stores carry frozen fruit bars, yogurt, pretzels, rice cakes, granola bars, trail mix, bottled water, juice, and milk.

At Your Destination

▲ Eat on schedule. The rhythm of your daily eating routine (breakfast, lunch, dinner, all served at approximately their accustomed times) shouldn't be uprooted when you are. If your vacation plans take you to three European cities in three whirlwind days (or your business plans take you to four Midwestern cities in four stress-filled days), make sure each of those days includes a regular morning breakfast, a midday lunch, and a dinner in the evening. By building time into your schedule for food, you ensure that your fetus is getting the regular nourishment it requires even while you're off taking in the sites or taking in the meetings. When you can't eat a full meal on schedule (you're in Madrid and the restaurants don't even open for dinner until eight), eat a sustaining snack to hold you over.

▲ Pack snacks (again). Because you never know when those hunger pangs may strike (and in case they hit when you're far from a restaurant or market), carrying easy-to-munch energy-boosting snacks is an away-from-home must.

▲ Request a mini-fridge. Don't rely on hotel mini-bars to satisfy your between-meal appetite; not only will the contents be high in price, but they'll be low in nutrition, as well.

Most hotels will provide guests with a small (empty) refrigerator upon request (sometimes for a small fee). Stock it with milk, cheese, fruits and vegetables, and snacks that need refrigeration. When those middle-of-the-night cravings hit, wholesome food will be an arm's reach away (instead of a trek to the hotel lobby or through unfamiliar streets searching for a twenty-four-hour grocery).

▲ Play it even safer. Eating carefully— avoiding raw fish and shellfish, under-cooked meats and eggs, soft cheeses —is even more important on the road, especially if the road has taken you to a foreign country. If it's a foreign country with poor sanitation, you'll have to avoid even more. Any food that hasn't been cooked could be contaminated, so steer clear of salads and raw fruits and vegetables that haven't been peeled by you (unless you're sure that they're safe). Stay away, also, from milk and milk products (like cheese) that you're not positive have been pasteurized. Thoroughly cooked foods that are still hot are generally safe to eat, though you shouldn't eat any food (hot or otherwise) that appears to have been prepared or stored under unsanitary conditions. If food that is served to you seems questionable, send it back and order something safer.

▲ Drink with caution when you're out of the country. Getting your quota of

fluids when you're traveling is important. But before you quench your
thirst with a glass of cold local water,
make sure it is safe to drink. (Visit
www.cdc.gov/healthywater/global
before you visit your destination.) If
the water is suspect, avoid ice cubes
and reconstituted juices or milks unless
they are made with bottled, boiled, or
sterilized water. (They will be in most
good hotels, but always ask.) Drink
bottled water instead.

▲ Don't ask for tummy troubles. For
most people, a case of traveler's diarrhea can be uncomfortable and incon-
venient. But stomach cramps and
diarrhea can do a lot more than spoil

your trip when you're expecting. They
can rob your baby of vital nutrition,
sap your energy, and lead to dehydration (which can lead to other problems). Besides, who needs another
reason for nausea when pregnant?

To make sure you don't pick up
anything but souvenirs at your destination, follow food-safety rules
scrupulously—especially if you're
traveling in a developing country. If
Montezuma does claim revenge, be
wary of self-treating. Many over-the-
counter diarrhea medicines are not
recommended for pregnant women.
Experts recommend, instead, putting
in a call to your doctor or midwife
back home for advice.

When Eating Out

WHETHER YOU'RE GRABBING A
quick bite at the food court or
lingering over four courses at a four-
star restaurant, entertaining a client
or date-nighting with your spouse,
eating out to celebrate or eating out
because you don't have the strength
to face the stove again, there will be
plenty of times during your pregnancy when you'll be feeding yourself and your baby away from home.
How to make sure good nutrition is
on the menu, even when cooking
isn't? It's easy, as long as you keep
these tips in mind:

▲ Choose a baby-friendly restaurant. It won't be high chairs you'll
be scouting for when you're taking
your baby out to dinner (at least not
yet)—it'll be healthy eating options.
Realistically, you won't always get to
pick the restaurant, but when you
do, be picky. Before you ask for a
table, ask for a menu and scan it for
nutritious offerings. (Most restaurants have at least some.)

▲ Order first. It might not be particularly polite to order your meal
first, but it can keep you from being

swayed by the less wholesome choices of others. ("Mmmm . . . fried clams! Sure could go for some of those myself!") Instead, you'll be able to set the nutritional standard for the table. See the box on page 186 for healthful choices at different types of restaurants.

▲ Be on portion patrol. Many restaurants serve portions that are much heftier than the recommended serving sizes for most foods. To avoid becoming too hefty yourself (especially if you're a frequent diner), eat only as much as you need to fill you up, not stuff you up. Take the rest home in a doggie bag (which—sorry, Fido—you'll be able to bring to work for tomorrow's lunch). Another option: Share an entrée (or an appetizer) with your dining companion, instead of ordering your own. Or skip the entrée entirely and select only a salad and appetizer (but make sure it's a high-protein one, like shrimp cocktail) instead of a full meal.

▲ Survey the bread scene. Before you leap into the basket mouthfirst, check out the contents for whole-grain options. If none turn up there, ask the waiter if there are any available from the kitchen (whole wheat sandwich bread, for instance). If you're still out of luck, go easy on the white stuff, saving your appetite for more wholesome foods still to come.

And try not to spread your bread with too much butter or dip it into too much olive oil. (Even if you order carefully, there'll be enough fat in the rest of your meal—in the salad dressing, on the fish; no need to add it on before the first course even arrives.)

▲ Think green. To make sure you fill your leafy green requirement, order a salad as a first course. Ask for the dressing on the side so *you* can choose how much dressing you want to pour on. Don't quite feel like a salad? Start with some grilled vegetables instead.

▲ Slurp your Daily Dozen. In many restaurants, some of the most nutritious dishes come in bowls (or cups). Look to lentil, bean, vegetable soups (from minestrone to tomato, sweet potato to winter squash), and don't forget to consider cold ones, too. (Gazpacho, for instance, is a veritable salad-in-a-soup-bowl.) Care for clam chowder? Take Manhattan when you have the chance; New England chowder and other cream-based soups are typically heavy on the fat.

▲ Keep it simple. In most cases, the less time the waiter has to spend describing your entrée ("and then after it's sautéed, it's finished with roasted shallot sauce and . . ."), the better your selection. Stick to lean

WHAT'S ON THE MENU?

▼ ▼ ▼

Sure, some restaurants make it easier to eat well when you're expecting than others. But even the local greasy spoon can dish out a nutritious meal for you and baby—if you order wisely. In restaurants that specialize in a certain type of cuisine, it helps to know what to look for and what to avoid: Use the following as a *general* guide, recognizing that cooking styles vary, even within a particular cuisine.

CUISINE	GO FOR	LIMIT
Seafood; steak house; American	■ Broiled or grilled fresh seafood, poultry, and lean meats ■ Specialties of the house served with baked potatoes, fresh vegetables, and salads* ■ Salad bar (but favor mostly raw choices)* ■ Pasta or legume dishes*	■ Refined breads in the bread basket; fries and onion rings
French	■ Roasted, braised, grilled, or poached fish, poultry, lean meats ■ Stews made with meat or poultry ■ Vegetables or beans; salads* ■ Vegetable-based soup	■ Classic French cuisine (often high in fat) ■ Rich sauces ■ Pastry shells *(en croute)* ■ Pâtés (they're held together with fat); sausages and duck confit (also prime sources of fat) ■ Organ meats ■ Rare or raw beef (steak tartare); rare duck
Chinese	■ Stir-fried fish, meats, poultry, and vegetables ■ Brown rice* ■ Broth-based soups ■ Steamed dumplings*	■ Extra soy sauce ■ MSG ■ Fried ("crispy") foods, including egg rolls ■ High-sugar, breaded, sweet-and-sour dishes ■ White rice and white noodles ■ Spicy dishes (if you get heartburn)

CUISINE	GO FOR	LIMIT
Italian	■ Grilled, roasted, or braised fish, chicken, veal, or lean beef entrées ■ Fresh cooked greens (spinach, broccoli, and broccoli rabe)* ■ Salads (especially those with nutritious dark greens, such as romaine or arugula)* ■ Pizza with tomato sauce, cheese, and fresh vegetables (such as peppers and broccoli)* ■ Pasta tossed with fish, seafood, chicken, and/or vegetables*; cheese and/or marinara sauce add extra nutrition. ■ Soups, especially minestrone, tomato, and bean varieties*	■ Cream sauces ■ Anything breaded, deep- or pan-fried
Japanese	■ Simmered (*nimono*), broiled (*yaki*), or grilled (*yalimono*) dishes ■ Sushi rolls made with cooked fish and/or vegetables* ■ Miso soups* ■ Vegetable sushi rolls; soybean dishes* ■ Seaweed salad, anything seaweed* ■ Stews (*domburi*) ■ Noodles (choose buckwheat soba)* ■ Edamame (steamed soybeans)*	■ Fried dishes (*agemono*, katsu, *agedashi*, tempura) ■ Avoid raw fish or seafood (sushi, sashimi)
Thai	■ Baked or grilled fish or poultry ■ Stir-fries ■ Hot-pot dishes ■ Soups with plenty of fish, poultry, meat, seafood, or tofu*	■ Deep-fried foods ■ Curries and other dishes made with coconut milk or cream ■ Sweet sauces

*Usually a good vegetarian choice

CUISINE	GO FOR	LIMIT
Indian	■ Baked and roasted (tandoori) fish or chicken (often marinated in yogurt) ■ Salads, soups, and vegetable dishes* ■ Whole-grain Indian breads (roti, chapati, and paratha)* ■ Lentil, pea, chickpea, cheese, and vegetable dishes*	■ Fried dishes
Cajun or Louisiana style	■ Boiled, steamed, broiled, and grilled fish or seafood ■ Seafood, poultry, and vegetable stews, such as jambalayas and gumbos	■ Fatty pork dishes ■ Fried dishes ■ White rice
Mexican, Spanish, and Tex-Mex	■ Dishes with low-fat cheeses, whole wheat tortillas, corn tortillas, and brown rice* ■ Gazpacho and black bean soups* ■ Asada (grilled chicken, meat, and seafood) ■ Chicken, beef, or shrimp fajitas, enchiladas, and burritos ■ Bean and cheese enchiladas, burritos, and quesadillas* ■ Veracruz-style dishes (made with tomato sauce) ■ Paella, a chicken-seafood stew (but don't let the white rice fill you up)	■ Fried taco shell ■ White rice ■ Taco chips ■ Refried beans
Southern; soul food; barbecue	■ Broiled, baked, barbecued, or grilled fish or chicken ■ Yams or sweet potatoes* ■ Steamed or sautéed greens (if made without animal fat)*	■ Fried foods ■ Healthy foods (such as vegetables) cooked in excessive fat or drippings ■ Biscuits, dumplings, and stuffings

CUISINE	GO FOR	LIMIT
Greek and Middle Eastern	■ Baked, grilled, and roasted fish, poultry, and lean meats (including shish kebab) ■ Dishes that combine vegetables with fish or meat and/or cheese (moussaka) ■ Lentil, broad bean, and chickpea dishes* ■ Yogurt-based soups* ■ Sautéed greens (horta)* ■ Vegetable salads* ■ Cooked whole grains, such as bulgur*	■ White rice and rice-stuffed dishes ■ Fried and phyllo-wrapped specialties
German, Russian, and Middle European	■ Broiled or grilled chops, chicken, or steak ■ Meat and vegetable stew like goulash or paprikash ■ Kasha or potatoes*	■ Breaded entrées ■ Dumplings ■ Noodles ■ High-nitrate, high-fat sausages and wursts
Pizzerias	■ Pizzas with vegetable topping (peppers and/or broccoli), thin crust (whole wheat even better), reduced or nonfat cheese (if available)* ■ Salad	■ Pizzas with extra cheese, pepperoni, or sausage
Health-food and vegetarian restaurants	■ Most everything, including dishes made with cheese, yogurt, tofu, legumes (beans, lentils, peas), fish or poultry, or fake meats (veggie burgers, hot dogs, and so on)*	

*Usually a good vegetarian choice

CUISINE	GO FOR	LIMIT
Coffee shops, diners, and delis	■ Hot oatmeal* ■ Omelets (especially with vegetable fillings) and other egg dishes* ■ Oat bran waffles* ■ Broiled fish and roasted chicken ■ Veggie burgers* ■ Turkey burgers ■ Freshly cooked vegetables* ■ Salads* ■ Vinegar-based slaws (lower in fat and calories than mayo-based), tomato and cucumber salad* ■ Vegetable* and chicken soups ■ Fruit and cottage cheese plate* ■ Melon, grapefruit, or fresh fruit salad* ■ Sandwiches (sliced fresh chicken or turkey, Swiss cheese, sliced egg on whole wheat or multigrain bread with lettuce and tomato)*	■ Slaw, if it's heavy on the mayo ■ Fried potatoes (French, hash browns, and home-style) ■ Extra pickles and sauerkraut ■ Rye and pumpernickel breads (unless they're whole grain) ■ Fatty and often nitrate-preserved fish, meats, and cold cuts (such as smoked salmon, white fish, pastrami, corned beef, frankfurters, salami, bologna, ham, and tongue) ■ Added mayo

meat, poultry, fish or seafood, and order them simply broiled, grilled, roasted, baked, steamed, or poached (preferably not sautéed or fried). Ask for sauces and gravies on the side. If you're looking for a vegetarian alternative for your main course, choose dishes with tofu, beans, peas, cheeses, or whole grains.

▲ Be side savvy. The company your meat (or fish) keeps is important, too. Since many restaurants offer a choice, choose wisely: Opt for steamed vegetables, beans, a baked potato, or if it's offered, brown or wild rice or another whole grain. Since veggie servings are often skimpy (are those two orange circles the carrots you

CUISINE	GO FOR	LIMIT
Fast-food restaurants	■ Grilled, broiled, or roasted chicken, grilled or barbecued chicken sandwiches (order with lettuce and tomato, without mayo, and add a slice of cheese if you're in need of calcium) ■ Turkey or chicken or cheese subs (pick the "wheat" bread over the white) ■ Wraps (especially whole wheat ones, with healthy fillings)* ■ Bean-and-cheese or chicken burritos or soft tacos* ■ Single cheeseburgers (consider the "protein style" option, wrapped in lettuce) ■ Thin-crust cheese pizza with vegetable toppings (skip the pepperoni)* ■ Pita sandwiches* ■ Baked potatoes ■ Salads (especially grilled chicken) ■ Veggie burgers* ■ Frozen yogurt*	■ Double, quarter-pounder, or bigger burgers; mayo-based "special sauce" ■ Fried chicken or fish ■ Fries ■ Shakes

*Usually a good vegetarian choice

ordered?), you might consider asking for an extra portion.

▲ Breathe when the desserts come your way. Remember, *desserts* spelled backwards is *stressed,* which may be the way you feel as the waiter rolls temptation your way. A few deep breaths may give you the power you need to say, "Fresh fruit and sorbet, please." When your cravings occasionally bring you to the edge of a dulce de leche cheesecake, share it with your dining partner instead of attacking it all by yourself. And (breathe!) slowly savor each creamy mouthful instead of inhaling your half of the slab in thirty seconds.

At Parties

So MAYBE YOU'RE NOT THE PARTY animal you used to be. (Those cocktail parties aren't quite as much fun without the cocktail, your eyelids can't stay open past ten, and your dancing feet are too swollen to fit in your dancing shoes.) But that doesn't have to make you a pregnant party pooper. You can still kick up your heels (just not those four-inch stiletto ones) and enjoy a few rounds (just not the alcoholic kind) on the social circuit—much as you did when your little black dress was actually little. Keep these tips in mind when stepping out on the town:

Have one for the road. Because you never know what'll be on the menu when you're not the one planning it, eat a healthy snack before you leave home to take the edge off your appetite without spoiling it entirely. Not running out the door on empty will minimize the chances that you'll belly right up to the buffet table upon arrival to stuff your starving self silly with what's available, good or not so good.

Party with care. Luckily, just about every party menu will have something with your name on it. Just be selective:

• At the bar. Obviously, your party spirit will have to come from within—not from alcohol—when you're expecting. But that doesn't mean you'll need to work the room without a cocktail in your hand. Order a sparkling water-and-twist, juice spritzer, virgin Bloody Mary, virgin blender drink, or sparkling cider.

• At the hors d'oeuvres. Nibble on cheese cubes, cooked seafood and cocktail sauce, meatballs, stuffed mushrooms, grilled chicken or beef on skewers, and other relatively healthy canapés, letting the really greasy ones (or those made with unsafe ingredients, such as raw oysters or smoked fish) pass you by. Make a beeline to the crudités, as well as any fruit platter. Spread cheese on whole-grain crackers or breads, if there are any—or skip the starchy stuff altogether and do your spreading on raw vegetables instead. (Remember to stay away from soft cheeses, such as Brie, unless you know they're pasteurized or they have been cooked until bubbly.)

• At the buffet. Help yourself from the healthier chafing dish selections—chicken breasts instead of fettuccine Alfredo, steamed asparagus instead of fried zucchini, a well-cooked beef stew instead of a slice of rare roast beef. Heap your plate high with salad and vegetables, if they're offered, leaving less room for sides that are beside the nutritional point. Skip over luncheon meats and smoked fish.

- At a sit-down dinner. Fill up with the predinner salad course or soup (which hopefully won't be cream-of-something). If dinner's preplated and you don't have a choice of entrée or sides, pick at or leave items that don't offer much more than calories; then dig in to the rest. If you have a choice, pass on or ask for small portions of the less nutritious offerings. (No one's going to question a pregnant woman's motives when it comes to food selections.)

- At dessert time. If dessert's served buffet style, you'll have more flexibility. (You can opt for fruit or slice yourself a small piece of cake to savor with your strawberries.) If dessert's presented already plated—and there's no fruit in sight—take enough bites to satisfy the host

(and your sweet tooth), but don't feel obligated to polish it off. Again, there's nothing strange about a pregnant woman watching what she's eating.

Pack your evening bag with more than lipstick. It's hard to be the life of the party when you're lightheaded with hunger. So on those rare occasions when the pickings will be slim enough to leave you starving (such as when you've been invited to a sushi party, or when "cocktails" means cocktails and the odd olive) you'll be glad you stashed a snack (a bag of trail mix, for instance) that you can discreetly munch on.

Be the guest with the mostest. Even if it's not a potluck you've been invited to, you may end up luckier (and better fed) if you offer to bring a dish—one that you'll be able to feast from should the rest of the menu prove less hospitable for pregnant women. No one has to be the wiser of your less-than-altruistic motives.

During the Holidays

'TIS THE SEASON TO BE JOLLY? No problem—and no need to get thrown off course. Eating well all year round is as easy as pumpkin pie, if you just remember these tips:

▲ There's room for tradition at your holiday table. Not only is healthy holiday eating possible, it usually doesn't require you to toss tradition. Most traditional favorites—from the

Thanksgiving turkey and sweet potatoes, to the Easter lamb, to the Fourth of July burgers, to the Jewish New Year chicken soup and roast— are good for you and your baby, so there's no need to eat around the holidays. Try not to overdo the high-calorie trimmings you pile on your plate, though; focus on the protein foods, salads, and veggies, and take just a small helping of stuffing or mashed potatoes instead of a heaping mound.

▲ Remain regular. Don't take a holiday from regular meals and snacks. Your baby still needs to eat breakfast, lunch, and a snack or two (though you can make them a little lighter than usual, especially as far as calories are concerned)—even if you'd rather save up for a big Christmas dinner or Thanksgiving feast.

▲ Don't be a Scrooge. Eating during pregnancy isn't about denying yourself—especially during the holidays. So while it's smart to be sensible, it's not necessary to play the expectant mother martyr. As long as you don't overindulge, there's no harm in enjoying the treats and sweets of the season. Make no exception, however, when it comes to safety; avoid alcoholic beverages, desserts with raw eggs (mousse, for example), raw seafood, and other potentially harmful foods (see Chapter Seven).

▲ Don't invite trouble. Enjoy the holidays, but keep sensible eating tips in mind as you do. Watch your overall caloric intake (so you don't end up with a ten-pound gain during a two-week holiday season), try not to overstuff yourself (so you don't pay the price in heartburn or gas pains), and favor healthier foods when you can. (Choose pumpkin pie over chocolate cream, dried apricots over candied ones, baked sweet potatoes in their jackets over a marshmallow-studded casserole.)

▲ Adapt yourself. Some holiday traditions will need a little modification while you're pregnant. You'll need to toast the New Year with sparkling cider instead of champagne, celebrate Passover with grape juice instead of wine, prepare your Christmas eggnog without the eggs (and without the rum).

▲ Look forward to next year (and years to come). If you feel a little deprived this season (and you probably will at some point, keep in mind that you have more unpregnant holidays ahead of you than pregnant ones. So take this year's holiday cheer with moderation, and look forward to being just a little jollier when next season rolls along.

On a Shoestring

WATCHING YOUR WALLET? DOESN'T mean you can't watch your diet, too. In fact, penny for penny, most wholesome foods cost less than most unwholesome ones—sometimes a lot less. And while a tight belt may not be the most comfortable accessory when you're expecting, there are plenty of ways to squeeze in good nutrition when you're feeling the financial pinch:

Go generic. While store brands and no-frills food items are generally not as pretty to look at as more expensive name-brand products (though, let's face it, unless you're using it to decorate with, the design on a box of oatmeal doesn't matter all that much), they're usually as nutritious as the costly ones. Practically every type of packaged food product is available in generic form—from breads and cereals to frozen and canned fruits and vegetables and fresh and frozen juices, from cottage cheese and other dairy products to raisins and nuts. And here's something the food-industry giants might not like you to know: In many instances, the store brand is actually a name brand with a store label.

Bring lunch. Need another reason why brown-bagging your lunch is such a good idea? It'll save you big bucks (see page 179 for all the other reasons). Instead of spending five dollars or more a day on a take-out lunch, spend considerably less on a delicious homemade salad, dinner leftovers (that extra hamburger patty and brown rice you wisely made), or a chicken breast sandwich on whole wheat baguette. Bag it, along with some fruit and a drink, and you'll probably save upwards of a thousand dollars over the course of your pregnancy. See page 279 for savvy sandwich ideas.

Drink on the cheap. You can save money eight times a day—every time, in fact, you fill your requirement for fluids. The least expensive drink in the house—water—is also one of the best fluid choices for you and baby. Not only will switching to water from soft drinks and sugar juice drinks save you a bundle (so you can save up for that bundle of joy)—it'll also save you plenty of empty calories. Save more, too, by buying frozen juice instead of fresh or reconstituted juice in cartons (it's at least as nutritious)—and even more by using nonfat dry milk, instead of fresh milk, in smoothies, soups, and desserts.

Stay seasonal. Buying fruits and vegetables in season isn't just healthier for you and baby, but healthier for your bank account. For instance, peaches and strawberries may be available year-round, but they're most nutritious and cheapest in the summer months. When the season is over for a certain fruit or vegetable, head to the frozen foods aisle, where the price and the nutrition are right year-round.

Keep it simple. Sauces add to the price and calorie count of a dish. Simpler preparations, such as broiling, steaming, poaching, roasting, and baking will result in a fatter wallet and a trimmer you.

Buy in bulk. Bigger is almost always better when it comes to budget grocery shopping. So buy economy sizes of nearly everything you can— from chicken breasts (cook and freeze all of them at once, and you'll have saved money and time) to oatmeal. (Just don't forget to eat it all.) Stock up on sale items, too, if they're not perishable and you're sure you'll be able to use them (that case of grapefruit might look like a good deal, until you realize you can't fit them all in your fridge).

Make life a little less convenient. It's certainly a lot easier to pop a frozen dinner in the microwave than it is to prepare a homemade meal from scratch. But convenience foods can put a big dent in your bank account without so much as scratching the surface of your Daily Dozen. Not only are frozen dinners, jars of salad dressing, and instant hot oatmeal more expensive than the homemade varieties, they're also higher in calories and lower in nutritional value.

When Time Is Tight

FEEL LIKE YOU'RE ALWAYS TRYING to run the eight-minute mile in four minutes flat? Like you're pulled in so many directions that you're stretched as thin as a woman sporting a belly as big as yours can possibly be? Like you barely have time to eat, never mind eat well? Not to worry. Even if time isn't on your side, good nutrition can be. Following these time-saving tips will help:

Stock up. No time to stop at the market after work? No problem—as long as your kitchen's well stocked. So keep your pantry, fridge, and freezer filled with all the ingredients you'll need to make quick healthy meals all week long.

Shop once. With a good preshopping plan and list in hand (see page 119), do a week's worth of staple shopping at once, supplemented, if necessary, by quick trips to the fish market for fresh fillets.

Equip yourself. So you got home from work at seven, have a class at eight—and somehow have to cook and eat dinner in between? The right kitchen equipment can shave many valuable minutes off your food-preparation time:

• A microwave. Use it to defrost frozen foods fast, reheat leftovers in no time, and even to cook a whole dinner. A microwave cookbook can show you how to make zap magic happen. See box, page 130.

• A slow cooker. Despite its name, a slow cooker can save more time than practically any appliance in your home. Chances are you got at least one for a wedding present; dust it off and get busy. Just toss some dried beans and meat or chicken, some vegetables and flavorful broth, and a few herbs into the slow cooker before leaving the house in the morning, and a delicious stew will be ready and waiting when you walk in the door. Instant dinner!

• A wok (or large frying pan). The secret of really speedy—and healthy—cooking is stir-frying. Throw some chunks of chicken, broccoli, carrots, and water chestnuts into the wok—and in less than five min-

utes, a delcicious dinner is served. Also try Ginger Beef Stir-Fry, page 340, or Broccoli and Tofu Stir-Fry, page 393.

• A blender. You can enjoy a breakfast smoothie in ten seconds flat. Recipes start on page 423.

• A food processor. Who has time to chop? Who would bother when there's a food processor to do the work for you? These handy appliances can dice, slice, mince, and puree onions, vegetables, potatoes, fruit, or just about anything else that would otherwise take time and elbow grease.

• A really good knife. Don't have the budget or the space on your kitchen counter for a food processor? Invest in the next best thing: a good-quality knife. A really sharp blade will chop hours off your food preparation time.

Cook fast foods. Instead of going out for fast food, choose foods that cook up fast. A fresh fillet of fish or a boneless chicken breast can be broiled or poached in minutes. Thinly sliced strips of lean beef or chicken (look for "fajita" cuts) can be stir-fried in moments. Vegetables can be steamed to just-tender more quickly than they can be boiled, and not only will you have saved time, you'll have saved the vitamins and minerals from going down the drain with the cooking water. Many recipes in this book can be prepared in twenty minutes or less.

Or don't cook at all. Serve vegetables raw. Eat leftover grilled chicken cold on a bed of greens. Enjoy some chunks of cheese and a pear straight from the refrigerator. Open a bag of baby carrots, snack on dry cereal, or peel a banana and slice it into a single-serving container of cottage cheese or yogurt. All nutritious fare—all in no time at all.

Concentrate on convenience. When feeding yourself and your baby is going to take more than just reaching into the refrigerator and chewing, look for ways to make cooking and preparing meals easier and faster. Instead of buying heads of lettuce that need to be torn, washed, and spun dry and vegetables that need to be peeled and chopped, open a precut, prewashed bag of greens, a bag of preshredded carrots or cabbage, and a rinsed box of cherry tomatoes, dump them all into a bowl, top with oil, vinegar, dried oregano, and some pre-grated Romano cheese. Presto—you've just made a fresh salad. (And that took how long?) Scan supermarket shelves for other time-saving ingredients: Shredded low-fat cheese, pasta-ready tomato sauces, prepeeled baby carrots, preshredded cabbage for coleslaw, bags of microwave-ready

vegetables, even prechopped garlic. Though these might cost more at the store, you'll find they're worth the price when time is at a premium. Look, also, to the grocer's freezer for frozen vegetables and fruit, as well as healthy frozen entrées (see page 123). And don't forget the take-out aisle, where you can pick up a roast chicken to go (a healthy choice once you've removed the skin, added that ten-second salad, a microwave-baked potato, and quick-cooked frozen vegetables).

Cook for an army. If you cook enough for two or more meals at once (which takes only a few moments longer) and tuck the extras, in meal-size portions, in the freezer for future use, you'll save loads of time. (Just mark the frozen meals carefully, so you won't be left with mystery meat.) Make a big batch of whole wheat pancakes or waffles on Saturday and freeze and reheat for quick weekday breakfasts. Any of the muffins starting on page 256 are also perfect for reheating.

Give leftovers a new lease on life. Roast a large turkey on Sunday, have warm turkey leftovers on Monday (along with leftover mashed sweet potatoes), turkey salad for lunch on Tuesday, Chinese turkey stir-fry with brown rice for dinner Tuesday night, and (because you're probably sick of turkey by Wednesday) freeze the rest for turkey cacciatore (just add ready-to-eat tomato sauce and some pasta) whenever the turkey mood strikes again. Or make a double batch of steamed broccoli, have it hot the first night and cold with a vinaigrette or warmed up in a pasta dish or casserole on the second.

Plan ahead. No time for breakfast? It'll take about a minute to toss some frozen fruit, some orange juice, a container of yogurt, and a couple of tablespoons of wheat germ into a blender to create a meal-in-a-glass smoothie (see pages 423 to 430 for more smoothie recipes). Or make a brown bag breakfast at night, and take it to work the next morning (like a Breakfast Burrito, page 244—just heat and go). Cut up vegetables and fruits in advance, and put them in plastic containers in the refrigerator for easy nibbling during the rest of the week; you'll lose a little of their nutritive value, but gain plenty of time. Boil a dozen eggs at week's start, then use them whole for quick snacks, chopped in egg salad, or sliced on a chef salad.

CHAPTER NINE

Eating Well in Every Situation

GRANTED, it's not always easy to eat well when you're experiencing the easiest pregnancy on the planet. It's even more difficult to follow a healthy eating plan when your appetite has flown with the flu; you're pregnant with twins (or more) and can barely stomach the requirements of a single baby, never mind a couple of them; gestational diabetes is limiting your already limited diet; or bed rest is keeping you out of the kitchen. And even if you're feeling fabulous, special eating considerations (you're lactose intolerant, or you're a vegan) can make getting your Daily Dozen especially challenging. Luckily, with a little nutritional know-how, you can eat well no matter what.

When You're Sick

IT DOESN'T SEEM QUITE FAIR, AND YET it's true. As an expectant mother—probably already saddled with a variety of uncomfortable pregnancy symptoms, from nausea and vomiting to heartburn and indigestion—

you're actually more likely to become sick than members of the nonpregnant population. That's because your immune system is slightly lowered during pregnancy (nature's way of ensuring that your baby—a foreigner to your system—won't be rejected by your body) leaving you particularly susceptible to infections, coughs, colds, gastrointestinal bugs, and the flu. And it's not just the glow that goes when illness strikes a pregnant woman. It's often her appetite and her ability to eat a regular diet, as well.

Should you find yourself sick in bed with more than just the usual pregnancy symptom suspects, be sure to call your practitioner for advice on how to combat your illness. While you're waiting for relief from whatever the doctor or midwife diagnoses, these dietary tips should come in handy:

Colds and flu. It's never a good idea to starve a cold or a flu, especially not while you're pregnant. Since your body needs energy (from food) to heal, you'll get better faster if you eat. And if you've got a fever to boot, you'll need still more calories to compensate for those being burned by the fever. Of course, that's easy to say, but not so easy to do when your nose is stuffy, your head achy, your mouth is always filled with a thermometer, and even your favorite foods taste like well-done wood chips. Under these conditions, when you're obviously not living to eat, but eating to live (and to nourish your baby), choose foods that are simple, palatable, and hopefully nutritious:

• Comfort foods. Now that you're practically a parent, start thinking like parents do. Those soothing, comforting, and warming dishes Mom or Dad used to make when you were sick as a child can provide the same comfort to you (and your baby) now. Hot oatmeal or other whole-grain cereal; scrambled eggs with whole wheat toast; chicken soup, made with plenty of carrots, celery, onion, parsnips, and parsley (pureed after cooking for an easy-to-swallow texture), and served with diced chicken; whole wheat English muffin; pasta with a little butter and a lot of cottage cheese; mashed potatoes and grated cheddar; or fruit-juice gels can all provide needed nutrients for your growing baby and some comfort to your aching body.

• Fluids. And remember how your parents pushed the fluids, too, when you were sick? They had a point. Not only do you need your usual quota of fluids to fill the Daily Dozen when you're laid up with a bug, you need extra fluids to replace those lost through a runny nose and fever, as well as to promote a quicker recovery. Staying hydrated keeps the mucous membranes that

WEIGHING IN ON THAT OUNCE OF PREVENTION

▼ ▼ ▼

The best kind of medicine—especially during pregnancy—is the preventive kind. Giving your immunity a shot in the arm—by keeping yourself well rested and well nourished—can keep you from coming down with mild infections in the first place, or help you recover from them faster when they do strike. Some of nature's finest immunity boosters also happen to be Daily Dozen hall-of-famers, including yogurt (the live cultures naturally found in them are believed to be excellent fighters against "bad" bacteria) and foods rich in vitamin C and beta-carotene.

On the other hand, you should probably not reach for some of the "natural" alternatives often used (though not scientifically proven) to boost immunity and prevent infection—such as zinc lozenges, echinacea, or megadoses of vitamin C. Though they may be effective in warding off colds or reducing the severity of their symptoms, they haven't been widely tested in pregnancy. Until they're proved safe in large-scale studies, it would probably be smarter to reach for a glass of OJ instead.

line your nose moist, helping to fight off viral attacks and reduce congestion. So keep a thermos next to your bed (or at your desk if you've brought your cold to work) and sip as often as you can. Soups, decaffeinated tea, diluted juices, and water (especially hot) are all good choices. And although milk has long been rumored to increase nasal congestion, there is no scientific evidence to back up that theory. So unless you find it makes you stuffier, there's no need to stop drinking the white stuff (or eating other dairy products) while a cold has you down.

• Vitamins. Getting enough vitamins and minerals can help keep

you from coming down with a cold or flu in the first place—or, if it's too late for that, help you fight off faster the illnesses you do succumb to. The extra nutrients in your prenatal vitamin supplement can also help you compensate nutritionally for the appetite-suppressing effects of whatever bug's bit you. When you do manage to get something (besides your supplement) down, make it count in the vitamin department. Concentrate on concentrated sources of nutrients—for instance, calcium-fortified orange juice, which gives you both vitamin C and calcium.

Sore throat. Cold germs have settled in the back of your throat, and it feels like they've started a fire, making swallowing a real pain in the neck? When you're pregnant, temporarily suspending swallowing until your throat cools down isn't an option, but eating foods that aren't so hard to swallow is. Turn to those cold and flu comfort foods—especially those that are soft enough to slide down with a minimum of effort (pureed soups, thinned-out hot cereals, fruit gel, for example). Warmth may be particularly soothing, but stay away from throat-irritating acidic foods; drink orange and grapefruit juices well diluted, or switch to less acidic juices or to decaffeinated tea with lemon and honey.

GI (gastrointestinal) distress. You finished weathering morning sickness, and thought you had nothing but smooth digestive sailing to look forward to. Then, those all-too-familiar rumblings began anew—this time, courtesy of a stomach virus or a mild case of food poisoning. While morning sickness can last for months (as probably nobody needs to tell a pregnant woman), fortunately, these GI conditions are blessedly brief—usually lasting no more than twenty-four or forty-eight hours. But because diarrhea and vomiting can rob your baby of vital nutrients and fluids—even in a short time—you'll need to pay as much attention as possible to your diet while you're waiting for the misery to pass:

• Fluids. You've heard it before (like when you were suffering from morning sickness), but it's worth repeating: In the short term, fluids are more important than solids. Even when you can't keep as much as a crust of bread down, you'll need to maintain an adequate fluid intake. Try plain water, sparkling water, or weak decaffeinated tea. If you're vomiting, taking small sips every fifteen minutes may give the fluids a fighting chance of staying down. If you can't stomach sipping, suck on ice chips or Popsicles. If symptoms are severe or you can't manage to get enough fluids into you (or both), your practitioner may recommend a rehydration fluid (or frozen rehydration pops) as a precaution. Once clear liquids (diluted fruit juices—particularly white grape, which is easier on the tummy—and clear broth) go down and stay down, you can add nutritious shakes or smoothies.

• Bland foods. If you can stomach solids, focus on those that are appealing (relatively), bland, and fat-free: thinned cream of wheat, unbuttered toast, mashed or baked potato (without the skin), bananas, applesauce, white rice or plain pasta with a little cottage cheese. As they start looking (and feeling) better to you, gradually add yogurt, chicken, fish, and then fruits and cooked vegetables.

• Vitamins. Try to take your pregnancy supplement daily at a time it's least likely to come back up, and never on an empty stomach.

But don't worry if you need to skip it for a day or two. Once the bug stops bugging you, you'll be able to make up those lost nutrients.

If You're Carrying Multiples

EXPECTING TWINS (OR MORE)? THEN you'll need to pay at least twice as much attention to your diet as a woman who is carrying just one baby. As it turns out, good nutrition during a multiple pregnancy has an even greater impact on baby birth weight than it does during a singleton pregnancy. And quality alone won't do it—you'll also need to add some quantity, too. For each extra baby you have on board, you'll have extra requirements above and beyond those of an expectant mother of one. Fortunately for you (and your belly, which will be stretched to capacity anyway during your multiple pregnancy), that doesn't mean you'll have to consume twice as many calories or vitamins for twins, or three times as much protein for triplets. Just keep in mind the extras you'll need when you're eating for three or more:

Extra weight. Not surprisingly, toting an extra baby means you'll have to tote around extra weight. Also not surprisingly, the healthier your weight gain (and your diet), the healthier your babies' weight gain is likely to be.

Most experts recommend that women of normal prepregnancy weight who are pregnant with twins should gain between 37 and 54 pounds—roughly 50 percent more than the recommended weight gain for a single pregnancy (for triplets, 50 to 60 pounds). And because you can expect your babies to arrive somewhat earlier than single babies (term for twins is usually considered thirty-seven weeks), you'll need to pack in that weight gain (and all those extra nutritional needs) in a shorter period of time. Challenging? You bet, especially because you're also likely to experience more nausea and vomiting in your first trimester and beyond than expectant moms of one. But with a little tummy-cramming, it can be done. See page 13 for tips on coping with morning sickness and page 51 for suggestions on putting on the pounds if you're having trouble gaining weight.

Extra calories. So how do you gain all that extra weight? The usual way—by piling on extra calories (about 300 to 500 per fetus; check with your practitioner to determine your magic number). Sounds like a chronic dieter's dream come true, right? Perhaps, but remember that the extra calories shouldn't come from the kinds of foods (candy bars, fries) most chronic dieters see in their dreams. Instead, you'll need to make sure those extra calories come from nutrient-dense foods that best nourish your babies and your pregnancy. Studies show that a high-calorie diet that's also high in nutrients significantly improves your chances of having healthy, robust full-term babies.

The prescription for these extra calories: Follow The Pregnancy Diet in Chapter Five and then add more food, more snacks, and bigger portions, keeping an eye on the scale to ensure your gain's on target. Rather than trying to squeeze the extra calories and nutrients into only three meals, try eating five or six small meals and several light snacks throughout the day. Another reason to eat more frequently: Research has suggested that women who eat at least five meals plus snacks a day are more likely to carry to term. Plus, you'll be less likely to be plagued by indigestion and heartburn. (See page 16 for mini-meal tips.)

Extra iron. Being pregnant means your body's in the blood-making business big-time, since blood volume must increase significantly to nourish the fetus. Naturally, the more fetuses (and placentas) that blood volume must support, the more it must increase. Enter extra iron—the mineral that helps manufacture red blood cells. Most women end up needing more iron than their diets can provide at some point in their pregnancy; you'll need lots more, lots sooner. To fill that need, your practitioner will probably prescribe an iron supplement early on in your pregnancy. Be sure to supplement that supplement by eating iron rich foods such as red meat and dried fruit. (And take iron sources with a vitamin C–rich food to aid absorption.)

Extra vitamins. More fetuses mean a greater need for nutrients. Though you won't have to take more than one prenatal supplement a day (unless otherwise recommended by your practitioner), you should try to increase your vitamin intake the old-fashioned way—by eating vitamin-rich foods.

Extra minerals. Your prenatals are a good place to start, but it won't provide you with all the extra minerals you'll need when you're building more than one baby. Many practitioners recommend, for instance, that women carrying twins supplement with magnesium and calcium—and for good reason. Magnesium reduces the risk of preterm labor—something most multiple pregnancies are at risk of. Calcium, of course, builds strong bones and teeth, and with at least two sets of each growing inside you, you'll need plenty of help from that essential mineral.

Extra fluid. Being dehydrated can also lead to preterm labor, so step up the fluids—drinking at least eight glasses daily. Drinking between meals (rather than attempting to sip with them) will keep the fluids from competing with the solids for coveted room in the closer and closer quarters of your stomach.

If You're a Vegetarian

IF YOU'RE A PREGNANT VEGETARIAN, chances are you've had at least one finger (or one steak) wagged your way by someone who felt compelled to warn you that babies can't grow without a good piece of meat. The fact is, those waggers are wrong. Babies born to vegetarian moms are just as healthy as those born to carnivores. With careful planning, you can follow a vegetarian diet that provides all the necessary vita-mins, minerals, protein, and other nutrients you and your growing baby need. There's no need to turn in your dietary principles for a healthier pregnancy (or turn in your soy burger for a beef one).

A vegetarian diet does, however, present some challenges for the pregnant mom-to-be, including:

Gaining weight. Some vegetarians find it difficult to gain enough weight during pregnancy because diets with no animal products tend to be low in fat and high in fiber. If you're having a hard time piling on the pounds, add more fat servings to your diet (see page 97), eat smaller amounts more often, and choose foods that are particularly dense in both calories and nutrition, such as nuts, dried fruit, and avocados.

Getting enough nutrients. You'll need to make sure you're getting enough of these important nutrients:

wisdom of 🌞 the ages?

Here are a couple of old wives' tales that may well have been generated by old vegetarians: Chinese folklore maintains that a woman should avoid eating both rabbit and chicken during her pregnancy—or else her baby will be born with a hoarse voice. Eating squid and crab are also discouraged, according to Chinese tradition. Squid, so the tale goes, is believed to cause the uterus to "stick" during delivery, and eating crab will result in a mischievous child.

• **Protein**. Vegetarians who include eggs and milk products in their diet usually have little trouble getting enough protein.* But vegans, who rule out all animal products, may need to work harder in the protein department. If you're a vegan, look to dried beans, peas, lentils, tofu, and other soy products (see page 84 for more vegetarian protein sources).

• **Vitamin B₁₂**. Since vitamin B_{12} is found only in foods that come from animals, vegetarians who eat no animal products will have to find other ways to get their B_{12}— usually in the form of supplements (ask your practitioner if you need more than what's provided in your prenatal vitamin), but also from vitamin B_{12}–fortified soy milk, fortified cereals, nutritional yeast, and fortified meat substitutes.

• **Iron.** It's not easy for anyone (except big meat eaters) to get enough iron from their diets. For those who stick to plant foods, it's next to impossible. If you're a vegetarian—and especially if you're a vegan—your practitioner

---

*It's important to keep in mind that eggs and dairy products, while excellent sources of protein, are not as efficient sources of protein as are fish and poultry. It takes only 4 ounces of halibut to fill a protein serving requirement, but 3 glasses of milk, 4 medium eggs, 3 ounces of Swiss cheese, or 2 cups of yogurt to do the same. Fat-free cottage cheese, however, is at least as efficient a source of protein as fish, filling a full protein requirement with just one 1-cup (160-calorie) serving.

VEGETARIANS, FEAR NOT

▼ ▼ ▼

With just a few tweaks, many of the recipes (including the salads, sandwiches, pastas, and stir-fry entrées) in this book can be easily adapted to suit your vegetarian lifestyle. Just leave out the meat, fish, or poultry, and substitute a vegetarian protein you find complementary, such as soy "meat" or "poultry," tofu or tempeh, soy beans, beans, or extra grains and nuts. If it's dairy that's off your menu, simply sub a nondairy alternative—soy cheese or soy milk, for instance. And don't hesitate to adapt recipes from your standard vegetarian cookbooks; with a few adjustments (you'll need extra calcium and protein), they're sure to be healthy enough to fit a pregnant bill of fare.

will probably recommend that you take an iron supplement.

• **Calcium.** Though dairy products are the most well-known sources of calcium, they're not the only ones. Calcium-fortified juice, for instance, offers as much calcium as milk, ounce for ounce—making it a perfect source of this essential mineral for vegans. Other nondairy dietary sources of calcium include dark green leafy vegetables, sesame seeds, almonds, calcium-fortified soy products, including soy milk, soy cheese, flour and baked goods, tofu, and tempeh. Still, adding a calcium supplement is probably good insurance for pregnant vegans.

• **Vitamin D.** Since the best dietary source of vitamin D is milk, non-milk drinkers will have to depend on their supplements (or fortified soy milk, cheese, or juice) to provide them with all they need of this vital vitamin. Also look for breads and cereals that are fortified with it.

Creating an eating plan. Since vegan dietary needs are more complex, some experts recommend that you see a nutritionist early in your pregnancy (or, even better, before becoming pregnant) to develop a healthy eating plan that takes into account the special needs of that special baby of yours.

If You Can't Handle Dairy

MILK AND DAIRY PRODUCTS ARE nature's finest sources of the calcium you and your baby need when you're expecting. But if milk leaves you with more than a mustache (think gas, and lots of it), you may think twice before reaching for that tall white glass. For the lactose intolerant, alas, milk does not always do the body (or at least, the stomach) good.

Lactose intolerance results from a lack of (or inadequate supply of) lactase, the enzyme needed to digest the milk sugar, lactose. Those who are lactose intolerant experience a range of symptoms, including gas, bloating, indigestion, cramping that can range from mild to severely uncomfortable, and diarrhea. As prevalent as the condition is, however, studies show that many people who believe they are lactose intolerant actually aren't. (You can take the test in the box on the facing page to see if you really are.) Keep in mind, too, that there are degrees of intolerance. While some people can take up to a cup of milk without hearing from their stomachs, a few may be so lactase deficient that even a sip of milk triggers tummy tumult.

Fortunately, you don't have to suffer so your baby can grow healthy bones and teeth. If you're lactose intolerant, there are plenty of ways to get the calcium you need without the stomach upset you certainly don't need:

▲ Take it small. Try drinking only ½ cup of milk at a time, a small dish of cottage cheese, a thin slice of cheese. In general, small quantities of the offending dairy products spread out during the day may cause less distress than a couple of large doses.

▲ Take it with food. Lactose is easier to digest when mixed with other foods (particularly high-fiber foods, such as whole-grain breads or cereals). So pour your milk into your bran flakes, or melt your cheese on a whole wheat tortilla.

▲ Shop wise. Look for lactose-free milk at the grocery store—and to get more bang for your buck (and your glass of milk), choose lactose-free calcium-fortified milk, which offers two-thirds more calcium than regular.

▲ Drop it in. Add over-the-counter lactase drops to your milk (or other dairy products) to break down the lactose and help ease digestion. Or take lactase in pill form (chewables or capsules) whenever you eat or drink a problematic dairy product.

▲ Say cheese. Since milk itself is usually the major culprit, the closer a dairy product is to milk, the more likely it is

TEST YOUR INTOLERANCE

▼ ▼ ▼

Got a stomachache last time you got milk? That doesn't necessarily mean that you're truly lactose intolerant—in fact, many people who seem to develop tummy troubles after drinking milk actually aren't. To tell if you really are lactose intolerant, take this simple test: When your stomach is empty (two to three hours after a meal or first thing in the morning), drink two glasses of skim milk. If you experience the symptoms associated with lactose intolerance, it's likely you are unable to digest lactose.

Can't take that much milk straight—especially on an empty stomach? Try this test instead: For several days, have someone make you a smoothie with either regular or lactose-free milk—using the same milk for several days straight and not telling you which it is. Then, have them make you a smoothie using the other milk for several days straight. If you have symptoms only with the regular milk, you're probably lactose intolerant.

Need even more confirmation (just to make sure pregnancy symptoms aren't confusing the picture)? Abstain from all dairy products for two weeks. (Be sure to substitute adequate amounts of nondairy forms of calcium.) If all symptoms disappear, you have a pretty definite diagnosis. If you find your tummy's still acting up, you'll have to blame something else for your gastrointestinal unrest.

to offend. Aged cheeses (such as cheddar, Swiss, and Parmesan) may be easier on your stomach because more
than half the lactose is removed during
processing.

▲ Get active. Active cultures, that
is—the kind that's found in yogurt.
These active bacterial cultures (usually acidophilus) often help break
down lactose without the need for
supplements.

▲ Abandon the dairy case. If milk in
any form, even lactose reduced, is
intolerable, steer clear of any food
that contains dairy products. Read
labels carefully. The words *pareve* or
parve indicates that a product contains no dairy at all.

▲ Look elsewhere. Since it's more of a
challenge to get adequate calcium if
you're not eating any dairy products,
you'll need to scour the market for
alternatives. First stop should be the
juice aisle, where you'll find orange,
grapefruit, apple, grape, and other
juices fortified with calcium. Still not
satisfied? Turn to canned salmon with

bones, sardines with bones, tofu,
greens, broccoli, and calcium-enriched
soy milk and cheese—all good calcium sources.

▲ Seek sunshine. Calcium is not the
only nutrient milk provides. Milk is
one of the major sources of dietary
vitamin D, so if you're not getting
milk, you'll need to find alternative
methods of getting vitamin D. Just a
few minutes a day of bright sunshine
will help. (But stay out of the sun
during peak hours, since pregnant
skin is sensitive skin.) So will taking
a prenatal supplement that contains
vitamin D (which you're probably
already doing), eating enriched cereals and breads, or drinking vitamin
D–enriched soy milk or juice.

▲ Supplement. Ask your practitioner
about prescribing a calcium supplement if you're not getting enough
through your diet. If your pregnant
tummy gives you plenty of trouble
with or without dairy, you might want
to consider taking the supplement in
the form of a calcium-containing
antacid, such as Tums or Rolaids.

Gestational Diabetes

IF YOU'VE BEEN DIAGNOSED WITH gestational diabetes, you're not alone.
Between 3 and 8 percent of pregnant
women develop this condition,

which occurs when the body can't
regulate blood sugar levels. Call it a
glitch in Nature's otherwise inge-
nious system. Normally, the pancreas

makes a hormone called insulin, which allows cells to turn glucose, or sugar, into usable fuel. During pregnancy, as increasing hormone levels make the body more resistant to insulin, the body is challenged to produce extra insulin in order to keep blood sugar in check. When the body doesn't meet the challenge, gestational diabetes results.

Unlike other types of diabetes, gestational diabetes is temporary—blood-sugar levels generally return to normal after delivery. Like other types of diabetes, it's best controlled by carefully following a proper diet. (Though there are also many nondietary changes to make if you have gestational diabetes, such as getting regular exercise; see *What to Expect When You're Expecting*.) To keep your blood sugar under control, you'll need to consider the following factors:

Diet changes. It's likely that your doctor will instruct you to follow the nutrition guidelines set by the American Diabetes Association, which emphasize a good balance of healthy carbohydrates, fats, and protein in the right amounts (and which you'll find doesn't differ all that much from The Pregnancy Diet). But those guidelines are just general; to be most successful, your diet should be individually tailored for you based on your blood-glucose level, weight, exercise habits, and food preferences. Ask your practitioner to recommend a

registered dietician who has experience in gestational diabetes, contact your hospital for a referral, or speak to someone from your local chapter of the American Dietetic Association or the American Diabetes Association.

The typical recommendations encourage women with gestation diabetes to do the following:

• Shun sugar. What goes for most pregnant women goes more emphatically for you. To keep your blood-sugar levels from escalating, you'll need to stay away from foods that increase them. Not surprisingly, simple sugars (including sugar, honey, brown sugar, corn syrup, maple syrup, turbinado sugar, high-fructose corn syrup, and molasses) top that list. When scanning labels for sugar, keep in mind that ingredients that end in *ose* are always sugar (sucrose, dextrose, glucose). You can eat foods that contain a small amount of sugar in moderation, but try to steer clear of high-sugar standards, such as pies, cakes, cookies, ice cream, candy, and soft drinks. Sucralose (Splenda) makes a good sugar substitute.

• Forgo fruit juices. Even fruit sugar can raise your blood sugar, which means that naturally sweet 100 percent fruit juices will have to be limited, too. Your dietician or doctor may give you the go-ahead on occasional small amounts of juice (up to six ounces, taken with meals); mixing the juice with sparkling water will dilute the fruit sugar, while making your treat last longer. Tomato juice (which is technically a fruit juice) is a good choice because of its low-sugar content. Fresh fruit isn't a problem, since (unlike juice) it contains fiber, which slows the absorption of sugar into the blood (see below).

• Be less refined. In your choice of starches, that is. Too many refined starches (white rice, mashed potatoes, white bread), because they turn quickly to sugar when digested, can also raise blood glucose. Concentrate, instead, on high-fiber complex carbs (such as whole grains, beans and peas, and vegetables), which decrease the amount of insulin your body needs to keep blood sugars within normal range.

• Get a kick from chromium. This mineral has been shown to improve glucose tolerance in gestational diabetes, so be sure your diet contains some. (You'll find it in whole-grain products, spinach, carrots, and chicken.) Also ask your practitioner whether it would be smart to take a supplement.

• Stay low-fat. Everyone needs some fat in her diet—especially pregnant women. But a high-fat diet causes insulin to be less efficient—which means your body will need more of it to keep blood sugar levels within normal range. Focus on healthy fats, such as those in nuts.

Meal control. The grazing approach to eating works best for most pregnant women, but is essential for those trying to regulate their blood sugar. Aim for at least three meals and three snacks (including a bedtime snack) each day—spaced as evenly as possible. Another rule that applies to all pregnant women, but must be more strictly adhered to by those with gestational diabetes is: no meal skipping. Skipping meals (or snacks) can result in hypoglycemia (low blood sugar), which can make you feel miserable (irritable, shaky, headachy), and which may be harmful to the fetus.

Your most important snack of the day will come in the evening and will help ward off the lower-than-normal blood sugar levels that are common during the night in women with gestational diabetes. Before turning in, eat a snack that contains protein (such as low-fat cheese) and complex carbohydrates (such as whole wheat bread). The carbohydrates will stabilize your blood sugar level in the early night, while the protein acts as a long-acting stabilizer. (See page 106 for snack ideas.)

Weight control. Since too many pounds can send blood-sugar levels soaring, you'll have to pay even more attention to your weight gain than other pregnant women. You'll also need to pay extra attention to the rate of gain. Gaining too much weight too quickly (two or more pounds per week) results in extra body fat, which, in turn can produce an insulin-resistant effect. See Chapter Three for ways to ensure proper weight gain at a good rate during pregnancy.

When You're on Bed Rest

MOST BUSY PEOPLE DREAM OF BEING able to kick off their shoes, put up their feet, plump up their pillows, and lounge the day away in bed. But if you've been put on bed rest, that dream may seem more like a nightmare. Bed rest is no vacation—at least after the first twenty-four hours. And mealtimes? Not exactly the room service experience some might envision—especially if there's no one around all day to deliver it.

How can you stay off your feet and on The Pregnancy Diet at the same time? These tips might help:

▲ Keep a bedside (or couchside, if that's where you do most of your lounging) snack bar, so you don't have to make unnecessary trips to the kitchen. Stock it with

• Plenty of fluids (a cup and a container of water or a thermos of juice or milk); drinking often is especially important if you've experienced preterm contractions or you're just anxious to prevent them.

• Plenty of healthy snacks that don't need refrigeration, such as whole-grain crackers; soy chips; fresh and dried fruit; nut and seeds; trail mix; dry cereal.

• If possible, a cooler or small refrigerator, to keep perishable snacks (like single-serve yogurts and cheese sticks) and meals fresh—and keep cold drinks chilled.

• A small microwave to warm up ready-made meals, if you're not allowed on your feet at all, or for very limited periods of time.

▲ Have a sturdy bed tray on which to eat your meals (a couple of days of lying in crumbs, and you'll know why this is so important). You can also use the tray for reading, writing, supporting your laptop, making crafts, or whatever else you'll be doing to pass the time.

▲ To prevent heartburn (which is exacerbated by eating while lying

wisdom of the ages?

According to Filipino folklore, one should never take food from a pregnant woman for risk of being constantly sleepy. You might want to tell your spouse that next time he tries to lift a chicken strip off your plate.

down), prop yourself up with a few pillows and eat in a sitting position (if you're allowed to). Eating smaller, more frequent meals and snacks (instead of large, heavy ones) will also help minimize digestive miseries.

▲ Fight constipation (which you'll be more likely to experience when you're lying down) with extra fiber and fluids. (See page 27 for more.)

▲ Depend on deliveries (as long as someone is around to answer the door). Put all your favorite take-outs on speed-dial. Order your groceries online. If you can afford it, look into meal-delivery services. (They can often customize catered meals for those with special nutritional needs, albeit with a hefty price tag.)

▲ Accept all the help that's offered (and ask for what isn't). Let anyone who's willing (your spouse, your friends, your neighbors) cook meals for you. Or hire some paid kitchen help, if you can.

▲ Remember to account in your calorie count for all that lying around you're doing. Unfortunately, you won't be burning as many calories in bed—which means you won't need to be eating as many. Keep an eye on the scale to make sure you're not gaining too quickly, and emphasize efficient eating (see page 77). If you're prone (especially when you're prone) to boredom-eating, make sure the snacking you do is low-calorie (a bag of baked soy crisps, not a bag of fried cheese puffs).

▲ Entertain in bed, if you're not allowed out of it. Misery loves company—and you'll be less miserable if your spouse joins you for meals when he's home. Consider throwing dinner-in-bed parties for your friends, too. (Order in pizza or make the meals potluck to keep efforts to a minimum.)

Eating Well Postpartum

CONGRATULATIONS AGAIN! You've made it through those nine-plus months of pregnancy and those long, long hours of childbirth. Now with those challenges (including the challenge of eating nutritiously for two) behind you, you're looking forward to the postpartum period—which, you figure, has to be that proverbial piece of cake in comparison. And, speaking of cake, bring it on (and while you're at it, add some ice cream and fudge)! After all, you've minded your diet for nearly a year, and you have a beautiful baby to show for it. Isn't it time for your just desserts? (And fries, and chips, and wine, and . . .)

Whoa there, woman! While postpartum eating may be easy as pie compared with pregnancy eating (and while you may have room in your diet for more pieces of pie than you did before), it does not make sense to shed those good eating habits you worked so hard to earn while you were expecting (especially if you hope to shed some of those pounds you packed on, too). Besides, eating well can provide significant benefits long after you've hung up (or burned) those maternity clothes, including a healthier you and a healthier family.

The Postpartum Diet

FEELING A LITTLE (OR VERY) DEPRIVED after the last nine months? There's plenty of good news awaiting you at the dinner table. Postpartum eating allows for a lot more leeway than pregnancy eating does. Need that coffee to get the day started (especially since it's been starting at 5 A.M.)? Fire up the coffeepot! Love the way that wine with dinner winds you down after a hard day with baby? Uncork that bottle of pinot noir! Having sushi withdrawal? Whip out those chopsticks, and even pass the sake!

But the good news comes (as it so often does) with some fine print, and a few caveats. While it may seem that postpartum eating should be open season (and open bar), it really isn't. The fact is that you'll still need to pay attention to your diet so you can recover from childbirth, keep your energy up (how else will you rise for those middle-of-the-night feedings, followed by sleep-deprived morning-after diaper changes?); keep the baby blues at bay; protect against constipation, hemorrhoids, and other occupational hazards of the postpartum woman; gradually take off those extra pounds put on during the nine months of pregnancy; and, if you're breastfeeding, produce enough quality milk.

Nine Basic Diet Principles for New Mothers

These nine basic principles that steered you through nine months of healthy eating can continue to be your guide during the postpartum period and beyond—whether you're breastfeeding or not:

Bites still count. Sure, you won't be sharing every bite with your baby anymore (even if you're breastfeeding). But making many of the bites you take during the day count toward good nutrition is always a sensible principle. If you are nursing, it's an especially smart guideline. (After all, running a milk factory takes a lot of energy—energy that comes from healthy eating.)

All calories are not created equal. If you're looking to lose the pregnancy love handles you're not exactly loving, you'd be wise to watch where your calories come from. Calories eaten in the form of refined carbohydrates, for instance, are less likely to be burned as fuel and more likely to accumulate in those hard-to-trim areas. Take in the same number of calories through lean protein, fruits, vegetables, and whole grains, and you'll find those inches melting off faster. (You'll also have more energy to burn.)

Starve yourself, cheat your baby. Missing meals day after day (who has time for breakfast when baby needs to be fed, burped, diapered, dressed, and repeat?) can leave you with less energy when you need it the most—and when baby most needs you to have it. So can subscribing to the latest hyped diet. And if you're breastfeeding, inadequate nutrition can, in time, result in an inadequate milk supply.

Stay an efficiency expert. Because it's likely you'll want those months of weight gain to come to an end (and for the months of weight loss to commence, albeit slowly and sensibly), continue selecting foods that pack in the most nutrition for the calories.

Carbohydrates will always be a complex issue. Just because you're sporting a baby instead of a belly doesn't mean it's time to revisit refined grains. First, if by now you've developed a taste for the grainier side of life, why go back to white? Second, everyone (especially women plagued by postpartum constipation) can benefit from taking a complex view of carbohydrates—and from the fiber, vitamins, and trace minerals that are naturally found in whole-grain breads and cereals, brown rice, dried beans,

peas, and other legumes. And third, by continuing to fill your pantry with complex carbohydrates, you'll help ensure that your baby will be weaned on wholesome whole grains.

Sweet nothings are exactly that. Maybe you've heard there's nothing like a candy bar to give you the energy boost you so sorely need these days (and nights). But the truth is, sugary treats will lift you only briefly before sending you into an energy crash-and-burn. And while having the occasional sugary treat won't throw your postpartum eating plan into a tailspin, making them your most frequented food group will. Not to mention make weight loss elusive (and weight gain a definite possibility). And remember, sugar calories are empty calories whether you're pregnant or not.

Eat foods that remember where they came from. Foods that are highly processed have not only lost a lot of their natural nutrition and (more than likely) gained a lot of saturated fat, sodium, and sugar in the processing plant, but they also often contain chemical additives that can possibly contaminate breast milk (see page 229). So stick to foods that haven't ventured far from their natural state.

Make good eating a family affair. There's never been a better time to join nutritional family forces for a healthier future. After all, there's a new mouth to feed in the house. How that mouth will be fed (and how it will eventually choose to eat) will depend a lot on the nutritional example you set, as well as on how you continue to stock the kitchen. A child who's raised in a household where the bread's whole wheat, the snack of choice is fruit, and salad is friend not foe is likely to grow up thinking good nutrition is a given.

Don't sabotage your diet. A healthy lifestyle doesn't stop at healthy eating. Even if you're breastfeeding, you can enjoy an occasional alcoholic beverage (see page 226). But too much alcohol (or any illicit drug use) can definitely have an adverse affect on your health (and, because it can impair your parenting judgment, your baby's well being). And tobacco use is harmful not only to you, but to baby, as well. (An infant is put at greater risk for SIDS, respiratory infections, and other serious problems if you or anyone in the home smokes.)

The Daily Dozen for Postpartum and Breastfeeding

Since your old friend the Daily Dozen represents the framework for a sensible, balanced diet, you should stay old friends—not just during the postpartum period, but for a lifetime of healthy eating. Only the number of servings will change now that you're no longer expecting; you'll need to eat more of most if you're breastfeeding, less if you're not:

Calories. After months of putting weight on, chances are you're very much in the mood to start taking it off. But drastically slashing calories isn't the smart way to rediscover your waist. Instead, you'll need to strike a balance: enough calories to keep you on the go, not so many that the numbers on the scale don't start dropping.

If you're breastfeeding, you'll actually need more calories than when you were pregnant (after all, you're still feeding baby—only baby is much bigger now)—up to 500 more a day than you would need to maintain your prepregnancy weight (double that if you're breastfeeding twins, triple if you're the milk source for triplets). Best of all, since all those calories go toward milk production, they won't end up on your thighs. In fact, some lucky moms find breastfeeding helps melt the pounds away—even with all those extra calories. (If, after the first six postpartum weeks, you don't seem to be losing weight, you can reduce the number of extra calories a little, but don't take in fewer than 1,800 calories a day. Cutting too many calories can cut down on your milk supply).

If you're not breastfeeding, your days of needing extra calories are officially over—and you'll have to work a little harder to lose the pregnancy weight (see page 229). Serious calorie cutting, however, shouldn't begin until you're completely recovered from childbirth. So for the first six weeks, eat about as many calories as you would need to maintain your prepregnancy weight. Once you've gotten your practitioner's okay, the dieting can begin in earnest (but still, within reason); reduce your calorie intake by 200 to 500 a day, and you'll start to see a gradual, steady weight loss.

Protein: three servings daily if you're breastfeeding; two if you're not. See the list of protein choices on page 83, keeping in mind that many also double as a calcium serving. If you're breastfeeding twins or triplets, get ready to eat hearty: You'll need an extra serving of protein for each additional baby. Vegans should also add an extra protein serving daily (because the quality of vegetable protein is not as high as that of animal protein).

Calcium: five servings daily if you're breastfeeding; at least three if you're not. Whether you're making milk or not, you should still be drinking it (or taking the equivalent in other calcium sources) to strengthen your bones. Remember that many of the calcium choices on page 86 also serve up a considerable amount of protein, so take full advantage of this nutritional overlapping. If you're breastfeeding twins or triplets, you'll need an extra calcium serving for each additional baby. (Use calcium-enriched dairy products or calcium supplements to reach your quota.) An important note for breastfeeders—while baby won't suffer if you don't meet your calcium requirement, your bones might. In order to keep baby's supply calcium-rich, your body will draw this essential mineral from your bones for milk production, possibly setting you up for osteoporosis later on if you don't take in enough calcium from your diet.

Vitamin C foods: two or more servings daily whether you're breastfeeding or not. See page 89 for vitamin C choices (and remember that many vitamin C foods also fill the requirement for green leafy and yellow vegetables and yellow fruits).

Green leafy and yellow vegetables and yellow fruits: three to four servings daily whether you're breastfeeding or not. See page 91 for good food choices, keeping in mind that many of these also fill the requirement for vitamin C.

Other fruits and vegetables: one or more servings daily whether you're breastfeeding or not. See page 93 for good choices.

DON'T FORGET YOUR DHA

▼ ▼ ▼

In your quest to drop those post-baby pounds, remember that some fats are still your friends—namely, those DHA-supplying ones. DHA is just as important while you're breastfeeding as it is during pregnancy, and here's why. The DHA content of your baby's brain triples during the first three months of life, and getting enough of this vital nutrient through your milk (which already contains DHA) will help fuel that growth. Even if you're not breastfeeding, there's another good reason to keep the DHA coming: Experts suspect that there may be a connection between a low intake of DHA and postpartum depression. See box, page 98, for good sources of DHA.

Whole grains and other concentrated complex carbohydrates: three or more servings daily whether you're breastfeeding or not. See page 95 for good choices.

Iron-rich foods: one or more daily whether you're breastfeeding or not. You'll need iron to replenish your blood stores after delivery and to prevent fatigue caused by anemia (you'll be plenty tired without it). See page 96 for good choices.

High-fat foods: small amounts daily. Even though a breastfeeding mom needs fat (half of the calories of breast milk come from fat), you don't need as much as you did when you were pregnant. So limit the amount of fat in your diet to no more than 30 percent of your total calories. See page 97 for a list of fat servings, and focus, when possible, on sources of omega-3 fatty acids (also see box, page 98).

Salty foods: limited quantities. While salt restriction wasn't necessary in pregnancy, you may consider holding the pickles now. Too much salt isn't good for anyone, so as a sensible rule, limit highly salted foods (like the kind you'll run into at fast-food outlets), and salt lightly to taste at the table. Since iodine is an important nutrient if you're breastfeeding, nursing moms should use iodized salt, and shouldn't cut back too much. Other great sources of iodine to tap into: seafood and seaweed.

Fluids: eight cups daily whether you're breastfeeding or not. Here's one requirement you might expect to increase when you're in the milk production business. Yet the fact is that you need exactly as much fluids as an average adult does—about eight cups a day. Drinking a lot less than your quota, of course, might leave you dehydrated, and unable to produce adequate milk. Surprisingly, however, drinking a lot more than those eight cups can also decrease milk production (though you may need to adjust your fluid intake upward in very hot weather or if you're exercising). Since you'll be nursing at least eight times a day, one of the easiest ways to keep up with your requirement is to drink when baby drinks—keeping a bottle or glass of water close during breastfeeding sessions.

Whether you're breastfeeding or not, keep an eye on your urine output. If you're not taking enough fluids, your urine will become darker and more scant. And drink to your thirst—but before thirst strikes. Waiting until you're thirsty to drink means you're going too long without fluids.

Vitamin supplements: Continue to take your prenatal vitamin daily if you're breastfeeding. If you're not breastfeeding, take your pregnancy vitamins for at least the first six weeks postpartum, switching over to a standard multiple vitamin and mineral supplement afterwards.

Eating Well While Breastfeeding

What to Eat

Getting started breastfeeding isn't always easy, between mastering the technique, enduring sore nipples, and containing leaky breasts. Fortunately, there's one aspect of nursing that doesn't take much effort at all: eating well enough to produce a good milk supply. Because the basic composition of breast milk isn't directly dependent on what you eat, breastfeeding actually makes minimal demands on your diet (with the exception of some vitamins, see box, page 225). Quantity isn't affected, either, unless your diet is seriously inadequate (as it might be under famine conditions—or more likely in this society, famine conditions induced by a very restrictive fad diet). That's because Mother Nature puts a breastfeeding baby's needs first (unlike during pregnancy, when mom's nutritional interests got priority). Skimp on the calories, fall short on the protein, or come up behind on minerals, and your body will tap into its own stores of nutrients to make milk. In other words, your breast milk won't suffer, but you might. So be sure to stick to The Postpartum Diet (with adjustments for breastfeeding), no matter how eager you are to shed weight. Eating an adequate, well-balanced, well-varied diet while breastfeeding will ensure the continued health of both your baby and you—and it won't be nearly as challenging as when you were pregnant.

NEW BABY KEEPING YOU DOWN?

▼ ▼ ▼

Feeling more like a zombie than like a mother? Finding the little things in life—putting one foot in front of the other, keeping your eyes open without the help of toothpicks, remembering to pour milk into your cereal instead of your orange juice—harder and harder to accomplish as night after night of broken sleep begin exhausting that last tiny bit of energy you still had on reserve after delivery? Though there isn't much you can do about the broken sleep (at least not until your baby decides to start skipping those midnight feedings), there is a way to keep sleep deprivation from taking its toll: by fighting fatigue with food.

In general, the same tips that helped you (sort of) deal with pregnancy fatigue (see page 34) can help now, too. For instance, opt for grazing—eating small portions of food frequently throughout the day—over those three hearty squares (as if you had time to sit down for square one!). Mini-meals will help keep your blood sugar (and thus your

stamina) up. And because they don't put as much demand on your digestive tract, they won't tap into those energy stores as much as a gut bomb would. (The bigger the meal, the more energy it takes to digest, so the more tired it makes you feel.) Try, also, to include a combination of carbohydrates and protein in each mini-meal so that you get the energy-enhancing benefits of both nutrients.

Hold the simple sugars (like that chocolate bar you're thinking about right now), which pick you up only briefly before sending you crashing. Instead, graze on some of the following:

■ **Trail mix.** You don't need to be planning a hike to munch on a combo of dried and/or freeze-dried fruit, nuts, and seeds; it has a good balance of complex carbs and protein—plus it's high in iron, which helps combat the fatigue caused by anemia. Toss in some dry cereal, too.

There's yet another reason to eat a well-varied healthy diet while nursing—and believe it or not, it's got nothing to do with nutrition. Because what you eat affects the taste and smell of your breast milk, your breastfed baby is exposed to different flavors well before he or she is ready to sit down at the dinner table. In fact, studies have shown

that babies fed breast milk are more accepting of new foods when they start on solids than babies who are formula-fed—probably because they've gotten a taste for them well before that first spoonful heads their way. Enjoy a lot of highly flavored foods while nursing, and your baby's more likely to grow into a child with a set of adventurous taste

■ **Whole-grain cereal with low-fat milk or oatmeal.** Chock-full of B vitamins that help break down food into fuel, whole-grain cereal is a great way to energize your day (after a nightmare all-nighter). And don't save the cereal for breakfast. It makes a high-energy lunch or snack, too.

■ **Egg salad on whole wheat toast.** A tasty way to combine carbs and protein.

■ **Half a whole wheat bagel, topped with melted Swiss.** Ditto on the carbs and protein—an energy boost with a calcium bonus.

■ **Hummus in a whole wheat pita.** Garbanzo beans (also called chickpeas, the main ingredient in hummus) are a good source of protein; the whole wheat pita provides your carbohydrates.

■ **Fruit and yogurt sprinkled with chopped walnuts or sliced almonds.** Complex carbohydrates in the form of fruit provide sugar the way nature intended, supplying longer-lasting energy for our body. The nuts deliver protein and healthy, brain-boosting fats, and the yogurt adds protein and calcium.

buds. (Forget the chicken fingers, Ma—pass the curry!) Eat your vegetables now, and you'll have a better shot at getting junior to eat his vegetables later. Load up on the candy and cookies, and you may find the first tooth baby cuts is a sweet one. (For more on what you eat and how it affects your breast milk, keep reading.)

▲ ▲ ▲

Q *"My breastfeeding baby seems to have a lot of gas. Could it have anything to do with the beans I ate last night? I know they made me gassy."*

A Gas can't be passed through breast milk. (It's produced in the intestines.) So you can't blame your baby's tummy troubles on yours. And while many mothers claim that eating gas-producing foods (such as broccoli, cabbage, onions, cauliflower, brussels sprouts, and beans) triggers gas attacks in their nursing babies, researchers have yet to back up this anecdotal evidence.

Still, those scientific studies don't amount to a hill of beans when it's your baby who's gassy and uncomfortable after you've eaten a plate of beans. While it's true that all babies—whether they're breast-fed or formula-fed—have days when they're gassy, fussy, or spitting up a lot, it is possible that your baby is showing sensitivity to something in your diet.

It takes between two and six hours from the time you eat a certain food until it affects the taste and odor of your milk. So, if you find your baby is gassy, spits up more, rejects the breast, or is fussy a few hours after you eat a certain food, try eliminating that food from your diet for a few days, and see if your baby's symptoms disappear.

wisdom of the ages?

As long as there have been breast-feeding mothers, there have been old wives (and others) telling them which foods, drinks, and herbal brews will help them make more milk. A short list of their recommendations includes:

- Cow's milk

- Beer

- Garbanzo beans (chickpeas)

- Licorice

- Potatoes

- Olives

- Carrots

Though it's never been scientifically proved that any of these proposed milk-producing potions actually do the trick, some women do find they work. The reason? Probably the power of the mind, a powerful force indeed—if a mother believes that what she eats or drinks will make milk, she'll be relaxed. If she's relaxed, she'll have a good let-down, leading her to believe she has more milk. Abracadabra—the potion works its magic after all.

If you want to stick with science, though, here's the best—and only proven—prescription for increasing milk production: Nurse your baby frequently, right from the start.

Q *"Is it true that if I eat garlic, my baby won't nurse well because of the taste of my breast milk?"*

A That probably depends on how much garlic you ate when you were pregnant. A baby who became used to that pungent flavor through garlic-infused amniotic fluid is likely to lap up breast milk after mom's been hitting the pesto. A baby whose mother steered clear of spices during pregnancy might turn up his or her button nose when presented with a breast full of garlic milk. It's all a matter of taste—baby's. And the only way to discover what baby's taste buds can handle is to experiment. Next time you sample the scampi, watch to see your baby's reaction to your milk in two to six hours (which is how long it takes for the garlic to make its way to baby's feed). No fuss? No need to skimp on the garlic.

Q *"I ate some asparagus earlier today and was shocked to see that my breast milk looked a little green. Is that normal?"*

A You don't have to be Irish to celebrate St. Patrick's Day with a touch of the green breast milk—all you have to do is eat a plateful of asparagus. What you eat can change the color of your milk (though it doesn't always), and from there, even the color of your baby's urine. And it's easier being green than you might think; kelp, green Gatorade, seaweed (in tablet form), and some other natural supplements have been associated with green breast milk. Green not your color? Consider a case report that linked a mom's orange soda to pink-orange breast milk and bright pink urine from her baby (and you thought you were alarmed when you saw green). Fortunately, a change of breast milk color doesn't mean there's been a change in breast milk quality. So, unless your green milk bothers your baby's tummy or your sensibilities, there's no need to pass on the asparagus while you're nursing.

Q *"My mother says my baby is colicky because he's allergic to my breast milk. She suggested I stop eating dairy products. Will that work?"*

A Unfortunately, not all of what you eat will necessarily have a happy ending in baby's tummy. While most babies tolerate just about anything their moms consume, colic in some babies has been linked to dairy products, caffeine, onions, cabbage, or beans in their mother's diet. A maternal diet that's heavy on melons, peaches, and other fruits can cause diarrhea in some babies. Red pepper can cause a rash in some breastfed infants.

But even such reactions to your milk doesn't mean that your baby is allergic to your breast milk. Babies are never allergic to their mother's milk, though they can occasionally be allergic or sensitive to foods in their mother's diets. Some of the more common offenders are cow's milk, eggs, fish, citrus fruits, nuts, or wheat. Check with your baby's pediatrician if you think your baby might

VITAMINS AND THE NURSING MOTHER

▼ ▼ ▼

When it comes to most nutrients, your diet doesn't make a difference in your breastfed baby's diet (though it can make a big difference in your own short- and long-term health). Vitamins (particularly B vitamins) are an exception; miss your vitamins, and baby will miss his or hers, too. Fortunately, most women in this country get all the vitamins they need to make good quality milk without any special dietary effort. Still, following The Postpartum Diet and taking a prenatal supplement will provide you and baby with extra vitamin insurance. Nursing vegans, whose diets may be low in several important nutrients, will definitely need to supplement; see box, page 228. And since too much of a good thing can end up in your milk (and, in the case of vitamin A, become a toxic addition), don't take any supplements besides your prenatal unless they've been prescribed by your practitioner.

be allergic (having symptoms such as excessive crying, stuffy nose, vomiting, diarrhea, diaper rash, or blood in the stools) to something you're eating. You'll be able to screen for such an allergy simply by eliminating common food allergens from your diet one at a time. If baby's symptoms improve dramatically, chances are you've found your culprit.

But here's another very important fact to keep in mind as you look to your diet for a cause (and a cure) for your baby's colic: Most cases of colic in breastfed babies have nothing to do with what their moms have been eating. Crying alone—without any of the symptoms listed above—is not a sign that a baby is sensitive to something in your milk.

▼ ▼ ▼

wisdom of ☼ the ages?

Old wives are fond of passing down this less than wise tale: Eating onions and garlic will help with weaning. Obviously, this tale is rooted in another tale—that babies don't like the taste of garlic, onions, or other strong flavors in their milk. But studies have shown that this is likely to be the case only when mom's been a bland eater throughout her pregnant and lactating days. If she's a fan of Chicken with Forty Cloves of Garlic, it's likely baby will be, too.

What to Avoid

As you know by now, eating when you're breastfeeding is definitely that proverbial piece of cake compared with eating when you're expecting. It's also that glass of wine. And those few cups of coffee. But while you've got lots more leeway now when it comes to your diet and your lifestyle than you did when you were pregnant, there are still a few caveats to observe and a few substances to avoid—or at least, cut back on—while you're nursing. Luckily, most of them (such as cigarettes and certain medications) are substances you're already probably all too used to avoiding. Here's a list of foods and drinks you'll have to watch out for when breastfeeding:

Alcohol. Whether you celebrated the birth of your baby with champagne or sparkling apple cider doesn't matter. The fact is that champagne is now—after nine teetotaling months—an option. But don't get carried away. Any alcohol you consume finds its way into your breast milk, though the amount your baby gets is considerably less than the amount you drink. While it's not known what the safe alcohol limit is for breastfeeding moms, some researchers suggest that as little as one glass of wine a day could *temporarily* slow both large and small motor development in nursing infants. To be on the safe side (always the best side to be on when it comes to your baby), it's probably best to limit yourself to one or two glasses of wine or beer a week.

Heavy drinking, on the other hand, has other drawbacks, as well. In large doses, alcohol can make baby sleepy, sluggish, unresponsive, and unable to suck well. In very large doses, it can interfere with breathing. Too many drinks can also impair your own functioning (whether you're nursing or not), making you more susceptible to depression, fatigue, and

PACKED WITH PEANUTS?

▼ ▼ ▼

They may be satisfying, filling, and pretty nutritious (even when they're packed into your favorite candy bar), but if you have a family history of allergies, should you think about avoiding peanuts and foods that contain them while breastfeeding? Some research suggests peanut allergens may be passed through breast milk from the mother to the nursing baby. It has been theorized that this early exposure to peanut allergens may cause the baby to become sensitized to them, eventually leading to potentially serious allergies later in childhood. But because this research isn't conclusive, be sure to ask the pediatrician whether pulling the plug on peanuts—and giving up your PB&J—is really necessary.

lapses in judgment. (You certainly don't need that in the early postpartum months.) Large amounts of alcohol can also weaken your let-down reflex and make you less able to nourish your baby.

If you do choose to have an occasional drink, take it right after you nurse, rather than before, to allow a couple of hours for the alcohol to metabolize. That way, far less will reach baby.

Caffeine. During those early, sleep-deprived postpartum weeks, a little jolt from your local coffee bar may be just the ticket. Fortunately, that ticket doesn't come with a price—at least, as long as you continue to limit your caffeine consumption. A couple of cups of caffeinated coffee, tea, or cola won't affect your baby or you (and may actually allow you to stay vertical when you'd really rather be horizontal). Much more than that, however, can make you, your baby, or both of you jittery, irritable, and unable to sleep (something you definitely don't want). Keep in mind, too, that babies can't process caffeine as efficiently as adults can, which means it can build up quickly in their systems. Another downside to the triple espresso drink: Caffeine also acts as a

wisdom of ☼ the ages?

Here's one more for the old wives' hall of fiction: According to folklore, if you get scared, your breast milk will go sour. While it's true that stress hormones (produced when you're scared, for instance) may temporarily suppress the let-down reflex, your milk won't taste any different to baby. So go ahead and rent that horror flick. Then take a deep breath, relax, and don't get yourself worked up over spilled (or sour) milk.

THE BREASTFEEDING VEGETARIAN

▼ ▼ ▼

You don't have to drink milk to make milk. But if you're a nursing vegetarian (and especially if you're a nursing vegan), you will have to pay a little extra attention to your diet to make sure you consume enough calories (plant products are lower in calories than are animal products) and enough of the following nutrients:

■ Calcium

■ Protein (see page 84 for vegetarian proteins)

■ Vitamin D

■ Vitamin B₁₂

diuretic, drawing valuable fluids out of your body. So limit your caffeine while you're breastfeeding, or supplement with decaffeinated until you wean.

Herbs. Although herbs are natural, they aren't always safe, especially for breastfeeding mothers. They can be just as powerful—and just as toxic—as some drugs, and their chemical ingredients can end up in breast milk. Herbs like fenugreek (which has been used for centuries to increase a nursing mother's milk supply and is sometimes recommended by lactation consultants, though the scientific studies have been mixed) can have a very potent effect on blood pressure and heart rate in large doses. And other herbal preparations touted for their milk-producing properties, such as alfalfa, blessed thistle, or mother's milk tea can cause nausea or vomiting. Because the FDA doesn't regulate herbs and little is known about how herbs affect a nursing baby, play it safe and consult with your doctor before taking any herbal remedy.

Choose herbal teas wisely too. The FDA has urged nursing moms to be cautious about consuming many of them until more is known. For now, stick to reliable types of herbal teas that are thought to be safe during lactation—these include orange spice, peppermint, raspberry, red bush, chamomile, and rosehip—read labels carefully to make sure other herbs haven't been added to the brew, and drink them only in moderation.

Sugar substitutes. Aspartame is probably a better bet than saccharine (only tiny amounts of aspartame pass into breast milk), but since the long-term health consequences of the sweetener, if any, aren't yet known, excess is definitely not best. (Don't use aspartame at all if you or your baby has PKU.) Sucralose (Splenda), however, is made from sugar and is considered safe and a good all-round low-calorie sugar substitute.

Fish. Though the pregnancy ban on raw fish lifts when you're breast-feeding (sashimi lovers, rejoice!), the same EPA guidelines on fish safety that apply to pregnant women apply to nursing ones. See page 169 for complete guidelines.

Chemicals. Since you share the chemicals you eat with your nursing baby, it's smart to continue avoiding processed foods that contain long lists of additives, choosing organic products when possible to avoid pesticides, and opting for low-fat dairy products and lean meats (which will not only limit the amount of chemicals you'll ingest, but the number of calories, helping you shed those pregnancy pounds faster). That said, there's no need to drive yourself crazy about the chemicals in your diet;

in most cases, the concentrations that end up in your breast milk will be too small to be harmful to your baby.

NURSING TWINS (OR MORE)?

▼ ▼ ▼

Double (or triple) the mouths to feed? If you're nursing twins or triplets, you'll need extra rest and, yes, extra food—more calories, in fact, than when you were pregnant. (So put away those diet books until you wean your brood.) Be sure to follow The Postpartum Diet for breast-feeding (increasing your calorie requirement by 500 calories for each additional baby).

Shedding Pounds Postpartum

ONE OF THE GREATEST CHALLENGES of the postpartum period (besides concealing those undereye circles) is recovering your figure. After all, it's no fun being mistaken for a pregnant woman ("So when are you due?") three months after you've delivered. If you're lucky, you'll be zipping up those jeans again in no time. If you're not so lucky, extra pounds and inches may linger a lot longer

than you'd hoped, especially if you packed on plenty during pregnancy.

There's no one right way to win the battle of the baby bulge, but keeping these tips in mind can put you on the road to victory:

▲ **Take six.** Sure, you're in a hurry to see your waist again. But it's not smart to embark on a diet program until your body has a chance to recuperate from childbirth—usually about six weeks postpartum. If you're breastfeeding, you should probably wait longer before dusting off diet books, though you're likely to drop weight in the meantime (as long as you're not eating too many calories).

▲ Go slow. You didn't put on those pounds overnight, so you can't expect to lose them that quickly either. And especially if you're nursing, you shouldn't try to. Remember that much of the weight you put on during pregnancy was set aside as fat stores earmarked for lactation. Losing too much weight too quickly can interfere with milk production. Aim for no more than half a pound a week if you're nursing. (The average postpartum weight loss among breastfeeding women is one to two pounds per month for the first four to six months after delivery.) And never consume fewer than 1,800 calories daily while nursing; otherwise your milk (and baby) will suffer. If you're not nursing, you can look forward to losing one to two pounds per week after the first six weeks. (But keep in mind that everyone loses weight differently and at different rates.)

▲ Don't depend on breastfeeding. Although breastfeeding burns about 500 calories a day (the same as a daily five-mile run, and without even breaking a sweat), nursing alone will not guarantee weight loss. Though plenty of moms find the pounds melt away when they're breastfeeding, others have trouble losing weight. Some can't manage to lose an ounce until after baby's weaned (maybe because breastfeeding makes them so hungry, they end up eating much more than those 500 calories).

▲ Do the combo. Studies have shown what most of us have known all along (but, perhaps, have tried to deny): The best way to lose weight postpartum is by combining exercise and diet. Once your practitioner has given the green light, resume (or begin) an exercise program that can help you shed the pounds and inches that just seem to be hanging on (to your hips, your thighs, your belly, your arms . . .).

▲ Be patient. Again, it took nine months to gain them—allow yourself as long to lose them.

Eating Well for the Next Baby

IS THERE A BABY IN YOUR NEAR FUTURE? Whether you're thinking about a first pregnancy or planning an encore, there's a lot more to the preparations than feathering your nest (or hunting for a bigger nest). You'll also have to prepare baby's very first source of bed and board: you. And one of the best ways to whip yourself into tip-top baby-making shape during the preconception months is by improving your diet. Even before you start eating for two, you can start eating well for your baby's health.

Why Plan?

YOU MIGHT BE WONDERING: ISN'T the preconception period the perfect time *not* to worry about what I'm eating and drinking? After all, isn't it my last shot (at least for nine months) at large fries and Cokes? At breakfast doughnuts? At my three-a-day espresso habit? My last shot at . . . well, shots? Can't I just wait until sperm meets up with egg before taking up the healthy eating plan I fully intend to embrace?

Well, you could—and most women do (after all, many couples

THE CARB CONCEPTION CONNECTION

▼ ▼ ▼

Whether high-protein, low-carb diets are the next best thing for dieters is still open to debate. But whether they're the best thing if you're trying to conceive may not be, according to recent research. Low-carb diets aren't just low on carbs (from breads, cereals, fruits, and vegetables), but they're low on the valuable nutrients found in carbs (especially that most essential preconception nutrient, folic acid). So for best conception results, make your diet a baby-balanced one—even before baby's on board.

never plan for pregnancy at all), with absolutely no harm done. But there are plenty of pluses to getting a head start on healthy eating, if you have the luxury of planning time ahead of you. First, eating well now will help you get your nutrient stores up to snuff (if they've been depleted by pregnancy, dieting, or just plain lousy eating). Second, the better your nutritional status (and your partner's), the better your overall chances are of getting pregnant. Third, jumping cold turkey into a healthy eating plan can be tough—especially if you've spent years perfecting poor eating habits (meal skipping, produce avoidance, bingeing on sweets, and so on); wading in (weaning yourself onto breakfast and a few fruits and vegetables) can be an easier way to go.

But here's probably the most compelling reason why eating better before you're eating for two makes so much sense. Since conception has a way of sneaking up on couples, it's quite possible you won't be sure when the preconception period ends and the actual pregnant period begins. In fact, by the time an early pregnancy test comes back positive, your baby will already have been developing for two weeks. If you're nutritionally well stocked before conception, the bundle of cells you'll soon be calling baby will receive the best possible start beginning literally from day one.

Adding On

YOU'RE ABOUT TO BECOME A BABY-making factory, the supplier of a steady flow of nutrients essential to the development of a new life. In preparation, it's particularly important to build up reserves of certain important nutrients before baby starts tapping them, such as:

▲ Folic acid. Ensuring you've got enough of this important B vitamin before you get pregnant is so crucial that current guidelines recommend that all women of childbearing age get 400 mcg of folic acid daily—even if they're not planning for pregnancy. If you are planning, there's all the more reason. Studies show that taking folic acid both before and during the first trimester of pregnancy significantly reduces the risk of a neural tube defect (a defect of the brain or spinal cord, which forms during the first four weeks of pregnancy) in the baby. So start taking your prenatal vitamin (which will fill your folic acid requirement) now, and see page 65 for dietary sources of folic acid.

▲ Iron. It's not surprising that many women are iron deficient. After all, it's hard to keep those iron stores up when monthly periods deplete them (especially if your periods are heavy). But if you start off pregnancy with your iron stores drained, you'll have a harder time getting up to speed during pregnancy, when the demand for iron (to generate that increasing blood supply) will be at an all-time high. Another reason to start taking

FERTILE FOODS?

▼ ▼ ▼

You've heard of fertility gods, of course, but fertility foods? Sure enough, lore from over the centuries and around the world tells of a number of foods and herbs guaranteed to boost your baby-making powers, and those of your partner. They range from the fairly ordinary (yams, pine nuts, prunes, chocolate, and ginseng, though not necessarily all at one sitting) to the slightly bizarre (shark's fin or camel's hump—try finding a recipe for *those* on the Internet). There's plenty of symbolism on the list: Foods that look like sexual organs are said to improve those organs' functions (think eggs and figs); foods that are spicy are said to make you hot, literally—increasing sexual potency by raising your blood pressure and pulse rate. And, not surprisingly, topping the list is the old standard of aphrodisiacs, oysters (which, because they contain zinc—a mineral science has linked to fertility—may actually be everything they're shucked up to be).

But zinc-packed oysters aside, scientists have yet to find definitive links between any one food or herb and increased fertility. One thing that is certain, however, is that severe malnutrition (caused by famine, poor eating habits, or extreme dieting) does result in lower fertility rates, while good overall nutrition increases a couple's chances of baby-making success. Care for a salad with those oysters?

your prenatal supplement, and to eat plenty of iron-rich foods while you're in the planning phase.

▲ **Zinc.** The preconception period isn't just about preparing for pregnancy—it's about preparing for becoming pregnant. Being low on nutritional reserves can lower your fertility (and that of your partner); in fact, a deficiency in zinc has been linked to fertility problems. You'll find zinc in your prenatal vitamin, as well as in oysters, beef, turkey, lamb, pork, almonds, beans, chicken,

wheat germ, and fortified breads and cereals.

▲ **Other vitamins and minerals.** Taking a prenatal vitamin even before you get pregnant will help you fill in nutritional deficits you have in any vitamin or mineral before baby's around to miss them. And it's not just baby who stands to benefit from boosting your nutrient intake. Studies show that women who take vitamins before pregnancy (especially B vitamins) actually have less morning sickness than those who don't.

Cutting Back

NOT ONLY IS IT SMART TO START stocking up on the good things before you get pregnant—it's also wise to start cutting back on the not-so-good things. That includes giving

up smoking, recreational drugs, and certain medications (see *What to Expect When You're Expecting* for more on those topics), all of which will be easier to quit if you have time on your side—in other words, before pregnancy puts the heat on. It also means cutting back on the following:

PREPREGNANCY DIET

▼ ▼ ▼

So what should you eat when you're trying to conceive? It's simple. Follow The Pregnancy Diet outlined in Chapter Five (minus those extra 300 calories, and aim for only three calcium servings and two protein servings daily) and have fun making a baby!

Alcohol. There are a couple of reasons to consider cutting way down on—or better still, cutting out—alcohol now, before you're drinking for two. First, since alcohol is unsafe when you're expecting, you'll have to give it up anyway once you conceive. But since you may not know exactly when conception will take place, you could end up wining (or cocktailing) your way through the early weeks of pregnancy without even realizing it. Second, if you're a regular drinker, it may be easier for you to cut down gradually before cutting out alcohol completely; starting now gives you a chance to slow down on consumption before having to halt it entirely. And perhaps most important, drinking—especially heavy drinking—can lower your fertility and that of your partner, making conception itself more elusive.

Caffeine. If your idea of a cup of coffee is a twenty ounce espresso drink (and especially if you can't get through your day without several of them), now's a good time to start cutting down, for a couple of reasons.

wisdom of the ages?

Believe it or not, those old wives even have a system worked out for selecting your baby's sex—and, as those tales tell it, it's as easy as selecting the right menu for dinner. In the market for a baby girl? Stop at the market for foods high in calcium and magnesium, such as yogurt, nuts, and green, leafy vegetables. Have your heart set on a boy? Go bananas over foods high in potassium, such as fish, meat, apricots, and of course, bananas.

In case you're wondering, scientists have yet to verify that your baby's sex can be determined by your diet, and it's unlikely they ever will. Still, in all fairness to old wives everywhere, it's also true this system is likely to have a 50 percent success rate. (Actually slightly better if you're trying for a boy, since 105 boys are born for every 100 girls.)

KICK THE COLA HABIT

▼ ▼ ▼

Are you a cola junkie? Now that you're trying for a baby, it's time to cut back on the amount of sugar-sweetened cola you drink. That's because drinking just a few servings (more than five) of sugary cola per week now—while you're trying to conceive—significantly raises your risk of developing gestational diabetes during pregnancy. So can the cola and toast your growing family with a nice, cold glass of water.

First, more than three to four cups of coffee a day has been linked to decreased fertility. (Though it's unclear whether it's the coffee that causes the fertility problems, or the stressful lifestyle that often accompanies a four-cup-a-day habit.) Second, most practitioners advise limiting the amount of caffeine you get while you're pregnant—usually to about two cups of coffee a day, or the equivalent (see page 175). Slowing down on consumption now will spare you any withdrawal symptoms you might encounter later when you actually are pregnant (and when early pregnancy fatigue, morning sickness, and other symptoms are more than enough for one woman to handle).

Getting Weight Under Control

IS YOUR WEIGHT WHERE YOU WANT IT to be? Being significantly under- or overweight is never in your body's best interest. Before pregnancy, either can reduce your chances of actually becoming pregnant; during pregnancy either can be responsible for a number of complications (see pages 44 to 45). Being overweight before and during early pregnancy comes with a particularly long list of drawbacks, including an increased risk of gestational diabetes and pregnancy-induced hypertension, a longer labor, and C-section delivery. What's more, newborns whose mothers were obese during pregnancy are more likely to have heart defects and to be obese themselves by four years old.

Your best bet is to get your weight under control before you become pregnant (gaining weight if you're underweight, or gradually losing weight if you're overweight). If getting closer to your target weight before conception isn't practical, ask your practitioner to help devise (or recommend a nutritionist who can help devise) a pregnancy eating plan that takes into account your individual needs.

PART TWO

COOKING WELL

What makes a pregnancy-perfect recipe? Though you can open up any cookbook and boil, fry, roast, grill, sauté, bake, or braise away, it's likely that many standard recipes are underperformers when it comes to pregnancy nutrition—because they're high in the wrong kinds of fat, low in the right kinds of vitamins and minerals, or just heavy on sugar and refined carbs. Chances are, even the healthiest recipes in your repertoire might need some fiddling to fit the pregnancy-perfect profile.

Luckily, in the chapters that follow you'll find recipes for dishes that are carefully designed to provide all the nutrients you need to feed yourself and your baby well—and all the good taste you want so you can enjoy yourself while you're at it.

Are you craving those comfort foods that your mom used to make? You'll find plenty to take comfort in. Or are your tastes distinctly grown-up these days? There are dishes to satisfy the most contemporary palate. Favor international flavors? Send your taste buds globe-trotting from Mexico to Milan to the East and back? Like to veg out in the kitchen? You'll find many ways to go meatless. Got a sweet tooth that won't quit? Discover cakes, cobblers, and a host of amazing muffins that will allow you to have your healthy desserts and eat them, too.

Best of all, each and every recipe fits the pregnancy profile exactly, which means you'll get the right bal-ance of the Daily Dozen nutrients wrapped neatly (and deliciously) in your favorite dishes. And most of the recipes can be prepared in fewer than twenty minutes (many in only five), giving you the best nutrition without forcing you to spend hours in the kitchen (an especially good thing when nausea is leading you out of the kitchen and into the bathroom).

Eating for two, but cooking for more? These recipes were definitely developed with the very special needs of a pregnant diner in mind, which explains why you'll see many dishes featuring pregnant-centric ingredients, such as ginger (to quiet a queasy tummy), and plenty of red bell peppers and mangoes (for their off-the-charts levels of vitamins A and C) and salmon (omega-3 fatty acids, baby!). But you definitely don't have to be pregnant to enjoy these dishes. Expectant fathers and siblings (and unexpectant guests of all ages) will find them a treat to eat, too.

Breakfast

Mom said it first and best (and most often, probably repeating it every time you tried to sneak out to the school bus without your cereal, toast, and OJ): Nothing starts the day off like a good breakfast. And that's especially true now that you're on your way to being a mom yourself. A healthy breakfast will ensure that both you and your baby will start the day off right. Plus, it can mean the difference between a day filled with nausea, heartburn, and fatigue and a day filled with . . . well, less nausea, heartburn, and fatigue. Still sneaking out the door without breakfast these days? Whether you're a breakfast phobic or time challenged, the recipes in this chapter are tempting and quick enough to lure you back to the table. From a quick Mellow Yellow Omelet and a sumptuous Tomato and Roasted Red Pepper Frittata to portable Breakfast Burritos and Stuffed French Toast, you'll have no problem braking for breakfast. Having trouble keeping that nutritious breakfast down? Try drizzling Gingered Pancake Syrup on Whole Wheat Buttermilk Pancakes, on yogurt and cottage cheese, or on your fingers!

Mellow Yellow Omelet

An egg-ceptionally nutritious way to start your morning, this omelet packs a healthy punch of protein, vitamins, and flavor. Sweet yellow bell pepper, mushrooms, and Swiss cheese combine to create a satisfying one-dish breakfast or brunch, or even a light supper.

1½ teaspoons olive oil
½ medium-size yellow bell pepper,
    thinly sliced
¼ cup sliced white button mushrooms,
    wiped clean
1 scallion, white part only, trimmed
    and sliced
Pinch of dried tarragon
2 large eggs
Salt and black pepper
2 slices Swiss cheese
    (about 1½ ounces total)

1. Heat ½ teaspoon olive oil in an 8-inch skillet over medium heat. Add the bell pepper, mushrooms, scallion, and tarragon and cook until tender, 2 to 3 minutes. Remove the vegetables, leaving some of the liquid in the skillet. Set the vegetables aside.

2. Place the eggs in a small bowl and add a pinch each of salt and black pepper and whisk to mix.

3. Heat the remaining 1 teaspoon of olive oil in the skillet over medium heat. Pour the egg mixture into the skillet and increase the heat to high. Once the eggs begin to set on the bottom, gently lift the edge to let the uncooked egg run underneath.

4. Cook the eggs until they are set, about 3 minutes, then place the Swiss cheese on top. Spoon the cooked vegetables onto one half of the omelet. Using a broad spatula fold the other half of the omelet over the filling. Slide the omelet onto a plate and serve hot.

SERVES 1

Nutrition Info
1 PORTION PROVIDES:

Protein: 1 serving

Calcium: 1 serving

Vitamin C: 2 servings

Other fruits and vegetables: ½ serving

Fat: ½ serving

MORE 'EGG'CELLENT FILLINGS

▼ ▼ ▼

Any combination of vegetables (or fruit, if veggies make you queasy) can be folded into an omelet. It's not only a delicious way to start your day but a great chance to get a head start on those Daily Dozen servings. Don't even have ten minutes to spare in the morning? Use last night's cooked vegetables as this morning's omelet filling. Here are some other yummy ways to fill an omelet.

MARGHERITE PLUS MORE OMELET: Chopped tomato, spinach, or kale (cooked, fresh, or frozen that has been thawed and drained well), chopped fresh basil or dried basil, grated Parmesan cheese, and shredded mozzarella cheese

RED, WHITE, AND GREEN OMELET: Chopped tomato, grated Parmesan cheese, steamed asparagus, and fresh dill

BROCCOLI AND CHEDDAR OMELET: Cooked broccoli florets and grated sharp cheddar cheese

CHEDDAR AND FRUIT OMELET: Sliced cheddar cheese and thinly sliced ripe pear or apple

BANANA SWISS OMELET: Shredded Swiss cheese and sliced ripe, but firm, banana—as odd as this combination sounds, it's really quite tasty

Diner Eggs

Home fries and eggs rolled into one, minus the greasy spoon heartburn—plus, you get an added healthy does of vitamin A from the red bell pepper.

1½ teaspoons olive oil
2 small cooked red potatoes,
    with their skin, diced (about ¼ cup;
    see box on page 253)
½ small onion, chopped
¾ teaspoons fresh thyme leaves,
    or ¼ teaspoon dried thyme

Salt and black pepper
2 large eggs
½ medium-size red bell pepper,
    diced
¼ cup finely shredded cheddar cheese
    or Monterey Jack cheese

1. Heat the olive oil in an 8-inch skillet over medium heat. Add the potatoes, onion, and thyme to the skillet and cook until browned, about 4 minutes, stirring occasionally. Season with salt and pepper to taste.

2. Meanwhile, place the eggs in a small bowl and whisk. When the potatoes and onion are browned, add the bell pepper to the skillet and cook until slightly softened, about 1 minute. Pour the eggs into the skillet but do not stir them. Lower the heat to low and cook until cooked through, about 3 minutes.

3. Sprinkle the cheese over the eggs and serve.

SERVES 1

FROM THE TEST KITCHEN **LOOKING TO SCORE** another yellow vegetable serving with your Diner Eggs? Substitute sweet potato for the red potatoes. Want something more adventurous to toss into your morning skillet? Try any of the following (depending, of course, on your tastes and your morning nausea status): diced apple, chopped avocado, diced tomatoes, steamed broccoli florets, sliced mushrooms, or jalapeño peppers.

IT'S NO YOLK

▼ ▼ ▼

Cholesterol's not a worry for most pregnant women. But if you're in the market for a particularly low-calorie omelet (or you're feeding someone who's watching his or her cholesterol), just leave out the yolks. To make a basic egg white omelet, whisk four egg whites with two teaspoons of water. Then cook them as you would a regular omelet and add your choice of fillings.

Nutrition Info

1 PORTION PROVIDES:

Protein: 1 serving

Calcium: 1 serving

Vitamin C: 2½ servings

Green leafy and yellow vegetables and fruits: 1 serving

Other fruits and vegetables: ½ serving

Fat: ½ serving

Tomato and Roasted Red Pepper Frittata

A brunch-worthy dish that cooks up in minutes—especially if you use leftover or store-bought roasted red peppers.

4 large eggs
4 teaspoons milk
1/2 cup grated Parmesan cheese or
   sharp provolone cheese
1 clove garlic, minced
Salt and black pepper
2 small tomatoes, seeded and
   chopped
1 tablespoon chopped fresh basil or
   1 teaspoon dried basil
1 tablespoon olive oil
1/2 cup coarsely chopped roasted red
   bell pepper (about 1 large pepper;
   leftover or from a jar)
1 tablespoon chopped fresh parsley,
   or 1 teaspoon dried parsley (optional)

1. Place the eggs, milk, cheese, and garlic in a medium-size bowl. Add a pinch each of salt and black pepper and whisk to mix. Add the tomatoes and basil and stir gently to combine.

2. Heat the olive oil in a medium-size skillet over medium-low heat. Pour the egg mixture into the skillet and cook until nearly set, 5 to 8 minutes, lifting the edge to let the uncooked egg run underneath.

3. Sprinkle the roasted red pepper on top of the frittata and cook until completely set, 1 to 2 minutes longer.

4. Slide the frittata onto a plate and sprinkle the parsley on top before serving.

SERVES 2

FROM THE TEST KITCHEN

HAVE SOME leftover steamed broccoli from last night's dinner? Toss it in the skillet along with the eggs and buy yourself an extra serving of green leafies and C.

Nutrition Info

1 PORTION PROVIDES:

Protein: 1 serving

Calcium: 1 serving

Vitamin C: 2 1/2 servings

Green leafy and yellow vegetables and fruits: 1 1/2 servings

Fat: 1/2 serving

Breakfast Burritos

The ultimate in portable breakfasts, a Breakfast Burrito brimming with avocado, tomato, black beans, eggs, and salsa can find its way to your mouth almost as quickly as the fast food variety (more quickly if there's a wait at the drive-thru) but contains much less fat and is much more nutritious.

Olive oil cooking spray
¼ cup canned black beans,
   rinsed and drained
2 tablespoons store-bought
   tomato-based salsa
1 scallion, both white and
   light green parts, trimmed
   and thinly sliced
1 tablespoon chopped fresh cilantro
2 large eggs, lightly beaten
1 whole wheat tortilla or wrap
   (each 12 inches in diameter)
¼ medium-size avocado (optional),
   preferably Hass, peeled and
   chopped
½ plum tomato, seeded and
   chopped
¼ cup shredded cheddar, Monterey
   Jack, or Colby cheese

1. Coat a medium-size skillet with olive oil cooking spray and heat over medium heat. Add the black beans, salsa, scallion, and cilantro and cook until heated through, about 2 minutes. Add the eggs and cook, stirring gently, until completely set, about 3 minutes. Remove from the heat.

2. Place the tortilla on microwave-safe paper towels and heat for 15 seconds in the microwave.

3. Place the tortilla on a work surface or on plates. Spoon the egg and black bean mixture in the center. Sprinkle the avocado, if using, tomato, and cheese on top.

4. Fold the top and bottom of the tortilla into the center. Then, starting at one side, roll up the tortillas, enclosing the filling. Wrap a burrito in aluminum foil if you'll be taking it with you.

SERVES 1

Nutrition Info

1 PORTION PROVIDES:

Protein: 1 serving

Calcium: 1 serving

Other fruits and vegetables: 1 serving

Whole grains and legumes:
  2½ servings

Iron from the beans

BEANS AREN'T EXACTLY what the doctor (or the guy who sits next to you at work) ordered? If tummy troubles have you avoiding gas makers, skip the beans and toss in ½ cup of cooked edamame (soybeans); you'll be getting some additional protein in the bargain. For that matter, you can roll up just about any steamed or sautéed veggie (think last night's leftovers) in a breakfast burrito.

Baby's Big Bite

Egg on a muffin without the McFat, but with plenty of grains and calcium. Pack one of these quick and convenient babies to go tomorrow morning.

1 whole grain English muffin, split,
   or 2 slices whole grain bread
1 tomato, sliced
2 slices Swiss cheese or cheddar
   cheese (about 1 to 1½ ounces total)
1 large egg
1 tablespoon milk
1½ teaspoons olive oil

1. Toast the English muffin.

2. Place the muffin halves split side up on a microwave-safe plate and arrange half of the tomato slices on each. Top each half with a slice of cheese. Microwave on high power until the cheese is slightly melted, about 30 seconds.

3. Place the egg and milk in a small bowl and whisk until well combined. Heat the olive oil in a small skillet over medium-high heat. Add the egg mixture and cook, stirring gently, until completely set, about 1 minute.

4. Spoon the scrambled egg on a muffin half and top with the other half. If you are packing the muffin to go, wrap it in aluminum foil.

SERVES 1

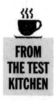

EXTRA HUNGRY this morning? Heat diced turkey breast or cooked crumbled vegetarian "sausage," then add them to the egg while it cooks.

Nutrition Info
1 PORTION PROVIDES:

Protein: 1 serving

Calcium: 1 serving

Vitamin C: ½ serving

Whole grains and legumes: 2 servings

Fat: ½ serving

Stuffed French Toast

Want a sandwich that eats like breakfast (only neater)? Slices of whole-grain bread stuffed with fresh peaches or banana and fruit preserves hit the spot when you're craving something sweet.

1 tablespoon almond butter or
    soy butter (see Note)
2 slices whole grain bread
2 teaspoons all-fruit preserves
    (any flavor)
1/2 fresh yellow peach or banana,
    very thinly sliced
1 large egg
1/4 cup milk
1/2 teaspoon vanilla extract
1/2 teaspoon ground cinnamon
1 1/2 teaspoons canola oil
    or butter

1. Spread 1½ teaspoons of the almond butter on one side of each slice of bread. Spread the preserves over one buttered slice of bread. Arrange the peach slices over the preserves, then top with the other slice of bread to make a sandwich.

2. Place the egg, milk, vanilla, and cinnamon in a shallow bowl and whisk to mix.

3. Place the almond butter and fruit sandwich in the milk mixture and let soak for 1 minute on each side.

4. Heat the oil in a small skillet over medium-high heat. Cook the sandwich until browned, 2 to 3 minutes per side.

5. Cut the sandwich in half and serve warm. Wrap it in aluminum foil if you're taking it to go.

SERVES 1

NOTE: Both almond butter and soy butter are available at health food stores. If neither you nor the baby's dad has a history of allergies, you can substitute peanut butter.

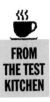

FROM THE TEST KITCHEN **NOT IN THE MOOD** for sweet? Make a savory Stuffed French Toast instead. Substitute turkey breast (protein) and Swiss cheese (calcium), or Swiss and thinly sliced tomato, for the almond butter and fruit.

Nutrition Info

1 PORTION PROVIDES:

Protein: 1/2 serving

Green leafy and yellow vegetables and fruits: 1/2 serving if made with a peach

Other fruits and vegetables: 1/2 serving if made with a banana

Whole grains and legumes: 2 servings

Fat: 1/2 serving

Any Day Breakfast Parfait

G etting your Daily Dozen doesn't get any easier than this. Or any cooler—a nice plus if you're carrying through a long, hot summer. This parfait teams fresh fruit, yogurt, and granola for a refreshing breakfast at home or on the go.

1 ripe yellow peach or nectarine,
   or $^1/_2$ mango, coarsely chopped
1 cup yogurt, any flavor
$^1/_2$ cup granola
$^1/_2$ cup blueberries or sliced
   strawberries
Mint sprig (optional)

Arrange the chopped peach, yogurt, granola, and berries in alternating layers in a parfait glass or stemmed glass. Top with a mint sprig, if desired. Want to take the parfait with you? Skip the parfait glass and layer the ingredients in a plastic container or cup.

SERVES 1

FROM THE TEST KITCHEN

ANY FRUIT THAT SUITS your fancy—or fills your fridge—can be layered into a yogurt parfait. Try raspberries, blackberries, plums, cherries, pineapple, or bananas, too. If winter leaves you with slim pickings in the produce department, opt for frozen fruit—it's at least as nutritious and some are even organic—but thaw and drain it first. And there's always room for some chopped dried fruit, or crunchy freeze-dried fruit, especially when it's extra nutritious, like dried apricots. Toasted nuts make a great toppng, too.

Nutrition Info

1 PORTION PROVIDES:

Protein: $^1/_2$ serving

Calcium: $1^1/_2$ servings

Vitamin C: 1 serving if made with strawberries; 2 if made with strawberries and mango

Green leafy and yellow vegetables and fruits: 1 serving

Other fruits and vegetables: 1 serving if made with blueberries

Whole grains and legumes: 1 serving

Fruit-and-Oat Meal

Turn same-old oatmeal into a crunchy, chewy, nutrition-packed treat. A mixture of grains, dried apricots, and nuts makes this a satisfying bowlful.

¼ cup water, or ¼ cup apple juice,
   if you like your oatmeal supersweet
1 cup milk, plus milk for serving
½ cup old-fashioned rolled oats
6 dried apricot halves, chopped
1 tablespoon oat bran, wheat germ,
   or flaxseed
Pinch of ground cinnamon
1 tablespoon chopped nuts, such as
   walnuts, pecans, or almonds
Low-fat vanilla yogurt (optional),
   for serving

1. Place the water in a small saucepan over medium heat and let come to a boil. Add 1 cup milk, and cook until just heated through, about 2 minutes. Stir in the oats, apricots, oat bran, and cinnamon and let come to a slow boil. Reduce the heat to medium-low and cook, stirring occasionally, until the oatmeal is thick enough for your taste, about 5 minutes.

2. Remove the oatmeal from the heat and add the nuts. Serve with vanilla yogurt or more milk, if desired.

SERVES 1

FROM THE TEST KITCHEN

HAVING A LAZY MORNING? Preparing oatmeal takes no time at all if you pop it into the microwave. Place the milk, water, oatmeal, oat bran, apricots, and cinnamon in a microwave-safe bowl. Microwave on high power until thickened, 2½ to 3 minutes (if your microwave does not have a turntable, rotate the bowl a quarter turn after about 1½ minutes). Add the nuts and stir well before serving.

Got a sweet tooth that just won't quit? Sweeten the oatmeal to taste with Splenda, honey, or a spoonful of all-fruit preserves.

Nutrition Info

1 PORTION PROVIDES:

Protein: ½ serving, more if you use walnuts and wheat germ

Calcium: 1 serving, more if you use yogurt

Green leafy and yellow vegetables and fruits: 1 serving

Other fruits and vegetables: ½ serving if made with apple juice

Whole grains and legumes: 1½ servings

Whole Wheat Buttermilk Pancakes

Pancakes made with only white flour just can't stack up to these. Plus, you won't have to give up fluffiness for nutrition—these pancakes have plenty of both. Make them sweet or spicy to suit your taste.

1¼ cups whole wheat flour
½ cup all-purpose white flour
3 tablespoons ground flaxseed,
    oat bran, or wheat germ
1 teaspoon baking powder
1 teaspoon baking soda
Splenda (optional), to taste
1 teaspoon cinnamon (optional)
Pinch of nutmeg (optional)
Pinch of salt (optional)
1¾ cups buttermilk
¼ cup milk
½ cup white grape juice concentrate
    or honey
2 large eggs
1 teaspoon vanilla extract
2 tablespoons plus 2 teaspoons
    canola oil

1. Place the whole wheat and white flour, flaxseed, baking powder, baking soda, Splenda, if using, and the cinnamon, nutmeg, and/or salt, if using, in a medium-size bowl and stir to combine.

2. Place the buttermilk, milk, grape juice concentrate, eggs, vanilla, and 2 tablespoons of oil in another bowl and whisk to mix. Pour the buttermilk mixture into the flour mixture and beat just until smooth. If possible, let the batter rest for

PANCAKE ADD-INS

▼ ▼ ▼

Make basic whole wheat pancakes anything but basic by tossing in:

- Finely chopped apple or pear

- Chopped banana

- Blueberries—fresh, thawed frozen, dried, or freeze-dried

- Dried or freeze-dried cranberries or cherries

- Raisins

- Chopped dried apricots or peaches

- Chopped dried pineapple or mango

- Chopped pecans, almonds, or walnuts

up to 30 minutes at room temperature before cooking the pancakes.

3. Heat the remaining 2 teaspoons of oil in a 9-inch skillet over medium-high

QUICK FRUIT SYRUPS

▼ ▼ ▼

Feeling fruity? Warm some all-fruit preserves in the microwave on medium-high power, then serve the preserves syrup-style over pancakes. If you like your syrup thinner, add some fruit juice after heating the preserves.

heat. Cook the pancakes two at a time, using ¼ cup of the batter per pancake, until the batter bubbles on top and the pancakes are firm on the bottom, about 3 minutes. Turn the pancakes over and continue cooking until the second side is brown, about 3 minutes. Repeat with the remaining batter.

4. Serve the pancakes warm. The buttermilk pancakes can be frozen for up to 2 weeks. Let them cool completely, then wrap them in a single layer or individually in aluminum foil. To reheat, unwrap a pancake and microwave it on high power for 2 minutes or heat it in a 350°F oven for 10 minutes.

MAKES ABOUT 12 PANCAKES

Nutrition Info
1 PORTION (ABOUT 3 PANCAKES) PROVIDES:

Protein: 1/2 serving

Calcium: 1/2 serving

Whole grains and legumes: 2 servings

Fat: 1/2 serving

Ginger-Blueberry Whole Wheat Pancakes

F eeling a little green this morning? Try some blues. These pancakes, infused with ginger and packed with blueberries and whole wheat, make a soothing and nutritious morning meal. What's better still is that these pancakes are surprisingly light—even with the whole wheat flour.

1½ cups whole wheat flour
1 teaspoon ground ginger
1 teaspoon ground cinnamon
Pinch of ground allspice
1 teaspoon baking soda
1 cup apple juice concentrate or
    white grape juice concentrate
⅓ cup milk
3 tablespoons butter, melted
2 medium-size eggs
1½ cups fresh or frozen (unthawed)
    blueberries, or 1 cup freeze-dried
2 teaspoons canola oil
Gingered Pancake Syrup (recipe follows)

1. Place the whole wheat flour, ginger, cinnamon, allspice, and baking soda in a large bowl and stir to combine. Set aside.

2. Place the apple juice concentrate, milk, butter, and eggs in a medium-size bowl, and whisk to blend. Add the juice mixture to the flour mixture and whisk until blended. Add the blueberries and stir gently to combine.

3. Heat the canola oil in a 9-inch skillet over medium-high heat. Cook the pancakes 2 at a time, using ¼ cup of the batter per pancake, until they are golden brown on the bottom, 2 to 3 minutes. Turn the pancakes over and continue cooking until the second side is golden brown, about 2 minutes. Repeat with remaining batter.

4. Serve the pancakes warm, with the Gingered Pancake Syrup. The ginger-blueberry pancakes can be frozen for up to 2 weeks. Let them cool completely, then wrap them in a single layer or individually in aluminum foil. To reheat, unwrap a pancake and microwave it on high power for 2 minutes or heat it in a 350°F oven for 10 minutes.

MAKES ABOUT 12 PANCAKES

Nutrition Info

1 PORTION (ABOUT 4 PANCAKES) PROVIDES:

Vitamin C: 1 serving if made with vitamin C–fortified white grape juice concentrate

Other fruits and vegetables: ½ serving

Whole grains and legumes: 2 servings

Fat: 1 serving

Gingered Pancake Syrup

Spicy and sweet, this syrup is tops for pancakes. But don't stop there; you'll want to drizzle it over French toast, yogurt, and fresh fruit, too.

1 cup pomegranate juice or
    blueberry juice (see Note) or
    apple juice
1/2 cup orange juice
1/2 cup white grape juice
    concentrate
1 piece (2 inches) fresh ginger,
    peeled and thinly sliced
1 teaspoon vanilla extract
2 teaspoons cornstarch

1. Place the pomegranate and orange juice, grape juice concentrate, ginger, and vanilla in a small saucepan over medium-high heat and let come to a boil. Reduce the heat and let simmer until slightly reduced, about 10 minutes.

2. Place the cornstarch in a small bowl, add 3 tablespoons of the pomegranate juice mixture, and whisk to mix, then stir into the remaining pomegranate juice mixture. Increase the heat to high and let the syrup come to a boil. Reduce the heat and let the syrup simmer until slightly thickened, about 3 minutes.

3. Remove the syrup from the heat and let cool to room temperature. If you like, pour the syrup through a strainer set over a bowl to remove the slices of ginger. The syrup can be refrigerated, covered, for up to 1 week. Let it come to room temperature or warm it slightly before serving.

MAKES 1 CUP

NOTE: Pomegranate and blueberry juice are available in the refrigerated section of supermarkets and health food stores.

Nutrition Info

1 PORTION (1/4 CUP) PROVIDES:

Vitamin C: 1 serving

Other fruits and vegetables: 1/2 serving

Salmon Hash Patties

A n omega-3-rich twist on a brunch classic combines salmon with potatoes and bell peppers to form patties worth sinking your teeth into. Using canned fish shaves time off your prep, plus it rewards you with a calcium serving (mash the salmon, bones and all—you won't taste them).

1 can (14³/₄ ounces) pink salmon,
   drained and mashed with a fork
2 medium-size cooked russet potatoes
   (see box on this page), peeled and
   diced
1 medium-size yellow bell pepper, diced
¹/₂ medium-size green bell pepper, diced
4 scallions, white parts only, trimmed
   and thinly sliced
1 large egg
1¹/₂ teaspoons chopped fresh dill
Grated zest of 1 lemon
2 tablespoons olive oil

1. Place the salmon, potatoes, yellow and green bell peppers, scallions, egg, dill, and zest in a mixing bowl and stir to mix.

2. Divide the mixture into 4 equal portions and shape each into a patty that's about ½ inch thick.

3. Heat the olive oil in a 9-inch skillet over medium-high heat. Add the salmon patties and cook until golden brown and heated through, about 4 minutes per side. Insert a knife in the center of a salmon patty; if the knife feels hot when removed, the patty is done. Serve hot.

SERVES 4

HOT POTATO

▼ ▼ ▼

I f you don't have any leftover cooked potatoes for these recipes, use the microwave. Dice raw potatoes and place them in a microwave-safe dish. Add 1 tablespoon of low-sodium broth for each potato. Cover the dish with microwave-safe plastic wrap, folding back one corner to allow the steam to escape. Microwave the potatoes on high power until cooked through, 3 to 4 minutes. If your microwave does not have a turntable, rotate the dish a quarter turn after 1¹/₂ minutes.

Nutrition Info

1 PORTION (1 PATTY) PROVIDES:

Protein: 1 serving

Calcium: 1 serving if the salmon has bones

Vitamin C: 2 servings

Other fruits and vegetables: ¹/₂ serving

Fat: ¹/₂ serving

Power Breakfast Bars

These pack a lot more nutrition than the bars you buy. With a side of yogurt or cheese, they're the perfect take-along breakfast or snack.

8 tablespoons (1 stick) butter, melted
¹⁄₄ cup Splenda, fructose, or brown sugar
³⁄₄ cup white grape juice concentrate
2 large eggs
1 teaspoon vanilla extract
2¹⁄₂ cups old-fashioned rolled oats
1 cup whole wheat flour
¹⁄₂ teaspoon baking soda
1 teaspoon ground cinnamon
2 tablespoons wheat germ, oat bran,
    or ground flaxseed
1 cup chopped walnuts or almonds
1 cup chopped raisins, or 1 cup mixed
    dried fruit, such as chopped apricots,
    blueberries, cranberries, and/or
    cherries

1. Preheat the oven to 375°F.

2. Place the butter, Splenda, grape juice concentrate, eggs, and vanilla in a mixing bowl and beat until well mixed.

3. Place the oats, whole wheat flour, baking soda, cinnamon, wheat germ, walnuts, and raisins in another mixing bowl and stir to mix. Add the oat mixture to the butter mixture and stir until thoroughly combined.

4. Line a baking sheet with parchment paper. Shape heaping tablespoons of the batter into bars that are roughly 2 by 4 inches, arranging them about 1¹⁄₂ inches apart on the baking sheet. Bake the bars

until the bottoms are brown and the tops are golden brown, about 15 minutes. For crisper bars, reduce the oven temperature to 200°F and let the bars bake 10 minutes longer.

5. Let the bars cool completely before sliding them off the cookie sheet. The bars can be stored in an airtight container for 3 days at room temperature or frozen for up to 1 month.

MAKES 20 BARS

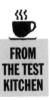

FROM THE TEST KITCHEN   THE POWER BREAKFAST BARS crumble when warm but firm up as they cool, so they travel great. Pop one or two in your bag for some extra energy to go.

Nutrition Info

1 PORTION (2 BARS) PROVIDES:

Protein: ¹⁄₂ serving

Vitamin C: ¹⁄₂ serving

Green leafy and yellow fruits and vegetables: ¹⁄₂ serving if made with apricots

Other fruits and vegetables: ¹⁄₂ serving

Whole grains and legumes: 1¹⁄₂ servings

Fat: 1 serving

Muffins

Mad about muffins but wondering whether there's a place for these sweet breakfast treats now that you're trying to eat healthier? Good news! While many store-bought or bakery muffins may be lightweights when it comes to nutrition (and heavyweights when it comes to calories), the sugar-free muffins in this chapter are tasty and nutritious. Start a queasy morning with a Ginger and Carrot Muffin. Spice up a snack with a Pumpkin Pie Muffin or linger over brunch with a Triple Blueberry Muffin. Whatever flavor you're craving, there's a muffin here for you.

So many muffin cravings, but so little time? Bake a few batches at once, and freeze the extras for munching later on. And don't stop with breakfast. A wholesome muffin (especially when teamed with a piece of cheese) makes the perfect pick-me-up when your blood sugar starts to take a midmorning or midafternoon dive. And, with a glass of milk, there's no better bedtime snack.

Triple Blueberry Muffins

Triple the blueberries—preserves, frozen, and dried—means triple the taste in these moist muffins. The addition of old-fashioned rolled oats gives this classic breakfast favorite a chewier texture and nuttier taste, plus some extra fiber.

¾ cup whole wheat flour
¼ cup ground flaxseed or oat bran
2 teaspoons baking powder
1 teaspoon baking soda
1½ cups old-fashioned rolled oats
1 cup white grape juice concentrate
½ cup all-fruit blueberry preserves
2 large eggs, lightly beaten
3 tablespoons canola oil
2 teaspoons vanilla extract
¾ cup frozen blueberries
½ cup dried or freeze-dried blueberries

1. Preheat oven to 400°F. Line a standard-size 12-cup muffin tin with paper liners.

2. Place the whole wheat flour, flaxseed, baking powder, and baking soda in a mixing bowl and stir to mix. Add the oats and stir until well combined.

3. Place the grape juice concentrate, blueberry preserves, eggs, oil, and vanilla in another mixing bowl and stir to mix well. Add the blueberry mixture to the flour mixture and stir gently just until thoroughly blended; be careful not to overmix.

4. Gently fold in the frozen and dried blueberries.

5. Spoon the batter into the prepared muffin tin, dividing it evenly among the muffin cups.

6. Bake the muffins until a toothpick inserted into the center of a muffin comes out clean, about 20 minutes.

7. Transfer the muffins to a wire rack and let cool completely. The muffins can be stored in an airtight container for 3 days or individually wrapped in plastic wrap and frozen for 3 months.

MAKES 12 MUFFINS

Nutrition Info
1 PORTION (1 MUFFIN) PROVIDES:

Vitamin C: ½ serving

Whole grains and legumes: ½ serving plus

FROM THE TEST KITCHEN

NOT FEELING BLUE? Make triple cherry muffins instead. Just substitute cherry preserves for the blueberry, chopped frozen cherries for the frozen blueberries, and dried cherries for the dried ones. Or make cranberry and apricot muffins using apricot preserves, ½ cup unsweetened frozen or fresh cranberries (if they're in season), and ½ cup each chopped dried apricots and dried cranberries.

MUFFINS NOW, MUFFINS LATER

▼ ▼ ▼

Are twelve muffins eleven muffins too many? Fortunately, the muffins you bake today can be enjoyed tomorrow and next week—and even for months to come. To store muffins at room temperature, place them in an airtight container or zipper-lock bag; they'll keep for up to three days. Still haven't polished them off? Wrap each muffin individually in plastic wrap or aluminum foil and freeze them for up to three months. To thaw, simply take a muffin out of the freezer and allow it to come to room temperature. Prefer a muffin that tastes fresh out of the oven? Wrap the thawed muffin loosely in foil and place it in a preheated 350°F oven for 7 to 10 minutes until it's warmed through.

Banana Muffins

Have some very ripe bananas that you don't know what to do with? Here's a delicious way to put them to good use. You'll go ape over these healthy banana muffins, especially once you discover their sweet surprise: a spoonful of strawberry preserves in the center of each.

2 medium-size ripe bananas,
   cut into chunks
1 cup white grape juice concentrate
3 tablespoons canola oil
2 large eggs, lightly beaten
2 teaspoons vanilla extract
1 cup whole wheat flour
1/4 cup ground flaxseed or oat bran
1/2 cup old-fashioned rolled oats
1 teaspoon ground cinnamon
1/4 teaspoon ground nutmeg
   (optional)
2 teaspoons baking powder

1 teaspoon baking soda
1/2 cup chopped toasted pecans
   (see page 272)
1/2 cup all-fruit strawberry
   preserves

1. Preheat oven to 400°F. Line a standard-size 12-cup muffin tin with paper liners.

2. Place the bananas, grape juice concentrate, oil, eggs, and vanilla in a blender or food processor and blend until smooth.

GOING FRUITY? GETTING NUTTY?

▼ ▼ ▼

Add an additional 1/4 cup of all-fruit preserves (any flavor) to any muffin batter, or better still, cut baked muffins in half and slather them with the preserves. Are you tired of raisins? Explore the dried fruits and freeze-dried fruits for more exciting options. Most supermarkets carry figs, pears, apples, peaches, pineapple, cranberries, cherries, blueberries—you get the picture. And don't forget to go nutty—add 1/2 cup of whatever chopped nuts you like (almonds, hazelnuts, pecans, walnuts, to name a few) to the muffin batter. Toast them first for even more flavor (see page 272 for toasting tips).

FLOUR POWER

▼ ▼ ▼

Any muffin batter can benefit from the addition of omega-3-rich (and constipation-combating) ground flaxseed. Substitute ¼ cup of flaxseed for ¼ cup of flour. If it's fiber you're looking for, substitute ¼ cup of wheat bran for ¼ cup of flour (although flax will give you the same results, more nutritiously). Want a nuttier flavor, protein boost, and some healthy fatty acids? You can use ¼ cup of ground nuts to take the place of ¼ cup of flour. For extra nutrients substitute ¼ cup of wheat germ or oat bran for ¼ cup of flour. For more protein use soy flour in place of up to a third of the flour in your recipe. Want to lighten things up? Substitute ½ cup of unbleached white flour for ¼ cup of the whole wheat flour.

3. Place the whole wheat flour, flaxseed, oats, cinnamon, nutmeg, if using, baking powder, and baking soda in a mixing bowl and stir to mix.

4. Pour the banana mixture over the dry ingredients, and stir gently just until thoroughly blended; be careful not to overmix.

5. Gently fold in the pecans.

6. Spoon the batter into the prepared muffin tin, dividing it evenly among the muffin cups.

7. With your index finger or the back of a spoon, make an indentation in each muffin, and fill each with 2 teaspoons of strawberry preserves.

8. Bake the muffins until a toothpick inserted into the center of a muffin comes out clean, about 20 minutes.

9. Transfer the muffins to a wire rack and let cool completely. The muffins can be stored in an airtight container for 3 days or individually wrapped in plastic wrap and frozen for 3 months.

MAKES 12 MUFFINS

FROM THE TEST KITCHEN

TO MAKE "BERRY GOOD" banana muffins, fold ⅔ cup of dried or dehydrated blueberries, or coarsely chopped dried strawberries, or cherries into the batter instead of the nuts (or be "berry good" and "berry nutty" and include both). Use a matching flavor of all-fruit preserves to top the muffins.

Nutrition Info

1 PORTION (1 MUFFIN) PROVIDES:

Vitamin C: ½ serving

Whole grains and legumes: ½ serving

Ginger and Carrot Muffins

S nappy and nutritious, these muffins also boast enough ginger to quell the queasies. (Taking a whiff of the fresh ginger as you cook may also be soothing.)

1 cup whole wheat flour
¼ cup oat bran
¼ cup ground flaxseed
1 tablespoon ground ginger
1 teaspoon ground cinnamon
½ teaspoon ground cloves
2 teaspoons baking powder
1 teaspoon baking soda
2 large eggs, lightly beaten
4 tablespoons canola oil
1¼ cups white grape juice
    concentrate
2 teaspoons peeled, grated fresh
    ginger
1 teaspoon vanilla extract
1¼ cups grated carrots
¾ cup golden raisins
½ cup chopped toasted walnuts
    (see page 272)

MUFFIN MATH

▼ ▼ ▼

T he recipes in this chapter call for standard-size 12-cup muffin tins. These have muffin cups that are 2 inches in diameter. Of course, if you have two 6-cup muffin tins, you can use those instead.

1. Preheat the oven to 400°F. Line a standard-size 12-cup muffin tin with paper liners.

2. Place the whole wheat flour, oat bran, flaxseed, ground ginger, cinnamon, cloves, baking powder, and baking soda in a mixing bowl and stir to mix.

3. Place the eggs, oil, grape juice concentrate, grated ginger, and vanilla in another mixing bowl and whisk to mix. Add the egg mixture to the flour mixture and stir gently just until the batter is smooth; be careful not to overmix. Gently fold in the carrots, raisins, and walnuts.

4. Spoon the batter into the prepared muffin tin, dividing it evenly among the muffin cups.

5. Bake the muffins until a toothpick inserted into the center of a muffin comes out clean, about 20 minutes.

6. Transfer the muffins to a wire rack and let cool completely. The muffins can be stored in an airtight container for 3 days or individually wrapped in plastic wrap and frozen for 3 months.

MAKES 12 MUFFINS

FROM THE TEST KITCHEN

DON'T LIKE YOUR GINGER quite that snappy? Omit the fresh grated ginger—or leave all the ginger out, and substitute 2 teaspoons of ground cinnamon. Like it even snappier? Increase the grated ginger to 1 tablespoon.

Nutrition Info

1 PORTION (1 MUFFIN) PROVIDES:

Vitamin C: 1/2 serving

Green leafy and yellow vegetables and fruits: 1/2 serving plus

Whole grains and legumes: 1/2 serving

THE ART OF CONCENTRATION

▼ ▼ ▼

Many of the dishes in this book were tested using white grape juice concentrate, which lends a more pronounced sweet flavor—more sugary, less fruity—than other kinds of juice concentrates. It also comes fortified with vitamin C, which means you'll be getting a nutritional bonus that doesn't often come in a muffin or slice of cake. But don't let that stop you from exploring other juice concentrate options.

Experiment with apple juice concentrate, which is still very sweet but much more fruity than white grape juice concentrate. Try blueberry or cherry juice concentrate; these are very sweet, with a very intense flavor. Mango, pineapple, orange, and peach juice concentrates often come combined and add a sweet tanginess to baked goods, fruit desserts, and savory dishes—especially sweet-and-sour and Asian ones.

Pumpkin Pie Muffins

For a little taste of Thanksgiving any time of the year, here's the spicy, sweet taste of your favorite pie in a moist, wholesome muffin.

1 cup whole wheat flour
1/4 cup oat bran
1/4 cup ground flaxseed
2 teaspoons baking powder
1 1/2 teaspoons baking soda
2 teaspoons ground cinnamon
1/4 teaspoon ground ginger
1/4 teaspoon ground cloves
1/4 teaspoon ground nutmeg
3/4 cup solid-pack pumpkin purée
2 large eggs, lightly beaten
3 tablespoons canola oil
1 cup white grape juice concentrate
1/3 cup all-fruit apricot preserves
2 teaspoons vanilla extract
2/3 cup golden raisins or chopped
    dried apricots
1/2 cup toasted chopped walnuts
    (optional; see page 272)

1. Preheat the oven to 400°F. Line a standard-size 12-cup muffin tin with paper liners.

2. Place the whole wheat flour, oat bran, flaxseed, baking powder, baking soda, cinnamon, ginger, cloves, and nutmeg in a mixing bowl and stir to mix.

3. Place the pumpkin, eggs, oil, grape juice concentrate, apricot preserves, and vanilla in another mixing bowl and mix well. Add the pumpkin mixture to the flour mixture, and stir gently just until blended; be careful not to overmix.

4. Gently fold in the raisins and walnuts, if using.

5. Spoon the batter into the prepared muffin tin, dividing it evenly among the muffin cups.

6. Bake the muffins until a toothpick inserted into the center of a muffin comes out clean, about 20 minutes.

7. Transfer the muffins to a wire rack and let cool completely. The muffins can be stored in an airtight container for 3 days or individually wrapped in plastic wrap and frozen for 3 months.

MAKES 12 MUFFINS

Nutrition Info

1 PORTION (1 MUFFIN) PROVIDES:

Vitamin C: 1/2 serving

Green leafy and yellow vegetables and fruits: 1 serving if using raisins; 1 1/2 if using apricots

Whole grains and legumes: 1/2 serving

Raisin Bran Muffins

Sure, all that bran will get things going—but these muffins are so delicious, you'll want to eat them on a regular basis even when you're regular.

1¹/₂ cups unprocessed bran
1 cup whole wheat flour
¹/₂ cup old-fashioned rolled oats
¹/₂ cup ground flaxseed
2 teaspoons ground cinnamon
¹/₂ cup chopped toasted nuts, such as
    walnuts, pecans, or almonds
    (see page 272)
2 teaspoons baking soda
1 teaspoon baking powder
1¹/₂ cups white grape juice concentrate
1¹/₄ cups buttermilk
2 large eggs, slightly beaten
3 tablespoons canola oil
2 teaspoons vanilla extract
³/₄ cup raisins

1. Preheat the oven to 400°F. Line a standard-size 12-cup muffin tin with paper liners.

2. Place the bran, whole wheat flour, rolled oats, flaxseed, cinnamon, nuts, baking soda, and baking powder in a mixing bowl and stir to mix.

3. Place the grape juice concentrate, buttermilk, eggs, oil, and vanilla in another mixing bowl and stir to mix well. Add the grape juice concentrate mixture to the bran mixture and stir gently just until thoroughly blended; be careful not to overmix.

4. Gently fold in the raisins.

5. Spoon the batter into the prepared muffin tin, dividing it evenly among the muffin cups. (You may have extra batter. If so, just bake a few more muffins.)

6. Bake the muffins until a toothpick inserted into the center of a muffin comes out clean, about 20 minutes.

7. Transfer the muffins to a wire rack and let cool completely. The muffins can be stored in an airtight container for 3 days or individually wrapped in plastic wrap and frozen for 3 months.

MAKES AT LEAST 12 MUFFINS

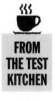

FROM THE TEST KITCHEN

TO PACK EVEN MORE FIBER into the Raisin Bran Muffins, fold in a diced apple or pear along with the raisins.

Nutrition Info

1 PORTION (1 MUFFIN) PROVIDES:

Protein: ¹/₂ serving

Vitamin C: 1 serving

Whole grains and legumes: ¹/₂ serving

JUST CAN'T CONCENTRATE?

▼ ▼ ▼

Juice-concentrate-sweetened treats can generally convert even confirmed sugar addicts, adding a bundle of nutrients in the bargain. But if you're having a hard time convincing your taste buds that juice sweetens like sugar, you can substitute refined sweeteners (such as sugar), honey, or the low-calorie sweetener Splenda for all or part of the juice concentrate in any recipe in this book. You'll still be reaping the benefits of all those whole grains (which might not be included in regular muffin, cake, and cookie recipes). If you want to use honey or another liquid sweetener, you'll need to add a little less (honey is sweeter): ¾ cup for every cup of juice concentrate. Make up the liquid difference (¼ cup in that case) with regular juice. If you're opting for a dry sweetener, you'll also need to replace that amount of liquid in the recipe with another, less sweet, one (milk, buttermilk, or regular apple juice, for instance). Use ¾ cup of dry sweetener for every 1 cup of juice concentrate.

Sandwiches

Lunchtime boredom sending you out for burgers? Stop filling your brown bag with the same old sandwiches. There's a lot more you can put between two slices of bread than turkey and cheese—in fact, sandwiches become even more interesting if you skip traditional bread altogether. So wrap your mouth around a tasty wrap (the perfect take-along lunch, since they're so neat to eat), stuff a pita or tortilla, layer a bagel, or fill a roll, and meet a surprising number of Daily Dozen requirements while you're at it. It's food to go that's good for you.

Chicken Burgers with Mango Relish

These chicken burgers are cheeseburgers with a twist—the cheese is combined with the ground chicken, giving the burgers extra flavor and keeping them moist. Topping the burgers with mango relish as they grill adds an unexpectedly exotic taste. And traditional burgers can't beat this: Each chicken burger contains a hefty serving of vitamin A, compliments of the carrot and mango.

1 pound ground white meat chicken or turkey or lean ground beef
1 cup grated or shredded carrot (packaged or from 1 large carrot)
1/2 cup shredded cheddar, Monterey Jack, or Colby cheese
1/2 teaspoon ground cumin
Salt and black pepper
Mango Relish (recipe follows)
4 whole-grain rolls

1. Preheat the broiler or set up the grill and preheat it to high.

2. Place the chicken, carrot, cheese, cumin, and salt and pepper to taste in a medium-size mixing bowl and stir to mix. Divide the chicken mixture into 4 equal portions and shape each into a burger.

3. Broil or grill the burgers until browned, about 6 minutes, then turn them over. Spread a spoonful of the Mango Relish over each burger and continue cooking until fully cooked through, 4 to 6 minutes longer.

4. Serve the burgers on whole-grain rolls with more spoonfuls of Mango Relish, if desired.

MAKES 4 BURGERS

Nutrition Info

1 PORTION (1 BURGER WITHOUT MANGO RELISH) PROVIDES:

Protein: 1 serving

Calcium: 1/2 serving

Green leafy and yellow fruits and vegetables: 1 serving

Whole grains and legumes: 2 servings

WHAT A SPREAD:
"NOT HONEY MUSTARD"

▼ ▼ ▼

Craving a sweet spread on your sand-wich? Try this Not Honey Mustard spread. It's sweet like honey mustard but has a more complex flavor. Yummy on chicken, turkey, or meat sandwiches—or anywhere else you'd enjoy honey mustard. Take a quarter cup of Dijon mustard and a quarter cup fruit-only apricot preserves. Mix them together and enjoy!

Mango Relish

A tropical departure from the standard condiments, this sweet and tangy relish can be spread on anything—from hamburgers and pork to fish fillets and shrimp.

1 tablespoon olive oil
1/2 medium-size red onion, finely
    chopped
1 teaspoon chopped garlic
    (from 2 cloves)
1 large ripe mango, cut into
    1/4-inch dice
1 teaspoon ground cumin
1 tablespoon chopped fresh oregano,
    or 1 teaspoon dried oregano
1 tablespoon chopped fresh cilantro
    (optional)
3 tablespoons orange juice
    concentrate
Juice of 1 lime

1. Heat the olive oil in a small skillet over medium heat. Add the onion and garlic and cook until beginning to soften, about 2 minutes. Add the mango, cumin, oregano, cilantro, if using, orange juice concentrate, and lime juice. Let come to a slow simmer and cook, stirring occa-sionally, until most of the liquid has evap-orated, about 15 minutes.

2. Remove the relish from the heat and let cool for 5 minutes. Place the relish in a food processor and purée it until it is the consistency of jam. The relish can be refrigerated, covered, for several days.

MAKES ABOUT 1 CUP

Nutrition Info

1 PORTION (1/4 CUP) PROVIDES:

Vitamin C: 1/2 serving

Green leafy and yellow vegetables and
    fruits: 1/2 serving

Hail Caesar Wrap

Next time you have a craving for chicken Caesar salad, leave the fork behind. Romaine, cheese, roasted red bell pepper, and chicken team up with a creamy dressing to create a salad that's high in flavor but low in fat. And it gets better—rolled up, the tasty salad becomes a super sandwich to go, so you can satisfy those cravings on the road.

1 cup shredded romaine lettuce
¹⁄₄ cup shredded provolone cheese
2 tablespoons grated Parmesan cheese
1 tablespoon Creamy Caesar Dressing,
  or more to taste (page 332)
3 slices cooked chicken or turkey
  (about 3 ounces)
4 strips roasted red bell pepper
  (leftover or from a jar)
1 whole wheat tortilla, seasoned wrap,
  or whole wheat pita (12 inches
  in diameter)

1. Place the romaine, provolone and Parmesan cheeses, and the Caesar dressing in a bowl and toss to mix. Add more dressing if desired.

2. Layer the chicken and roasted pepper strips on the tortilla and top with the romaine salad. (If you're using a pita, trim ½ inch off an edge of the pita and stuff it into the bottom of the pita. Fill the pita with the chicken and roasted pepper strips, then add the romaine salad.)

3. Fold the sides of the tortilla over the filling. If you're packing the sandwich to go, wrap it tightly in plastic wrap.

MAKES 1 SANDWICH

ALL WASHED UP

▼ ▼ ▼

Many of these recipes call for greens, such as arugula, watercress, and romaine lettuce, and herbs like cilantro, parsley, dill, and basil. As with all fruits and vegetables, you'll need to thoroughly rinse the greens and herbs and pat them dry before adding them to sandwiches (even prewashed). See page 129 for more tips on washing lettuce.

Nutrition Info
1 PORTION (WITHOUT DRESSING)
PROVIDES:

Protein: 1¹⁄₂ servings

Calcium: 1¹⁄₂ servings

Vitamin C: 1¹⁄₂ servings

Green leafy and yellow vegetables and
  fruits: 1¹⁄₂ servings

Whole grains and legumes: 2 servings

Market Chicken Pita

A departure from the deli, this low-fat, creamy, Indian-inspired chicken salad sandwich really hits the spot when you're looking for something out of the ordinary. A cool combination of tomato, cucumber, and greens is tossed with diced chicken and spiced up with curry and cilantro. Stuffed into a pita, topped with a sprinkling of raisins and sunflower seeds, it makes a refreshingly different sandwich.

¾ cup diced cooked chicken or turkey (about 4 ounces)

3 tablespoons plain yogurt

2 teaspoons mayonnaise

¼ cup ¼-inch slices peeled hothouse (seedless English) cucumber

1 plum tomato, diced

1 teaspoon chopped fresh cilantro

½ teaspoon curry powder

Pinch of ground cumin

Hot red pepper sauce (optional)

Salt and black pepper

1 whole wheat pita

½ cup arugula or watercress, rinsed, patted dry, thick stems removed, or ½ cup coleslaw mixture

1 tablespoon raisins

1 tablespoon toasted sunflower seeds (see page 272)

1. Place the chicken, yogurt, mayonnaise, cucumber, tomato, cilantro, curry powder, and cumin in a mixing bowl and stir to mix. Season with hot sauce, if desired, and salt and pepper to taste.

2. Trim ½ inch off an edge of the pita and stuff it into the bottom of the pita. Fill the pita with the arugula, then add the chicken salad. Top with the raisins and sunflower seeds. If you're packing the sandwich to go, wrap it tightly in plastic wrap.

MAKES 1 SANDWICH

Nutrition Info

1 PORTION PROVIDES:

Protein: 1 serving

Vitamin C: ½ serving plus

Green leafy and yellow vegetables and fruits: ½ serving

Other fruits and vegetables: ½ serving

Whole grains and legumes: 2 servings

Fat: ½ serving

Wrap 'n' Roll

One part salad, one part sandwich, two parts delicious—toss cabbage, red bell pepper, tomato, kalamata olives, and cheddar cheese with turkey or chicken (the perfect place for last night's leftovers), then wrap it all up and you're ready to roll.

1 tablespoon olive oil
1 tablespoon fresh lemon juice or
   seasoned rice vinegar
1/8 teaspoon dried oregano
Salt and black pepper
1/2 cup cole slaw mix
1 plum tomato, chopped
1/4 medium-size red bell pepper,
   diced
4 pitted kalamata olives, chopped
1/4 cup cubed cheddar cheese
1 whole wheat tortilla or seasoned wrap
   (12 inches in diameter)
3 slices cooked turkey or chicken
   (about 3 ounces)

1. Place the olive oil, lemon juice, and oregano in a mixing bowl and whisk to mix. Season to taste with salt and pepper. Add the cole slaw mix, tomato, bell pepper, olives, and cheese and toss to combine.

2. Place the tortilla flat on a work surface. Arrange the turkey on top, then spoon the salad in the center. Fold the sides of the tortilla over the filling. If you are packing the sandwich to go, wrap it tightly in plastic wrap.

MAKES 1 SANDWICH

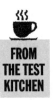

FROM THE TEST KITCHEN

NO WRAP IN SIGHT? Use a whole wheat pita pocket instead. Trim 1/2 inch off an edge of the pita and stuff it into the bottom of the pita. Fill the pita with the turkey slices, then add the salad. If you're packing the sandwich to go, wrap it tightly in plastic wrap before setting out.

Nutrition Info

1 PORTION PROVIDES:

Protein: 1 serving

Calcium: 1 serving

Vitamin C: 2 servings

Green leafy and yellow vegetables and fruits: 1 serving

Whole grains and legumes: 2 servings

Fat: 1 serving

Turkey Trio

Not your average turkey and cheese sandwich, this intriguing combo features turkey and avocado slices, arugula, and sharp cheese. The sandwich takes a turn for uptown with a zesty and sophisticated Arugula Pesto standing in for plain old mustard and mayo. Take a bite—you deserve it!

3 slices cooked turkey (about 3 ounces)
½ medium-size avocado, preferably
    Hass, sliced
½ cup arugula, thick stems removed
¼ cup shredded cheddar, Swiss, or
    Gouda cheese
2 slices whole-grain bread
2 tablespoons Arugula Pesto, or more to
    taste (recipe follows)

Layer the turkey, avocado, arugula, and cheese on a slice of the bread. Spread the Arugula Pesto on the remaining slice of bread and place it on top of the sandwich. Cut the sandwich in half and enjoy. Or, if you are packing the sandwich to go, wrap it tightly in plastic wrap.

MAKES 1 SANDWICH

FROM THE TEST KITCHEN

ARE YOU CRAVING a taste of childhood? Turn the Turkey Trio into an updated grilled cheese sandwich. Toast the sandwich in a toaster oven, on the grill, or in a hot skillet (with a little melted butter or some olive oil spray) until the cheese melts and the outside of the bread is nicely toasted.

Nutrition Info
1 PORTION (WITHOUT PESTO) PROVIDES:
Protein: 1 serving
Calcium: ½ serving
Green leafy and yellow vegetables and fruits: ½ serving
Other fruits and vegetables: 1 serving
Whole grains and legumes: 2 servings

Arugula Pesto

This pesto has a lot of flavor, with very little fat. Use it as a sandwich spread or a veggie dip, or spoon it over fish or chicken before baking. And don't forget the traditional way to serve it: Toss it with pasta and cheese (and maybe some shrimp or chicken).

4 cups arugula, rinsed, patted dry,
    thick stems removed
1/2 cup grated Parmesan cheese
1/4 cup toasted pine nuts (see box below)
2 to 3 cloves garlic, minced (if raw garlic
    bothers you, see page 331)
2 tablespoons plain low-fat yogurt,
    or more to taste
1 tablespoon fresh lemon juice, or more
    to taste
2 tablespoons olive oil, or more to taste
Salt and cracked black pepper

Place the arugula, Parmesan cheese, pine nuts, and garlic in a food processor and process until finely minced. Add the yogurt, lemon juice, and olive oil and process until well blended. Too thick? Add a little more yogurt, olive oil, and/or lemon juice. Season with salt and pepper to taste. The pesto can be refrigerated, covered tightly, for up to 5 days.

MAKES ABOUT 2 CUPS

A TOAST TO TOASTING

▼ ▼ ▼

Tempted to skip the toasting when a recipe calls for toasted nuts or seeds? You'll be skipping more than you think. Toasting brings out the true nutty flavor, adding a memorably rich dimension to any salad, sandwich, pasta, poultry—you name it. There are several ways to toast nuts or seeds.

ON THE STOVE TOP: Sprinkle 1/2 cup nuts or seeds in an ungreased heavy skillet (don't use a nonstick one). Cook over medium heat, stirring frequently, until the nuts begin to brown, 5 to 7 minutes.

IN THE OVEN: Spread 1/2 cup nuts or seeds in an ungreased shallow pan. Bake uncovered in a 350°F oven, stirring frequently, until the nuts are light brown, about 10 minutes.

IN THE MICROWAVE: Spread 1/2 cup nuts or seeds evenly in a flat microwave-safe dish. Cook on high power until they are lightly browned, 3 to 4 minutes.

Toasted nuts will continue to darken after you remove them from the heat. A good test for doneness—along with color—is when you can smell a toasted (not burnt—that's overdone) aroma.

When toasting small seeds in a skillet, use a splatter screen, if possible. The seeds tend to pop around.

For ground nuts or seeds, you can grind toasted nuts or seeds in a food processor or minigrinder. Just be careful not to overprocess them, or you'll end up with nut or seed butter.

FROM THE TEST KITCHEN

FOR A MORE TRADITIONAL pesto, substitute ½ cup basil leaves for ½ cup of the arugula. For a zippier pesto, substitute watercress for the arugula. For a milder one, try baby spinach. For a creamier sandwich spread, add a table-spoon or two of mayonnaise to the pesto along with the yogurt.

Nutrition Info
1 PORTION (¼ CUP) PROVIDES:

Green leafy and yellow vegetables and fruits: ½ serving

Salmon Pocket

Looking for a home for leftover or canned salmon? How about this tasty Salmon Pocket, which combines greens, tomato, avocado, and pesto with salmon for a lunch (or dinner) that packs in not only protein but those baby-friendly omega-3 fatty acids.

1 whole wheat pita, or 2 slices whole-grain bread

½ cup flaked cooked salmon (fresh or canned)

2 tablespoons Pesto with Sunflower Seeds (page 309), or Arugula Pesto (page 271)

1 small plum tomato, thinly sliced

¼ medium-size avocado, preferably Hass, thinly sliced

½ cup arugula or similar greens

Trim ½ inch off an edge of the pita and stuff it into the bottom of the pita. Fill the pita with the salmon, then spoon the sauce over it. Top with the tomato, avocado, and arugula. If packing the sandwich to go, wrap it tightly in plastic wrap.

MAKES 1 SANDWICH

Nutrition Info
1 PORTION (WITHOUT SAUCE) PROVIDES:

Protein: 1 serving

Calcium: 1 serving if made with canned salmon with bones

Vitamin C: ½ serving

Green leafy and yellow vegetables and fruits: ½ serving

Other fruits and vegetables: ½ serving

Whole grains and legumes: 2 servings

A Better BLT

Here's a great way to get your BLT without the F (fat) but with plenty of F (flavor). The flavor comes from the mayo substitute—a white bean spread—that adds a tasty fifth dimension to the avocado, tomato, arugula, and vegetarian "bacon."

1 whole-grain roll
2 tablespoons (or more) White Bean
    Sandwich Spread (recipe follows)
1/2 cup arugula, watercress, or shredded
    red leaf lettuce, thick stems removed
1/4 cup shredded carrot
4 slices vegetarian "bacon"
    (about 4 ounces), cooked
1/2 medium-size avocado, preferably
    Hass, sliced
1 plum tomato, sliced

Cut the roll in half and spread both cut sides with the bean spread. Layer the arugula, carrot, "bacon," avocado, and tomato on one half of the roll, then top with the other half. If you're packing the sandwich to go, wrap it tightly in plastic wrap.

MAKES 1 SANDWICH

Nutrition Info
1 PORTION PROVIDES:

Protein: 1/2 serving

Vitamin C: 1/2 serving if made with watercress

Green leafy and yellow vegetables and fruits: 11/2 servings

Other fruits and vegetables: 1 serving

Whole grains and legumes: 2 servings

White Bean Sandwich Spread

Hold the mayo, and use this creamy spread on your sandwiches instead. Makes a great dip for crudités and pita strips, too.

2 tablespoons olive oil
1 large clove garlic (if raw garlic bothers
    you, see page 331), peeled and crushed
1 can (about 15 ounces) cannellini or
    Great Northern beans, rinsed and
    drained
2 tablespoons coarsely chopped fresh
    cilantro or flat-leaf parsley
Juice of 1 large lemon
Salt and black pepper

Place the olive oil, garlic, beans, cilantro, and lemon juice in a food processor and process until a smooth purée forms. Season to taste with salt and pepper. Serve at room temperature, or warm in the microwave or on top of the stove. The bean spread can be refrigerated, covered, for up to 5 days.

MAKES ABOUT 1 CUP

FROM THE TEST KITCHEN

FOR A SPICIER SPREAD, substitute chickpeas for the beans in the White Bean Sandwich Spread, add a teaspoon of ground toasted cumin seeds, and a dash of hot paprika and/or cayenne pepper (add both if you want the spread really hot). You can kick it up with more garlic, too.

Nutrition Info

1 PORTION (1/4 CUP) PROVIDES:

Whole grains and legumes: 1/2 serving

Iron: from the beans

Fat: 1/2 serving

Black Bean Quesadilla

Quesadillas—Mexican-style grilled cheese sandwiches—are quick to make and easy to customize. Packed with authentic Mexican flavor and an impressive array of nutrients, this Black Bean Quesadilla features Monterey Jack cheese, tangy black bean salsa, avocado, and tomato. Off to work? Take it cold, then heat it in the office microwave.

1 whole wheat tortilla or seasoned wrap (12 inches in diameter)

1/2 cup shredded Monterey Jack or cheddar cheese

1/3 to 1/2 cup Black Beans in Lime and Cumin Vinaigrette (recipe follows)

1/4 medium-size avocado, preferably Hass, sliced

1/2 medium-size tomato, chopped

1/2 medium-size red bell pepper, chopped

1/4 cup chopped fresh cilantro (optional)

1. Line a microwave-safe plate with a paper towel and place the tortilla on top. Sprinkle half of the cheese over half of the tortilla. Top the cheese with the Black Beans in Lime and Cumin Vinaigrette, avocado, tomato, and bell pepper. Sprinkle the remaining cheese on top.

2. Fold the bare half of the tortilla over the filling, covering it. Microwave the quesadilla on high power until the cheese melts, 1½ to 2 minutes.

3. Remove and discard the paper towel, then cut the quesadilla into wedges and sprinkle the cilantro over it, if desired, before serving.

MAKES 1 QUESADILLA

THERE'S MORE THAN ONE way to fill a tortilla—dozens, in fact. Here's one more: Spread 3 to 4 tablespoons of fat-free refried beans over a tortilla. Top these with 3 tablespoons of your favorite salsa. Sprinkle ¼ cup of your choice of shredded cheese over the salsa and microwave the tortilla on high power until the cheese melts, 1½ to 2 minutes. Roll the tortilla and enjoy it immediately or wrap it to go. Have leftover chicken, pork, steak, fish, or shrimp? Add it to the tortilla, too. And that's a wrap!

Nutrition Info

1 PORTION (WITHOUT BLACK BEANS) PROVIDES:

Protein: ½ serving plus

Calcium: 2 servings

Vitamin C: ½ serving; 2½ servings if made with red bell pepper

Green leafy and yellow vegetables and fruits: 1 serving if made with red pepper

Other fruits and vegetables: ½ serving

Whole grains and legumes: 2 servings

Black Beans in Lime and Cumin Vinaigrette

These marinated black beans show off bold Southwestern flavors. Try using them in your next burrito.

1 can (about 15 ounces) black beans, rinsed and drained
1 medium-size red bell pepper, finely chopped
1 medium-size tomato, finely chopped
4 scallions, both white and light green parts, trimmed and sliced
2 tablespoons chopped fresh cilantro
1 tablespoon chopped fresh flat-leaf parsley
2 tablespoons fresh lime juice
1 tablespoon olive oil
½ teaspoon ground cumin, or more to taste
Salt and black pepper

Place the black beans, bell pepper, tomato, and scallions in a salad bowl and stir to mix. Add the cilantro, parsley, lime juice, olive oil, and cumin and toss to mix. Taste for seasoning, adding salt and pepper and more cumin if necessary. The beans can be refrigerated, covered, for up to 2 days.

SERVES 4

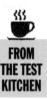

Beans are a great source of protein—but they can also be a great source of gas. Keep the protein and skip the gas by substituting cooked edamame.

Nutrition Info

1 PORTION PROVIDES:

Protein: ½ serving

Calcium: ½ serving

Vitamin C: 1 serving

Green leafy and yellow vegetables and fruits: ½ serving

Whole grains and legumes: 1 serving

Dilled Egg Salad

The humble egg salad has filled sandwiches and lunch boxes for generations. But this Dilled Egg Salad is a far cry from that cafeteria fixture. Eggs (with an extra egg white) are dressed up with mustard, yogurt, celery, onion, dill, and carrot for loads of flavor and nutrition. Try the egg salad with crackers, too.

3 hard-cooked eggs, chopped
2 hard-cooked egg whites, chopped
1 small rib celery, minced
2 tablespoons grated or shredded carrot
1 tablespoon chopped red onion
   or minced fresh chives
1 tablespoon plain yogurt, or more to
   taste
1 tablespoon mayonnaise
1 teaspoon minced fresh dill,
   or more to taste
1 teaspoon Dijon mustard,
   or more to taste
1/2 teaspoon fresh lemon juice,
   or more to taste
Salt and black pepper

Place the hard-cooked eggs and egg whites, celery, carrot, onion, yogurt, mayonnaise, dill, mustard, and lemon juice in a bowl and stir to mix. Taste for seasoning, adding more dill, mustard, and/or lemon juice as necessary, and salt and pepper to taste. The egg salad can be refrigerated in an airtight container for up to 2 days.

**MAKES ENOUGH FILLING FOR
1 LARGE SANDWICH**

Nutrition Info
1 PORTION PROVIDES:

Protein: 1 serving

Green leafy and yellow vegetables and
  fruits: 1/2 serving

Other fruits and vegetables: 1/2 serving

Fat: 1 serving

Fruity Turkey Salad

A chewy (and vitamin-packed) surprise—dried apricots—makes this salad a treat for the taste buds. Nuts add crunch and important fatty acids. Serve the turkey salad with red leaf lettuce in pitas or on whole-grain bread. And try it with chicken, too.

1¼ cups chopped cooked turkey or chicken breast (about 7 ounces)
1 medium-size celery rib, thinly sliced
6 dried apricot halves, coarsely chopped
2 tablespoons coarsely chopped toasted pecans or walnuts (see page 272
2 tablespoons chopped red onion or scallion
3 tablespoons plain yogurt (whole-milk yogurt will make a creamier dressing)
1 tablespoon mayonnaise
1 tablespoon whole-grain mustard
1 tablespoon apricot all-fruit preserves, finely chop any pieces of fruit
1 tablespoon fresh lemon juice, or more to taste
1 tablespoon chopped fresh parsley
Salt and black pepper

1. Place the turkey, celery, apricots, nuts, and onion in a bowl and stir to mix.

2. Place the yogurt, mayonnaise, mustard, apricot preserves, lemon juice, and parsley in a small bowl and stir to mix. Taste for seasoning, adding more lemon juice as necessary, and salt and pepper to taste.

3. Add the yogurt mixture to the turkey mixture, and stir to coat well.

MAKES 2 SERVINGS

Nutrition Info
1 PORTION PROVIDES:
Protein: 1 serving
Green leafy and yellow vegetables and fruits: 1/2 serving
Other fruits and vegetables: 1 serving
Fat: 1/2 serving

FILL 'ER UP

▼ ▼ ▼

Tired of the same old sandwich? Throw a few of these into your brown-bag rotation. Don't be afraid to mix and match:

■ Roast beef, whole-grain mustard, arugula or spinach, fresh basil leaves, and tomato slices on a whole grain roll

■ Roast beef, sun-dried tomato pesto, or Pesto with Sunflower Seeds (page 309), fresh basil leaves, roasted red pepper, and roasted red onion wrapped in a whole wheat tortilla

■ Grilled chicken breast, Not Honey Mustard (page 267), Swiss cheese, romaine lettuce, and thinly sliced cantaloupe or mango in a pita

■ Chicken, Pesto with Sunflower Seeds (page 309) or whole grain mustard, shaved Parmesan cheese, fresh basil leaves, and roasted red pepper on a whole wheat roll

■ Turkey breast, watercress, tomato slices, Swiss cheese, and Dijon mustard on whole wheat bread

■ Turkey breast, sharp cheddar cheese, watercress, and all-fruit cranberry sauce on a whole-grain roll

■ Sliced hard-cooked egg, shaved Parmesan cheese, baby spinach leaves, and tomato slices on a whole wheat English muffin

■ Egg salad, whole-grain mustard, shaved Parmesan cheese, watercress, and tomato slices on a whole wheat bagel

■ Cheddar cheese, Not Honey Mustard (page 267), thinly sliced apple, and watercress on whole-grain bread

■ Provolone cheese, Arugula Pesto (page 271), tomato slices, fresh basil leaves, and arugula in a whole-grain pita

■ Mozzarella cheese (use pasteurized only), sun-dried tomato pesto, tomato slices, roasted red pepper, and a roasted portobello mushroom on a whole wheat roll

■ Grilled portobello mushroom, roasted red pepper, Pesto with Sunflower Seeds (page 309), red onion slices, arugula, and provolone cheese in a whole wheat tortilla

■ Grilled eggplant, shredded romaine lettuce, hummus, and shredded Swiss cheese in a whole wheat pita

Soups and Chilies

"**S**oup's on" can mean lots of things! For a cool, elegant start to a summer brunch, think Tomato Soup with Avocado. For a hearty, soul-warming meal in a bowl on a winter's evening, there's Beef and Barley Soup or Turkey Chili. And for a nourishing pick-me-up in the middle of a long afternoon, pick Vegetable and Edamame Soup or Red Lentil and Tomato Soup. But there's one thing that all the soups and chilies here serve up: Plenty of delicious nutrients in a soothing form, a definite plus for tummy-trouble sufferers who find sipping easier than chewing.

Broccoli and Cheese Soup

Broccoli, cheese, and potatoes are friends from way back; this velvety smooth and vitamin-rich soup brings them together for a delicious reunion. You'll never miss the cream—or the calories it would add. Save time by using a package of broccoli florets.

1 tablespoon butter or olive oil
½ medium-size onion, chopped
1 clove garlic, minced
2 cups broccoli florets
1 medium-size Yukon Gold potato, diced
2½ cups low-sodium chicken broth or vegetable broth
¾ cup finely shredded cheddar cheese
¼ cup buttermilk, or more to taste
Salt and black pepper

1. Melt the butter in a large saucepan over medium heat. Add the onion and garlic and cook until softened, about 5 minutes.

2. Add the broccoli, potato, and chicken broth, raise the heat to high, and let come to a boil. Reduce the heat, cover the saucepan, and let simmer until the broccoli and potato are softened, about 7 minutes.

3. Let the broccoli mixture cool slightly, then transfer it to a blender or food processor and, working in batches if necessary, purée it until satiny smooth.

4. Return the soup to the saucepan, add ¼ cup of the cheese and the buttermilk.

BURN, BABY, BURN?

▼ ▼ ▼

If pregnancy indigestion has you feeling the burn, try omitting garlic and/or onion from your soups.

Cook the soup over low heat until the cheese melts (do not let the soup come to a boil), about 3 minutes. Season with salt and pepper to taste. Pour the soup into serving bowls and top each with 2 tablespoons of the remaining cheese.

SERVES 2

Nutrition Info

1 PORTION PROVIDES:

Protein: ½ serving

Calcium: almost 2 servings

Vitamin C: 2 servings

Green leafy and yellow vegetables and fruits: 2 servings

Other fruits and vegetables: ½ serving

Fat: ½ serving

Ginger and Carrot Soup

Ginger and carrot soup makes a soothing way to take your vitamins, especially when morning sickness outlasts the morning.

2 teaspoons olive oil or butter

1 medium-size sweet onion, chopped

1 clove garlic, minced

1 package (16 ounces) baby carrots
   (about 3 cups)

2-inch piece of fresh ginger, peeled and
   thinly sliced

4 cups low-sodium chicken broth
   or vegetable broth

Fresh lemon juice

Salt and black pepper

Plain low-fat yogurt or buttermilk,
   for serving

1. Heat the olive oil in a large saucepan over medium heat. Add the onion and garlic and cook until softened, about 5 minutes. Add the carrots and ginger and cook until the ginger is fragrant, about 2 minutes, stirring frequently.

2. Add the chicken broth, raise the heat to medium-high, and let come to a boil. Cover the saucepan, reduce the heat, and let simmer until the carrots are very soft, about 15 minutes.

3. Let the soup cool slightly, then, working in batches if necessary, transfer it to a blender or food processor and purée it until velvety smooth.

4. Return the soup to the saucepan and season it with lemon juice, salt, and pepper

to taste. Let the soup come to a simmer over medium-low heat and cook until heated through. Pour the soup into serving bowls and top each with a large spoonful of yogurt or a tablespoon of buttermilk (drawing a knife through the buttermilk will create an attractive pattern). The soup can be refrigerated, covered, for 2 days.

SERVES 4

FROM THE TEST KITCHEN

DON'T HAVE THE TIME—or the stomach—to sauté the onions and carrots for Ginger and Carrot Soup? Place the carrots, onion (you don't even have to chop it, quartering will do, and you can leave out the garlic), and ginger in a pot with the broth. Bring it to a boil and let simmer until the carrots are soft, then purée it. Add a little lemon juice and some salt and pepper and you've got a lighter soup without that lingering onion odor in your kitchen.

Nutrition Info

1 PORTION (1 BOWL) PROVIDES:

Vitamin C: 1/2 serving

Green leafy and yellow vegetables and
   fruits: 3 servings

Other fruits and vegetables: 1/2 serving

Butternut Squash and Pear Soup

Fragrant and elegant, this bisque only looks like it took a lot of effort. It's easier and faster to cook than you'd think, and you reap powerful nutritional rewards. The sweet and subtly spiced combination of squash and pears will reward your taste buds, too.

1 small butternut squash
   (about 1½ pounds), diced
3 cups low-sodium vegetable broth
   or chicken broth
Salt
1 tablespoon butter or canola oil
1 small onion, very thinly sliced
2 red pears, peeled, cored, and
   coarsely chopped
1½ teaspoons curry powder
¾ teaspoon ground turmeric
½ teaspoon ground ginger (optional)
⅓ cup plain whole-milk yogurt
White pepper
½ cup finely shredded cheddar cheese

1. Place the squash, 2½ cups of the vegetable broth, and a pinch of salt in a large saucepan over medium-high heat and let come to a boil. Reduce the heat and let simmer until the squash softens, about 35 minutes. Set the squash, with its cooking liquid, aside.

2. While the squash is cooking, melt the butter in a large skillet over medium heat. Add the onion and cook, stirring frequently, until softened, about 5 minutes. Add the pears and cook, stirring frequently, until softened, about 5 minutes. Add the curry powder, turmeric, and ginger, if using, and the remaining ½ cup of vegetable broth and let come to a simmer. Cover the skillet and let cook until the flavors blend, about 10 minutes.

3. Add the onion and pear mixture to the cooked squash. Let the squash mixture cool slightly, then working in batches if necessary, transfer it to a blender or food processor and purée until smooth.

4. Return the soup to the saucepan, add the yogurt, and season to taste with salt and pepper. Place the saucepan over low heat and let the soup heat through, 2 to 3 minutes. Do not let it boil. Pour the soup into serving bowls and top each with 2 tablespoons of the cheddar cheese.

SERVES 4

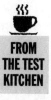

FROM THE TEST KITCHEN

ONLY SERVING TWO (and a half) for dinner tonight? Make the Squash and Pear Soup through Step 3, then divide it in half. Continue with Step 4, using 3 tablespoons of yogurt and ¼ cup of cheddar cheese. The rest of the soup can be refrigerated, covered, for up to 2 days. Reheat it before continuing with Step 4.

Nutrition Info

1 PORTION (1 BOWL) PROVIDES:

Calcium: ½ serving

Green leafy and yellow vegetables and fruits: 2 servings

Other fruits and vegetables: 1 serving

Sweet Potato Vichyssoise

With more flavor and nutrition than the traditional vichyssoise, making the soup with sweet potatoes is an elegant way to serve up your yellow vegetables.

1 tablespoon olive oil

2 large leeks, trimmed, rinsed well, and thinly sliced

2 medium-size sweet potatoes, peeled and chopped

3 cups low-sodium chicken or vegetable broth

¼ cup chopped fresh flat-leaf parsley

Salt and black pepper

1. Heat the olive oil in a saucepan over medium-high heat. Add the leeks and cook until they soften, about 3 minutes. Add the sweet potatoes and cook until they begin to soften, about 5 minutes. Add the chicken broth and parsley and let come to a boil. Reduce the heat and let simmer until the sweet potatoes are completely soft, about 10 minutes.

2. Let the soup cool slightly, then working in batches if necessary, transfer it to a blender or food processor and purée it until smooth. Season the soup with salt and pepper to taste. The soup can be served either hot or cold. Reheat it over low heat after puréeing, if desired. The soup can be refrigerated, covered, for up to 4 days.

SERVES 4

FROM THE TEST KITCHEN

IF YOU'D LIKE THIS SOUP a little thinner, add some milk or buttermilk after it cools. You'll get a creamier taste and a calcium bonus.

Nutrition Info

1 PORTION (1 BOWL) PROVIDES:

Vitamin C: ½ serving

Green leafy and yellow vegetables and fruits: 1 serving

Other fruits and vegetables: ½ serving

Tomato Soup with Avocado

This versatile soup is delicious hot and refreshing chilled, a cornucopia of flavor and nutrition.

2 teaspoons olive oil
3 scallions, both white and light
   green parts, trimmed and
   thinly sliced
1/2 teaspoon coarsely chopped
   garlic (from 1 clove)
4 medium-size ripe tomatoes,
   seeded and coarsely chopped,
   or 1 1/2 cups canned crushed
   tomatoes, with their juices
4 cups tomato juice or vegetable
   juice, such as V8
1/4 cup fresh basil leaves,
   thinly sliced, or 2 teaspoons
   dried basil
Salt and black pepper
Diced avocado, for serving
1/2 red bell pepper, finely chopped
   for serving
4 lime wedges, for serving

1. Heat the olive oil in a saucepan over medium heat. Add the scallions and garlic and cook until softened, about 2 minutes.

2. Add the tomatoes, tomato juice, and basil, raise the heat to medium-high, and let come to a boil. Reduce the heat and let the soup simmer until the flavors are well blended, about 15 minutes. Season to taste with salt and pepper.

3. Pour the soup into serving bowls, sprinkle avocado and bell pepper on top and serve the lime wedges alongside. The soup can also be served chilled. It can be refrigerated, covered, for up to 2 days.

SERVES 4

Nutrition Info

1 PORTION (1 BOWL) PROVIDES:

Vitamin C: 2 1/2 servings if made with tomato juice; 3 if made with vegetable juice

Green leafy and yellow vegetables and fruits: 1 1/2 servings if made with vegetable juice

Red Lentil and Tomato Soup

Besides being prettier to look at than green or brown lentils, red lentils have a creamier texture and a milder taste. Teamed with chunky tomatoes, carrot, and celery, they make a rich-tasting, nutritious, and sustaining soup that's gentle on the stomach.

1 tablespoon olive oil
1 medium-size onion, chopped
½ teaspoon ground cumin
½ teaspoon ground turmeric
½ teaspoon ground allspice
½ tablespoon minced peeled fresh ginger
2½ cups vegetable broth or
　low-sodium chicken broth
½ cup red lentils
1 large rib celery, chopped
1 medium carrot, chopped
4 plum tomatoes, coarsely chopped
　(set aside 1 chopped tomato)
Salt and black pepper

1. Heat the olive oil in a large saucepan over medium heat. Add the onion and cook until softened, about 5 minutes.

2. Add the cumin, turmeric, allspice, and ginger and cook, stirring freuently, until fragrant, about 1 minute.

3. Add the vegetable broth, lentils, celery, carrot, and 3 of the chopped tomatoes, raise the heat to medium-high, and let come to a boil. Reduce the heat and let simmer until the lentils are tender, about 30 minutes.

4. Add remaining tomato and season with salt and pepper to taste. Let the soup simmer

until the fourth tomato is heated through, about 3 minutes (see Note). The soup can be refrigerated, covered, for up to 2 days.

SERVES 2

NOTE: If you are serving only half of the soup now, add half of 1 chopped plum tomato at this stage. Add the second half after the rest of the soup has been reheated.

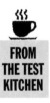

FROM THE TEST KITCHEN

IF YOU HAVE A HARD TIME finding red lentils (they are usually available in health food stores), you can substitute regular brown lentils. They'll take more simmering time—45 minutes to 1 hour.

Nutrition Info
1 PORTION (1 BOWL) PROVIDES:

Protein: ½ serving

Vitamin C: 1 serving

Green leafy and yellow vegetables and fruits: 1 serving

Other fruits and vegetables: ½ serving

Whole grains and legumes: 1½ servings

Fat: ½ serving

Roasted Vegetable Soup

Rich and thick, this soup is filled with fall vegetables and vitamins but there's not a drop of cream or butter. Roasting the vegetables does take a little bit of time, but it's less than an hour and the payoff's in the deliciously complex flavor.

Cooking oil spray
2 medium-size carrots, cut into
   1-inch chunks (about 1½ cups)
2 medium-size parsnips, cut into
   1-inch chunks (about 1 cup)
1 small rutabaga, cut into
   1-inch chunks (about 1 cup)
1 small red onion, quartered,
   each quarter cut in half
1 tablespoon olive oil
Salt and black pepper
4 teaspoons fresh thyme leaves
3 to 4 cups chicken broth
Toasted pumpkin seeds
   (see page 272)
Chopped fresh flat-leaf parsley

1. Preheat the oven to 400°F. Spray a large rimmed baking sheet with cooking oil spray.

2. Place the carrots, parsnips, rutabaga, and onion in a large bowl, add the olive oil, and toss to coat evenly. Spoon the vegetable mixture in an even layer onto the prepared baking sheet. Sprinkle some salt and pepper and 3 teaspoons of the thyme leaves on top.

3. Bake the vegetables until tender, about 45 minutes, stirring occasionally.

4. Transfer the roasted vegetables to a large saucepan and add 3 cups of the chicken broth and the remaining 1½ teaspoons of thyme leaves. Let come to a boil over high heat, then reduce the heat and let simmer until very tender, about 15 minutes.

5. Let the soup cool slightly, then working in batches if necessary, transfer it to a blender or food processor and purée it until slightly chunky or smooth (as you prefer). If the soup is too thick, add additional chicken broth to thin it. Taste for seasoning, adding more salt and/or pepper as necessary.

6. If the soup has cooled down too much, return it to the saucepan and gently reheat it over low heat. Sprinkle pumpkin seeds and parsley on top just before serving. The soup can be refrigerated, covered, for up to 2 days.

SERVES 4

Nutrition Info
1 PORTION (1 BOWL) PROVIDES:

Green leafy and yellow vegetables and fruits: 1 serving

Other fruits and vegetables: 1 serving

Spiced-up Gazpacho

Like a salad you can sip, this soup is especially pleasing on a hot summer's day. There's no cooking necessary, plus once you make it, you can enjoy it for several days, as a starter or a snack. Adding olive oil will make a richer gazpacho, but the soup is refreshing without it.

6 large plum tomatoes, or
   3 medium-size regular tomatoes,
   coarsely chopped
1 medium-size cucumber, peeled,
   seeded, and coarsely chopped
1½ large red bell peppers,
   chopped
1 small red onion, chopped
1 clove garlic, minced
3 tablespoons chopped fresh
   flat-leaf parsley
2 tablespoons chopped fresh basil
1 can or bottle (32 ounces; see Note)
   tomato juice, or vegetable juice,
   such as V8
3 tablespoons red wine vinegar
3 tablespoons olive oil
   (optional)
1 tablespoon fresh lemon juice, or
   more to taste
Salt and black pepper
Tabasco sauce

1. Place the tomatoes, cucumber, bell peppers, onion, garlic, parsley, basil, tomato juice, wine vinegar, olive oil, if using, and lemon juice in a food processor and pulse until finely chopped but not puréed.

2. Transfer the gazpacho to a large bowl and season it with salt, black pepper, and Tabasco sauce to taste. Add more lemon juice if desired. Refrigerate the soup, covered, until chilled through, at least 2 hours, or up to 3 days. Serve in soup bowls or in glasses. The soup can be refrigerated, covered, for up to 4 days.

SERVES 6

NOTE: Using 32 ounces of tomato juice will produce a thick gazpacho. If you like a more sippable soup, use a 46-ounce bottle. You'll get more nutrients, too.

FROM THE TEST KITCHEN **THERE ARE ANY NUMBER** of possible variations on this gazpacho. Here are just a few:

■ Replace the V8 with tomato juice.

■ For a chunkier gazpacho, don't run the vegetables through the food processor. Or just process half the veggies.

■ For a little taste of Mexico, substitute 2 tablespoons cilantro for the basil and fresh lime juice for the lemon juice; garnish the soup with chopped avocado.

■ Chop two hard-cooked eggs and add them just before serving.

■ For a more substantial soup, cut chilled cooked shrimp or scallops in half lengthwise and float them on top. Feeling really flush? Add chunks of chilled cooked crab or lobster.

Nutrition Info

1 PORTION (1 BOWL) PROVIDES:

Vitamin C: 2¹/2 servings

Green leafy and yellow vegetables and fruits: 2 servings

Other fruits and vegetables: ¹/2 serving

Fat: ¹/2 serving if using olive oil

Vegetable and Edamame Soup

This hearty but quick-cooking vegetable soup combines the best in beans—in this case white beans and protein-packed edamame (soybeans). The soup is half puréed, half chunky, so you get an interesting mix of textures, too. Provolone or cheddar cheese (your choice) adds even more flavor and a serving of calcium, too.

1 tablespoon olive oil
1 small onion, chopped
1 clove garlic, minced
4 plum tomatoes, coarsely chopped
2 medium carrots, coarsely chopped
3 to 4 cups vegetable broth
2 teaspoons fresh thyme leaves
¹/4 cup chopped fresh parsley
1 cup shelled cooked edamame
1 can (15¹/2 ounces) Great Northern
   beans, rinsed and drained
Salt and black pepper
1 cup shredded provolone or
   cheddar cheese

1. Heat the olive oil in a large saucepan over medium heat. Add the onion and garlic and cook until softened, about 5 minutes. Add the tomatoes and carrots and cook until the carrots are softened, about 10 minutes. Set aside 1 cup of the cooked vegetables.

2. Add 3 cups of the vegetable broth and the thyme and parsley to the saucepan. Raise the heat to medium-high and let come to a boil, then cover the saucepan and reduce the heat. Let the soup simmer until the vegetables are very tender, about 15 minutes.

3. Let the soup cool slightly, then transfer it to a blender or food processor, working in batches if necessary, and run the machine until the soup is puréed.

4. Return the soup to the saucepan and add the reserved cooked vegetables and the edamame and beans. If the soup is too thick, add additional vegetable broth to thin it. Bring the soup to a simmer over medium heat and cook until the beans are heated through, about 5 minutes. Season the soup with salt and pepper to taste. Sprinkle the cheese over the soup before serving. The soup can be refrigerated, covered, for up to 2 days.

SERVES 4

Nutrition Info
1 PORTION (1 BOWL) PROVIDES:

Protein: 1/2 serving

Calcium: 1 serving

Vitamin C: 1 serving

Green leafy and yellow vegetables and fruits: 1 serving

Whole grains and legumes: 1 serving

Iron: from the beans and edamame

Purée of Black Bean Soup

Soups don't get much easier than this, or more satisfying. Top the black bean soup with cheddar, serve a salad on the side, and call it lunch or dinner. Have the leftovers tomorrow.

1 tablespoon olive oil

1 small onion, chopped

1 teaspoon minced garlic
  or 2 chopped garlic cloves

1 medium-size yellow bell pepper,
  chopped

1 teaspoon ground cumin

1 can (about 15 ounces) black beans,
  rinsed and drained

1 can (14 1/2 ounces) low-sodium
  chicken broth

2 tablespoons chopped fresh
  cilantro

Black pepper

Tabasco sauce (optional)

Chopped avocado (optional),
  for serving

Chopped tomato (optional),
  for serving

1/2 cup shredded cheddar cheese
  (optional), for serving

3 lime wedges, for serving

MAKE SOUP A MEAL

▼ ▼ ▼

Topped with shredded cheese and served with a salad and some whole-grain bread, most soups make an easy but sustaining meal at the end of a long day. Or pack a thermos of soup, with cheese already melted on top, to take to work with you.

1. Heat the olive oil in a medium-size saucepan over medium heat. Add the onion, garlic, bell pepper, and cumin and cook until the vegetables are softened and turn golden brown, about 5 minutes. Add the black beans and chicken broth and cook until heated through, 3 to 4 minutes.

2. Let the soup cool slightly, then transfer it to a blender or food processor, working in batches if necessary, and add 1 tablespoon of the cilantro. Purée the soup until it is smooth.

3. Return the soup to the saucepan and season it with black pepper to taste. If you want some heat, add Tabasco sauce. Let the soup come to a simmer over medium-low heat and cook until heated through.

4. Pour the soup into serving bowls and sprinkle the remaining 1 tablespoon of cilantro on top. Top the soup with avocado and tomato, and cheese, if desired, and serve the lime wedges on the side.

SERVES 2

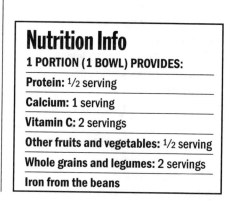

Nutrition Info

1 PORTION (1 BOWL) PROVIDES:

Protein: 1/2 serving

Calcium: 1 serving

Vitamin C: 2 servings

Other fruits and vegetables: 1/2 serving

Whole grains and legumes: 2 servings

Iron from the beans

Turkey Chili

Leaner than your average chili, but no less flavorful; you can adjust the amount of chili powder to sound as many (or as few) alarms as you (and your heartburn) can handle. Substitute beef for the turkey if you'd like to up your iron. Want to steer clear of tummy troubles? Use edamame instead of the black beans.

WRAP IT UP, I'LL EAT IT HERE

▼ ▼ ▼

Wrap up leftover turkey or vegetarian chili, along with a little chopped tomato and avocado and maybe a spoonful of salsa or low-fat sour cream, in a warm whole wheat tortilla for a quick but satisfying lunch or dinner.

1 tablespoon olive oil

1 medium-size onion, chopped

2 cloves garlic, minced

1½ pounds ground turkey breast

1 medium-size red bell pepper, chopped

1 medium-size yellow bell pepper, chopped

1 small jalapeño pepper (optional), seeded and diced

2 tablespoons chili powder

1 tablespoon ground cumin

1 can (about 15 ounces) black beans or red kidney beans, rinsed and drained

1 can (14½ ounces) diced tomatoes, with their juices

1½ cups shredded cheddar cheese

2 tablespoons chopped fresh cilantro

1. Heat the olive oil in a large saucepan over medium heat. Add the onion and garlic and cook until beginning to soften, about 2 minutes. Add the turkey, red and green bell peppers, and jalapeño, if using, and cook until the peppers begin to soften, about 3 minutes. Stir in the chili powder and cumin and cook until fragrant, about 2 minutes.

2. Add the beans and tomatoes and let come to a simmer. Reduce the heat and let simmer until the flavors are blended, about 10 minutes.

3. Spoon the chili into serving bowls and top with some cheese and cilantro. The chili can be refrigerated, covered, for up to 3 days. Garnish it with cheese and cilantro just before serving.

SERVES 6

Nutrition Info

1 PORTION (1 BOWL) PROVIDES:

Protein: 1 serving plus

Calcium: 1 serving

Vitamin C: 2 servings

Green leafy and yellow vegetables and fruits: ½ serving

Whole grains and legumes: ½ serving

Iron: from beans

Vegetarian Chili

Y ou don't have to be a vegetarian to enjoy this meatless chili, you just have to be hungry for a hearty meal. Again, substitute edamame (soybeans) for the beans if gas has got you down.

2 teaspoons olive oil
1 medium-size red bell pepper,
  chopped
1 carrot, cut into 1/2-inch chunks
1 small onion, chopped
1 clove garlic, minced
2 teaspoons chili powder,
  or more to taste
1 1/2 teaspoons ground cumin
1 can (14 1/2 ounces) diced
  tomatoes, with their juices
1 can (about 15 ounces) kidney beans
  or black beans, rinsed and
  drained
1/2 cup granular textured soy protein
  (see pages 142–143)
1/2 cup water
1 cup shredded cheddar cheese
  or soy cheese

1. Heat the olive oil in a large saucepan over medium heat. Add the bell pepper, carrot, onion, and garlic and cook until the vegetables soften, about 5 minutes. Stir in the chili powder and cumin and cook until fragrant, about 2 minutes.

2. Add the tomatoes, beans, textured soy protein, and water to the saucepan. Let come to a simmer and cook until the flavors are blended, about 10 minutes. Taste for seasonings, adding more chili powder as necessary.

3. Spoon the chili into serving bowls and sprinkle 2 tablespoons of cheddar cheese over each. The chili can be refrigerated, covered, for up to 3 days.

SERVES 4

Nutrition Info

1 PORTION (1 BOWL) PROVIDES:

Protein: 1/2 serving plus

Calcium: 1 serving

Vitamin C: 1 1/2 servings

Green leafy and yellow vegetables and fruits: 1 serving

Whole grains and legumes: 1 serving

Iron: from beans

Mexican Tortilla Soup

This authentically flavored meal in a bowl will take you south of the border in twenty-five minutes or less. Leaving the garlic unpeeled produces a heady flavor, without the burn—plus it saves chopping time.

4 corn tortillas (each 6 inches
  in diameter)
1 large head garlic
2 tablespoons olive oil
2 medium-size onions, finely chopped
1 pound skinless, boneless chicken
  breasts, cut into 1-inch strips
2 medium-size carrots, finely chopped
2 bay leaves
1 teaspoon ground cumin
4 cups low-sodium chicken broth
1 can (14½ ounces) diced tomatoes
3 tablespoons chopped fresh cilantro
4 lime wedges, for serving

1. Preheat the oven to 300°F.

2. Cut the tortillas into ½-inch-wide strips and place them flat on a rimmed baking sheet. Bake the tortillas until they are crisp, about 20 minutes. (Baked tortilla strips can be stored in an airtight container for up to 1 week.)

3. Meanwhile, remove and discard the loose paper skin on the outside of the head of garlic. Place the head of garlic on its side on a work surface and, holding it steady, use a sharp knife to cut it in half crosswise. Set the head of garlic aside.

4. Heat the olive oil in a large saucepan over medium heat. Add the onions and cook until they begin to soften, about 2 minutes. Add the chicken, carrots, bay leaves, cumin, and the 2 half heads of garlic and cook until the chicken browns and the carrots begin to soften, about 3 minutes.

5. Add the chicken broth and tomatoes, raise the heat to medium-high, and let come to a boil. Reduce the heat and let simmer until the flavors are well blended, about 10 minutes.

6. Remove and discard the head of garlic and the bay leaves. If you will be serving only half of the soup, set aside the rest (the soup can be refrigerated, covered, for up to 3 days). Pour the soup into serving bowls and sprinkle cilantro over each. Squeeze some lime juice on each serving, then scatter strips of tortilla on top.

SERVES 4

FROM THE TEST KITCHEN

YOU CAN ADD EVEN MORE flavor, texture, and nutrition to the tortilla soup with any of the following:

- Diced avocado (Other Vegetables)
- Diced red bell pepper (Green Leafy and C)
- Minced pickled jalapeño peppers
- Shredded Monterey Jack cheese (Calcium)

Nutrition Info

1 PORTION (1 BOWL) PROVIDES:

Protein: 1 serving

Vitamin C: 1/2 serving

Green leafy and yellow vegetables and fruits: 1 serving

Other fruits and vegetables: 1 serving

Whole grains and legumes: 1 serving

Fat: 1/2 serving

THE CREAM OF THE CROP

Love cream soups but don't love all the calories that come with them? Get creamy the low-fat way.

CALLING ALL VEGANS: Adding 4 ounces of well-drained, puréed soft tofu to a warm puréed soup will lend creaminess without the cream, and no noticeable taste.

YOU SAY POTATO: Adding a diced Yukon Gold potato to a soup before cooking it will result in a very creamy texture for a puréed soup that's creamless.

MILK IT FOR ALL IT'S WORTH: Evaporated skim milk and evaporated low-fat milk are more concentrated than regular milk and will make soup creamier. Buttermilk also adds more creaminess than regular milk—along with a tangier taste. Add evaporated milk or buttermilk just before you are ready to serve; gently bring the soup back to a simmer over very low heat, then whisk it.

LAST BUT NOT LEAST: Adding yogurt will make soup creamier and thicker. For a richer flavor, use whole-milk yogurt, which while higher in fat still has far less than cream. Whisk yogurt into hot soup, then serve it immediately.

Hearty Fish and Potato Chowder

You can chow down on this creamy but creamless chowder without guilt. Add a green salad, and you have an elegant and nourishing meal.

1 tablespoon olive oil
1 medium-size onion, chopped
1 rib celery, chopped
1 medium-size carrot, chopped
1¹/₂ cups low-sodium chicken broth
 or vegetable broth
1 cup buttermilk
4 small red potatoes, scrubbed and
 quartered
Salt and black pepper, to taste
¹/₂ pound salmon, tilapia, or red snapper
 fillet, cut into 1-inch cubes
1 tablespoon chopped fresh dill,
 or 1 teaspoon dried dill
¹/₂ medium-size red bell pepper
 (optional), finely diced

1. Heat the olive oil in a large saucepan over medium heat. Add the onion, celery, and carrot and cook until softened, about 5 minutes.

2. Reduce the heat to low, add the chicken broth and buttermilk, and let the soup come to a simmer.

3. Add the potatoes, let the soup return to a simmer, and cook until the potatoes are tender, about 10 minutes. Season the soup with salt and black pepper to taste. The soup can be prepared up to this point and

refrigerated, covered, for 1 day. Reheat the soup gently over low heat before proceeding with Step 4.

4. Add the fish and dill and let simmer until the fish is just cooked through (don't overcook it). Pour the soup into serving bowls and top with a sprinkling of bell pepper, if desired.

SERVES 2

FROM THE TEST KITCHEN

LIKE TO COVER EVEN MORE Daily Dozen bases in your bowl of fish chowder? Substitute cubes of sweet potatoes for the red-skinned ones.

Nutrition Info

1 PORTION PROVIDES:

Protein: 1 serving

Calcium: ¹/₂ serving

Vitamin C: 1¹/₂ servings

Green leafy and yellow vegetables and fruits: 1¹/₂ servings

Other fruits and vegetables: 1 serving

Fat: ¹/₂ serving

Beef and Barley Soup

I s it soup? Or is it stew? Who cares—this all-in-one meal is the perfect way to warm up a chill evening. It's delicious heated up the next day. Top with shreddded cheese to add a calcium serving.

1 tablespoon olive oil
1 pound lean beef, cut into
   1-inch cubes
1 small onion, chopped
4 cloves garlic, minced
1 package (16 ounces)
   baby carrots
2 teaspoons dried oregano
4 cups low-sodium beef broth,
   chicken broth, or vegetable
   broth
1 bay leaf
$1/2$ cup pearl barley
1 package (8 ounces) sliced mushrooms
   (about 3 cups)
Salt and black pepper, to taste

1. Heat the olive oil in a large saucepan over medium-high heat. Add the beef and brown on all sides, about 3 minutes. Add the onion, garlic, carrots, and oregano and cook until the onion is softened, about 5 minutes.

2. Add the beef broth and bay leaf. Let come to a boil, then reduce the heat and let simmer until well blended, about 45 minutes.

3. Add the barley and mushrooms and cook until the barley is tender, about 30 minutes. Remove and discard the bay leaf, then season the soup with salt and pepper to taste. The soup can be refrigerated, covered, for up to 2 days.

SERVES 4

Nutrition Info

1 PORTION PROVIDES:

Protein: 1 serving

Green leafy and yellow vegetables and fruits: 3 servings

Other fruits and vegetables: 2 servings

Whole grains and legumes: $1/2$ serving

Iron: from beef

Pasta

Nothing satisfies a carb craving or comforts a tumultuous tummy like a plateful of pasta. And there's good news these days for pregnant pasta lovers: Though pasta in the past was almost always made with refined wheat, you can now find an impressive selection of whole-grain, high-protein, and vegetable pasta alongside that white stuff. Not only are these pasta options usually more nutritious (with more fiber, more trace minerals, and more naturally occurring vitamins), their heartier bite and nutty taste give a new dimension to standard pasta recipes. They're also more colorful.

You can toss virtually anything—seafood, poultry, vegetables, cheese—with pasta and call it a meal. From Sautéed Shrimp and Linguine to Whole Wheat Spirals with Chicken, Tiny Tomatoes, and Spinach, there are plenty of delicious one-bowl ways to eat pasta while loving every nutritious bite.

Fettuccine with Turkey and Wild Mushrooms

Take a walk on the wild side, and explore the intriguing texture wild mushrooms add to fettuccine. Yogurt makes the sauce Alfredo-like, without Alfredo's fat.

¼ pound whole wheat, spinach, or soy fettuccine

1 tablespoon olive oil

½ pound turkey breast, thinly sliced across the grain

3 cups sliced mixed wild mushrooms such as shiitakes or portobellos (about ½ pound)

2 shallots, minced

1 teaspoon fresh thyme leaves

⅓ cup plain yogurt (whole-milk yogurt makes a creamier sauce)

3 tablespoons minced fresh dill

½ cup grated Parmesan cheese

Salt and black pepper, to taste

2 tablespoons toasted pine nuts (optional; see page 272)

1. Bring a large pot of water to a boil over medium-high heat. Add the fettuccine and cook it according to the directions on the package.

2. Meanwhile, heat the olive oil in a large nonstick skillet over medium heat. Add the turkey and cook until almost cooked through, about 3 minutes. Add the mushrooms, shallots, and thyme and cook until the mushrooms soften, 3 to 4 minutes. Add the yogurt and dill and toss to mix. Set the turkey and mushroom

mixture aside until the fettuccine is ready, covering it to keep warm.

3. Drain the fettuccine, shaking off any excess water. Toss the fettuccine with the turkey and mushroom mixture and the Parmesan cheese, then season with salt and pepper to taste. Sprinkle the pine nuts over the fettuccine, if desired.

SERVES 2

FROM THE TEST KITCHEN

SLICED CARROTS STEAMED until just tender would add a yellow vegetable, a bit of crunch, and a little color to the Fettuccine with Turkey and Wild Mushrooms. Toss them in after the mushrooms have cooked for about 2 minutes.

Nutrition Info

1 PORTION PROVIDES:

Protein: 1½ servings; 2½ if made with soy pasta

Calcium: 1 serving

Other fruits and vegetables: 3 servings

Whole grains and legumes: 2 servings

Fat: ½ serving

Whole Wheat Spirals with Chicken, Tiny Tomatoes, and Spinach

Chicken, cherry tomatoes, and spinach make a colorful and nutritious combo for a light yet zesty sauce that's a flash in the pan to prepare.

¼ pound whole wheat or soy spirals, rotelle, or rotini
1 tablespoon olive oil
½ pound skinless, boneless chicken breasts or turkey cutlets or tenderloins, thinly sliced
2 shallots, thinly sliced
1 clove garlic, thinly sliced
1 cup cherry or grape tomatoes
1 bag (about 6 ounces) baby spinach, thick stems removed, or
1 package (10 ounces) frozen whole-leaf spinach, thawed and drained well
2 tablespoons sliced fresh basil (optional)
½ cup shredded mozzarella cheese
¼ cup grated Parmesan cheese
Cracked black pepper
Grated zest of 1 medium-size lemon

1. Bring a large pot of water to a boil over medium-high heat. Add the pasta and cook it according to the directions on the package.

2. Meanwhile, heat the olive oil in a skillet over medium-high heat. Add the chicken and cook until cooked through (there should be no pink), 5 to 7 minutes. Remove the chicken from the skillet and set aside.

3. Add the shallots and garlic to the skillet and cook over medium heat until softened, about 3 minutes. Add the tomatoes and cook until they soften, about 3 minutes. Return the chicken to the skillet, then add the spinach and basil, if using. Cover the skillet and cook until the spinach wilts, about 1 minute. Set the chicken sauce aside until the pasta is ready, covering it to keep warm.

4. Drain the pasta, shaking off any excess water. Toss the pasta with the mozzarella, Parmesan cheese, and cracked black pepper. Divide the pasta between 2 serving bowls. Spoon the chicken sauce over it, then sprinkle the lemon zest on top.

SERVES 2

Nutrition Info
1 PORTION PROVIDES:

Protein: 1$\frac{1}{2}$ servings if made with whole wheat pasta; 2$\frac{1}{2}$ if made with soy pasta

Calcium: 1$\frac{1}{2}$ servings

Vitamin C: 2 servings

Green leafy and yellow vegetables and fruits: 3 servings

Whole grains and legumes: 2 servings

Iron: from the spinach

Fat: $\frac{1}{2}$ serving

PASTA PRIMER

▼ ▼ ▼

Don't know fusilli from fettuccine? Not to worry. Most recipes will work no matter what pasta you pick. Still, some pasta shapes are better suited to certain types of dishes than others. Here's a handy guide:

■ Regular spaghetti is typically served with light tomato-based sauces. The skinniest pastas, such as angel hair and vermicelli, work best in broths or with thinner sauces.

■ Long, flat pastas, like fettuccine and linguine, stand up to thicker, creamier sauces.

■ Specialty pasta shapes, such as bow ties, shells, corkscrews, rotelle, radiatore (radiators), and so on, can help trap a chunkier sauce and hold it as it travels from plate to mouth (so you won't end up with quite so many stains on your belly). Most are also sturdy enough to use in pasta salads and baked casseroles.

■ Tubular pasta, like penne or ziti, are the pasta of choice for salads, thick sauces, and casseroles. Tubes with grooves on the exterior, like fusilli, penne rigate, and rigatoni do a better job of securing sauces.

Alotta Broccoli with Chicken and Penne

A plateful of broccoli never tasted so good. Not surprising, consider-ing the tasty company it keeps: chicken, cheese, and crunchy wal-nuts. The result is a lightly sauced but flavor-filled pasta dish.

¹/₄ pound whole wheat or soy penne

2 cups broccoli florets

1 tablespoon olive oil

1 small onion, chopped

1 clove garlic, minced

¹/₂ pound skinless, boneless chicken
   breast, cut into ¹/₂-inch strips

¹/₄ cup low-sodium chicken broth,
   or more if necessary

¹/₂ teaspoon dried oregano

¹/₂ cup grated cheddar or
   Asiago cheese

¹/₂ cup grated Parmesan cheese

1 tablespoon chopped fresh
   flat-leaf parsley

2 tablespoons coarsely
   chopped toasted walnuts
   (see page 272)

Cracked black pepper

1. Bring a large pot of water to a boil over medium-high heat. Add the penne and cook it according to the directions on the package.

HOW MUCH PASTA?

▼ ▼ ▼

The recipes here usually call for ¹/₄ pound of pasta to serve two people or ¹/₂ pound for four. If a 2-ounce serving of pasta sounds small, bear in mind that the kinds of pastas being used are whole wheat, spinach, or high-protein (such as soy or lentil), and so are more substantial than regular pasta made with semolina.

Don't have a kitchen scale? Most whole wheat and spinach pastas come in 1-pound packages, so boil a quarter of the pasta for two. (Some pasta comes in 8-ounce packages, in which case, use half.) High-protein pastas are often sold in 12-ounce packages; boil one third of the pasta for two.

CHICKENED OUT?

▼ ▼ ▼

You can substitute turkey cutlets or tenderloins, sliced lean beef, scallops, or peeled and deveined shrimp in almost any pasta recipe that calls for chicken. Shrimp and scallops won't need to cook as long; simmer or sauté it only until it's firm and opaque—don't let it overcook.

For a vegan alternative, substitute chunks of well-drained extra-firm tofu for the chicken. Add the tofu after the other ingredients have cooked through. If you have the time, it will pick up more flavor if you let it cook briefly.

For extra spice, add ½ teaspoon (or more) crushed red pepper flakes to chicken sauces.

2. Meanwhile, steam the broccoli following the instructions on page 391 until crisp-tender, about 7 minutes.

3. Heat the olive oil in a large nonstick skillet over medium-low heat. Add the onion and garlic and cook, stirring, until they begin to soften, about 3 minutes. Add the chicken and cook until it is no longer pink, about 4 minutes. Add the chicken broth and oregano and cook until heated through, about 1 minute.

4. Remove the broccoli from the steamer and add it to the chicken mixture. Reduce the heat to low and cook, stirring frequently, until the flavors blend, about 2 minutes. Set the broccoli mixture aside until the penne is ready, covering it to keep warm.

5. Drain the penne, shaking off any excess water. Add the penne and the cheddar cheese, ¼ cup of the Parmesan cheese, and the parsley to the broccoli

mixture and toss to mix. If the penne seems too dry, add more chicken broth.

6. Divide the penne among 4 serving bowls. Top it with the remaining ¼ cup of Parmesan cheese and the walnuts. Sprinkle cracked black pepper over the penne and serve at once.

SERVES 2

Nutrition Info
1 PORTION PROVIDES:

Protein: 1½ servings; 2½ if made with soy pasta

Calcium: 1½ servings

Vitamin C: 2 servings

Green leafy and yellow vegetables and fruits: 2 servings

Other fruits and vegetables: 1 serving

Whole grains and legumes: 2 servings

Fat: ½ serving

Whole Wheat Penne with Chicken and Skillet Tomato Sauce

Why settle for pasta with tomato sauce from a jar when you can make a healthier and tastier version in just a few minutes? Want an extra serving of green leafy and C? Add a cup of steamed broccoli.

¼ pound whole wheat or soy penne
1 tablespoon olive oil
½ pound skinless, boneless chicken
   breast, thinly sliced
1 clove garlic, thinly sliced
½ small onion, finely chopped
1 medium-size red bell pepper,
   chopped
2 cups chopped canned Italian
   tomatoes
1½ teaspoons chopped fresh
   oregano, or ½ teaspoon dried
   oregano
1½ teaspoons chopped fresh basil,
   or ½ teaspoon dried basil
½ cup grated Asiago cheese
½ cup grated Parmesan cheese
2 tablespoons chopped fresh
   flat-leaf parsley

1. Bring a large pot of water to a boil over medium-high heat. Add the penne and cook it according to the directions on the package.

2. Meanwhile, heat the olive oil in a large nonstick skillet over medium heat. Add the chicken and cook it until no longer pink, about 4 minutes. Add the garlic and cook until the flavor releases, about 1 minute. Add the onion and bell pepper

and cook until they begin to soften, about 3 minutes. Add the tomatoes, oregano, and basil and let simmer until the flavors are well blended, about 4 minutes. Set the chicken sauce aside until the penne is ready, covering it to keep warm.

3. Drain the penne, shaking off any excess water. Toss the penne with the Asiago, ¼ cup of the Parmesan cheese, and the parsley. Divide the penne between 2 serving bowls and top it with the chicken sauce and the remaining ¼ cup of Parmesan cheese.

SERVES 2

Nutrition Info

1 PORTION PROVIDES:

Protein: 1½ servings; 2½ if made with soy pasta

Calcium: 2 servings

Vitamin C: 2 servings

Green leafy and yellow vegetables and fruits: 1½ servings

Whole grains and legumes: 2 servings

Fat: ½ serving

Sautéed Shrimp and Linguine

Elegant enough for company and easy enough for a speedy (and tasty) end to a busy day, here's a scampi that's skimpy on fat but generous in flavor. Chicken broth, enriched by provolone and Parmesan cheese, makes a light but creamy tasting sauce. Red bell pepper (as always) adds extra nutrients.

¹⁄₄ pound whole wheat or soy linguine
1 tablespoon olive oil
1 teaspoon chopped garlic, or 2 cloves garlic thinly sliced
1 medium-size red bell pepper, thinly sliced
¹⁄₂ pound large shelled and deveined shrimp
2 cups low-sodium chicken broth, or 2 cups fish or shellfish stock
¹⁄₂ cup grated provolone cheese

¹⁄₄ cup grated Parmesan cheese
Cracked black pepper
2 tablespoons chopped fresh flat-leaf parsley
¹⁄₄ teaspoon crushed red pepper flakes (optional)

1. Bring a large pot of water to a boil over medium-high heat. Add the linguine and cook it according to the directions on the package.

PASTA PRESTO

▼ ▼ ▼

Looking for a way to shave time off your pasta prep? Try this trick: Add the contents of an entire box of pasta to a pot of boiling salted water and cook it for five minutes. Remove half the pasta from the pot (or as much as you want to save for later) and drain it. Toss this pasta with about 2 tablespoons of olive oil (just enough to coat it lightly) and ¹⁄₄ cup chopped fresh flat-leaf parsley. Let the pasta cool to room temperature, then refrigerate it in an airtight container until you're ready for another pasta fest—up to one week (if you can wait that long). Continue cooking the remaining pasta until it's done and use it for tonight's dinner. When you're next in the mood for pasta, simply heat a sauce or broth in a saucepan and add the partially cooked pasta to the pan. Let the pasta simmer until it has finished cooking, then serve.

2. Meanwhile, heat the olive oil in a skillet over medium heat. Add the garlic and cook until just golden, 2 minutes. Add the bell pepper and cook until slightly softened, about 2 minutes. Add the shrimp and cook until it is cooked through and turns opaque, about 4 minutes. Remove the bell pepper and shrimp from the skillet and set aside, covered to keep warm.

3. Add the chicken broth to the skillet, let come to a simmer, then add the provolone and Parmesan cheese, and the parsley and pepper to taste.

4. Drain the linguine, shaking off any excess water. Divide the linguine between 2 serving bowls, spoon the broth mixture over it, and top it with the shrimp and bell pepper mixture. If you like a little spice, sprinkle the red bell pepper flakes on top.

SERVES 2

FROM THE TEST KITCHEN

YOU'RE NOT STILL SHELLING and deveining your shrimp, are you? Keep a bag of ready-to-cook peeled and deveined shrimp in the freezer. Or you can substitute scallops.

Nutrition Info

1 PORTION PROVIDES:

Protein: 1½ servings; 2½ if made with soy pasta

Calcium: 1½ servings

Vitamin C: 2 servings

Green leafy and yellow vegetables and fruits: 1 serving

Whole grains and legumes: 2 servings

Fat: ½ serving

Cozy at Home Macaroni and Cheese

Comfort food at its most nutritious, this macaroni and cheese is definitely different from the orange stuff you get in a box. It's a whole lot tastier, too. Four cheeses add flavor and calcium and broccoli adds vitamins—try finding those in that box! Plus you'll love the leftovers—they reheat in the microwave in minutes.

½ pound whole wheat or soy pasta,
    such as elbow macaroni, penne,
    or shells
2 tablespoons butter or margarine
1½ tablespoons whole wheat flour
1 cup milk
½ cup grated Gouda cheese
½ cup shredded mild cheddar cheese
    or Havarti cheese
1 cup shredded part-skim mozzarella
    cheese
Dash of hot pepper sauce, or more
    to taste (optional)
Salt and black pepper
1 cup cooked broccoli, or 1 cup
    cooked chopped kale
2 tablespoons grated Parmesan
    cheese
1½ tablespoons wheat germ or
    whole wheat bread crumbs

1. Preheat the oven to 350°F.

2. Bring a large pot of water to a boil over medium-high heat. Add the pasta and cook it according to the directions on the package.

3. Meanwhile, melt the butter in a non-stick saucepan over medium heat. Add the flour and cook until a paste forms, 1 to 2 minutes. Add the milk and let it come to a boil, stirring constantly. When the milk thickens slightly, remove it from the heat and add the Gouda, cheddar, and mozzarella cheese. Stir until the cheeses melt. Season the cheese sauce with hot sauce and salt and pepper to taste, then set it aside.

4. Drain the pasta, shaking off any excess water, then add the cheese sauce and stir to coat evenly. Add the broccoli to the pasta and stir to combine. Place the pasta mixture in a 9-by-13-inch baking dish or a 9-inch round casserole.

5. Place the Parmesan cheese and the wheat germ in a small bowl and stir to mix, then sprinkle this over the pasta.

6. Bake the pasta and cheese until hot and bubbly, about 10 minutes.

SERVES 4

FROM THE TEST KITCHEN

FOR A BIGGER PROTEIN punch, toss diced tofu, cooked chicken, or edamame into the macaroni and cheese. You can also add other vegetables or add more than one. Try 1 cup chopped roasted red bell peppers, yellow corn, green peas, or cooked spinach. To go white-on-white, use 1 cup chopped cooked cauliflower instead of broccoli. You won't even notice that you're eating your vegetables.

Nutrition Info

1 PORTION PROVIDES:

Protein: 2 servings; 3 if made with soy pasta

Calcium: 2½ servings

Vitamin C: ½ serving

Green leafy and yellow vegetables and fruits: ½ serving if made with broccoli; 1 serving if made with kale

Whole grains and legumes: 2 servings

Fat: ½ serving

Udon Noodles with Vegetable Stir-Fry

Udon are thick Japanese noodles with a chewy texture; they're a world away from regular spaghetti. You can add just about any quick-cooking vegetable or protein to this tasty skillet meal.

4 ounces *udon* noodles (preferably whole-grain)
1¹/₂ tablespoons low-sodium soy sauce
2 tablespoons seasoned rice vinegar
1¹/₂ teaspoons sesame oil
1 tablespoon grated peeled fresh ginger
2¹/₂ teaspoons olive oil
3 scallions (optional), both white and light green parts, trimmed and thinly sliced
1 cup sliced shiitake mushrooms
1 cup snow peas or sugar snap peas
¹/₂ cup small broccoli florets
¹/₂ cup shredded carrots
2 cups (16 ounces) firm tofu, drained well and diced
1 tablespoon chopped fresh cilantro

1. Bring a large pot of water to a boil over medium-high heat. Add the udon noodles and cook them according to the directions on the package, then drain them, shaking off any excess water, and set them aside.

2. Place the soy sauce, rice vinegar, sesame oil, and ginger in a small bowl and whisk to mix. Set the soy sauce mixture aside.

3. Place the olive oil in a large nonstick skillet over medium heat. Add the scallions,

if using, the mushrooms, snow peas, broccoli, carrots, and tofu. Stir-fry until the vegetables begin to soften, about 3 minutes.

4. Add the soy sauce mixture and udon noodles to the skillet and cook until the noodles are heated through and the flavors are blended, about 3 minutes. Sprinkle the cilantro over the noodles and serve.

SERVES 2

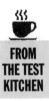

FROM THE TEST KITCHEN **NOT A TOFU FAN?** Stir-fry thinly sliced chicken breast, lean beef or pork, or some shelled and deveined shrimp instead. You'll net extra protein, too.

Nutrition Info

1 PORTION PROVIDES:

Protein: 1¹/₂ servings

Calcium: ¹/₂ serving

Vitamin C: 1¹/₂ servings

Green leafy and yellow vegetables and fruits: 1 serving

Other fruits and vegetables: 1 serving

Whole grains and legumes: 3 servings

Fat: ¹/₂ serving

Sauces

A t a loss for pasta sauce? You won't be if you make extra-large batches of any (or all) of these sauces. Most can be refrigerated, covered, for a week or frozen for up to three months. Toss with pasta, veggies, and chicken, fish, seafood, or tofu, and you'll have a meal in minutes!

◆◆◆◆◆

Pesto with Sunflower Seeds

Instead of the traditional pine nuts, this pesto gets its rich flavor—and healthy fatty acids—from sunflower seeds. Spoon it on pasta, in sandwiches, on poultry, or on anything else that could use a pesto pick-me-up.

2 cups loosely packed fresh
　　basil leaves
1/2 cup shelled sunflower seeds
11/2 teaspoons chopped garlic
2 tablespoons olive oil, plus more for
　　storing the pesto
Juice of 1 medium-size lemon
1/2 cup grated Parmesan cheese
Salt and black pepper

1. Place the basil, sunflower seeds, and garlic in a food processor and process until finely chopped.

2. With the motor running, add the olive oil and lemon juice in a steady stream through the feed tube.

3. Transfer the pesto to a small bowl. Fold in the Parmesan cheese, and salt and pepper to taste. To store, place the pesto in a small airtight container and float a thin layer of olive oil over the top to keep the basil from turning brown. To use, toss 2-ounce servings of hot pasta with several tablespoons of pesto. The pesto can be refrigerated for 2 weeks.

MAKES ABOUT 2 CUPS

Nutrition Info

1 PORTION (1/2 CUP) PROVIDES:

Calcium: 1/2 serving

Fat: 1/2 serving

Turkey Bolognese Sauce

Think of this as Bolognese sauce on a diet—lean and tasty, flavored with turkey instead of beef.

1 tablespoon olive oil
1 medium-size onion, chopped
3 medium-size carrots, chopped
2 ribs celery, chopped
2 cloves garlic, peeled and crushed,
   or 1 teaspoon chopped garlic
1½ pounds ground turkey or chicken
1 can (28 ounces) diced tomatoes
   with their juices
1 can (about 29 ounces) tomato purée
1½ teaspoons dried oregano
2 bay leaves
¼ cup chopped flat-leaf parsley
Salt and black pepper

1. Heat the olive oil in a saucepan over medium heat. Add the onion and cook until slightly softened, about 1 minute. Add the carrots, celery, and garlic and cook until the carrots and celery start to soften, about 2 minutes.

2. Add the turkey and cook, chopping up the pieces with a wooden spoon, until the turkey is cooked through, about 10 minutes.

3. Add the diced tomatoes, tomato purée, oregano, bay leaves, and parsley, let come to a simmer and cook until the flavors blend, about 15 minutes. Let the sauce cool to room temperature, add salt and pepper to taste, then discard the bay leaves and spoon the sauce into three 1-pint containers. The sauce can be frozen for up to 2 months. Let it thaw in the refrigerator overnight before reheating it.

MAKES ABOUT 6 CUPS

Nutrition Info

1 PORTION (1 CUP) PROVIDES:

Protein: 2 servings

Vitamin C: 2 servings

Green leafy and yellow vegetables and fruits: 1½ servings

Gazpacho Sauce

With tomatoes fresh from the garden (or your grocer's produce aisle), instead of from a jar, you can practically taste the sunshine in this gazpacho sauce. Use it on pasta, poultry, and fish or seafood dishes.

1 tablespoon olive oil
1/2 teaspoon chopped garlic
6 medium-size tomatoes, coarsely
   chopped, or 4 cups canned
   crushed tomatoes, with their
   juices
1 medium-size red bell pepper,
   coarsely chopped
3 scallions, both white and
   light green parts, trimmed
   and thinly sliced
1/4 cup fresh basil leaves, or
   2 teaspoons dried basil
1 teaspoon balsamic vinegar,
   or more to taste
Salt and pepper

Heat the olive oil in a large nonstick saucepan over medium heat. Add the garlic and cook until beginning to soften, about 1 minute. Add the tomatoes, bell pepper, scallions, and basil and cook until the tomatoes are saucelike and the bell pepper softens, about 10 minutes. Remove the sauce from the heat and add vinegar and salt and pepper to taste. You can serve this sauce as is or purée it in a food processor. To store, spoon the cooled sauce into two 1-pint airtight containers and refrigerate or freeze it. The sauce can be frozen for up to 2 months. Let it thaw in the refrigerator overnight before reheating it.

MAKES ABOUT 4 CUPS

Nutrition Info

1 PORTION (1 CUP) PROVIDES:

Vitamin C: 2 1/2 servings

Green leafy and yellow vegetables and fruits: 1/2 serving

SAUCY SECRETS

▼ ▼ ▼

Feel like you can't look at another carrot or red bell pepper or another piece of broccoli or cauliflower? Don't look at them—hide them in tomato sauce. Tomato sauces (or tomato and meat sauces) can camouflage just about any vegetable (which is why this is a trick you'll want to keep up your sleeve when you start feeding a picky toddler), and what you can't see or smell won't be off-putting to you.

If you're making sauce from scratch, add the chopped vegetable or vegetables when you sauté the onion and garlic. If you're opening up a jar, just simmer the vegetables in the sauce until they're tender enough to be inconspicuous. If you're adding chopped meat to store-bought sauce, add the veggies when you brown the meat (just make sure your meat is extra-lean).

Spicy Tomato Sauce

Dragging after a long day? This tasty tomato sauce (hot mamas and papas can add even more red pepper flakes if they like) will give you just the jolt you need. It's particularly good tossed with shrimp, scallops, or other seafood.

1 tablespoon olive oil
1 medium-size onion, finely chopped
3 cloves garlic, finely chopped
   (for 1¹/₂ teaspoons chopped garlic)
6 ripe medium-size tomatoes, chopped,
   or 4 cups canned diced tomatoes,
   with their juices
1 medium-size red bell pepper,
   coarsely chopped
1 small hot red chile pepper,
   seeded and minced
¹/₄ cup fresh basil leaves, or
   2 teaspoons dried basil
2 tablespoons chopped fresh oregano,
   or 2 teaspoons dried oregano
1 teaspoon crushed red pepper flakes
Salt and black pepper

Heat the olive oil in a large nonstick saucepan over medium heat. Add the onion and cook until softened, about 5 minutes. Add the garlic and cook until the flavors blend, about 2 minutes. Add the tomatoes, peppers, basil, oregano, and red pepper flakes. Reduce the heat and let simmer gently until the tomatoes are saucelike and the flavors are blended, about 15 minutes. Let the sauce cool to room temperature and season with salt and pepper to taste. Spoon it into two 1-pint containers and either refrigerate or freeze. The sauce can be frozen for up to 2 months. Let it thaw in the refrigerator overnight before reheating it.

MAKES ABOUT 4 CUPS

Nutrition Info

1 PORTION (1 CUP) PROVIDES:

Vitamin C: 2¹/₂ servings

Green leafy and yellow vegetables and fruits: ¹/₂ serving

Salads

Sure, you can fill a bowl with lettuce and tomato, douse it with bottled dressing, and call it a salad. But why settle for that when there are so many exciting salad combinations just waiting to be tossed your way? Whether a salad's a side dish or the main event, all the varieties you'll find here deserve a starring role on the table. From fruit salads to ones with cheese, from salads of cabbage to spinach salads, from seafood to poultry, there's a salad in here for everybody (any of the salads that serve two can easily be doubled).

Side Salads

Want a little salad with your dinner? Try one of these tasty side salads. Each crunchy serving will satisfy your taste buds and your nutritional requirements. Don't have room on the side? Side salads make an elegant first course, too—one that can take the edge off your appetite before you dig into the main course. Starting with a salad can also help you pace yourself at dinner, so that you don't get full—or eat—too fast. (Think of it as a meal within a meal.)

Spinach Strawberry Salad

Here's a summer treat that you can prepare in just minutes. Skip the onion if it offends your tummy (or if you'll be doing some after-dinner kissing)—the salad's just as yummy without it.

4 cups (packed) baby spinach
1 cup sliced fresh strawberries
   (about ¹⁄₂ pint)
¹⁄₄ cup sliced red onion (optional)
¹⁄₄ cup toasted sliced almonds
   (see page 272)
2 tablespoons distilled white
   vinegar or white wine vinegar
2 tablespoons canola oil

2 tablespoons white grape juice
   concentrate, apple juice concentrate,
   Splenda, honey, or brown sugar,
   to taste
¹⁄₂ teaspoon paprika
Salt and black pepper

1. Place the spinach, strawberries, onion, if using, and almonds in a salad bowl.

2. Place the vinegar, oil, grape juice concentrate, and paprika in a small bowl and whisk to mix. Season with salt and pepper to taste. Toss the salad with enough dressing to coat evenly. Divide the salad between 2 smaller salad bowls and serve.

SERVES 2

Nutrition Info

1 PORTION PROVIDES:

Vitamin C: 3 servings

Green leafy and yellow vegetables and fruits: 2 servings

Fat: 1 serving

ENOUGH IS LIKE A FEAST

▼ ▼ ▼

Salad eaters come in all kinds of packages—including the kind who can eat their way through a whole package of salad (and the kind who can barely make it through leaf one). The salad servings in this section are geared to that salad eater in the middle—the one who can happily manage about 2 cups of greens (which, when dressed, wilt down to considerably less). If the recipe makes too much salad for you, cut the servings in half or more (just realize you'll also have to cut the number of green leafy and vitamin C servings you'll net). If the recipe doesn't make enough salad, double the recipe—and double the nutrients you'll be able to score.

Crunchy Pear Salad

Pick a pear that's ripe enough to be fragrant, yet firm enough to lend crunchiness to this lovely fall salad.

1 ripe pear, halved, cored, peeled, and thinly sliced
4 cups (packed) baby spinach or arugula, thick stems removed
2 tablespoons balsamic vinegar
1 to 2 tablespoons olive oil
2 teaspoons Dijon mustard

1 shallot, minced
Salt and black pepper
1/2 cup Parmesan cheese shavings (about 2 ounces; see box on page 317)
1/4 cup toasted walnut pieces (see page 272)

1. Place the pear and spinach in a salad bowl and stir to mix.

2. Place the balsamic vinegar, olive oil, mustard, and shallot in a small bowl and whisk to mix, then season with salt and pepper to taste. Toss the salad with enough dressing to coat evenly. Divide the pear salad between 2 smaller salad bowls and top with the Parmesan shavings and walnut pieces.

SERVES 2

Nutrition Info

1 PORTION PROVIDES:

Protein: 1/2 serving

Calcium: 1 serving

Vitamin C: 1 serving if made with spinach; 1/2 serving if made with arugula

Green leafy and yellow vegetables and fruits: 2 servings

Other fruits and vegetables: 1/2 serving

Fat: 1/2 serving if made with 1 tablespoon oil; 1 serving if made with 2

A BETTER BALSAMIC VINAIGRETTE

▽ ▽ ▽

Looking for a balsamic vinaigrette without a lot of oil? Whisk together the following: 2 tablespoons balsamic vinegar, 1 tablespoon olive oil, 1 minced shallot, 1 minced garlic clove (optional, but if raw garlic bothers you, see page 331), 1 teaspoon Dijon or whole-grain mustard, and salt and pepper to taste. You can add any herb you like—fresh or dried tarragon, basil, or flat-leaf parsley would all be good. If you prefer a sweeter dressing, add enough fruit juice concentrate, Splenda, honey, brown sugar, or another sweetener to suit your sweet tooth.

Pomegranate Salad

Pomegranates are a delicious exception to the "Eat the fruit; throw out the seeds" rule. In this unusual twist on a standard salad, pomegranate seeds add crunch and a tangy sweetness to the greens, while the juice lends a rich flavor to the dressing. Both are great sources for vitamins and antioxidants. Salty Parmesan cheese complements the sweet combo.

A QUICK SHAVE

▼ ▼ ▼

Those fancy curls of Parmesan cheese only look like they take forever (and a culinary degree) to create. It's actually as easy as this: Let a chunk of Parmesan soften slightly at room temperature, then use a potato peeler to peel off thin shavings. That's all there is to it!

½ cup pomegranate juice (see Note)
1 tablespoon balsamic vinegar
1 tablespoon olive oil
1 teaspoon whole-grain mustard
1 shallot, minced
Fresh lemon juice
Salt and black pepper
4 cups (packed) baby greens
    (mâche, baby spinach, spring mix,
    watercress, or a combination)
Seeds from ½ pomegranate
½ cup Parmesan cheese shavings
    (about 2 ounces; see box)

1. Place the pomegranate juice in a small saucepan and bring to a boil over medium heat. Reduce the heat and let simmer until the juice is reduced to about 2 tablespoons, about 10 minutes. Remove the juice from the heat.

2. Add the balsamic vinegar, olive oil, mustard, and shallot to the reduced pomegranate juice and whisk to mix. Season with lemon juice, salt, and pepper to taste.

3. Place the greens and pomegranate seeds in a large salad bowl. Toss with enough dressing to coat evenly. Divide the pomegranate salad between 2 smaller salad bowls, sprinkle the Parmesan shavings on top, and serve immediately.

SERVES 2

NOTE: Pomegranate juice is available in the refrigerated section of supermarkets and health food stores.

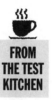

FROM THE TEST KITCHEN

TURN POMEGRANATE SALAD into a main dish by doubling the recipe and topping it with grilled shrimp or chicken.

Nutrition Info

1 PORTION PROVIDES:

Calcium: 1 serving

Vitamin C: ½ serving; 2 servings if made with watercress

Green leafy and yellow vegetables and fruits: 2 servings

Other fruits and vegetables: 1 serving

Fat: ½ serving

Ginger Melon Salad

Always save your fruit salad for dessert? This melon combo makes a refreshing first course or side for grilled chicken or fish. Best of all, it's a comforting way to tuck away vitamins—without vegetables.

2 tablespoons white grape juice
  concentrate, Splenda, honey,
  brown sugar, or another sweetener
1/2 tablespoon minced peeled fresh
  ginger
1/2 tablespoon chopped fresh mint
1/2 teaspoon grated lime zest
2 tablespoons fresh lime juice
1 cup 1-inch watermelon cubes
1 cup 1-inch cantaloupe cubes

1. Place the grape juice concentrate, ginger, mint, lime zest, and lime juice in a small bowl and stir to mix.

2. Place the watermelon and cantaloupe cubes in a large salad bowl, pour the lime and ginger mixture over them, and toss to coat evenly. Cover the salad and refrigerate for at least 1 hour before serving.

SERVES 2

FROM THE TEST KITCHEN FOR A TANGIER SALAD, substitute orange or pineapple juice concentrate for the white grape concentrate in the Ginger Melon Salad. For calcium, toss in or top with 1/2 cup pasteurized feta or goat cheese.

DRESSING IT UP

▼ ▼ ▼

A sweet yet tangy cider vinaigrette can dress up any simple green salad, but it's especially tasty tossed with a fruit and cheese combo, such as baby greens with sliced pear and cheese wedges or baby greens with figs and Parmesan shavings. Boil 3/4 cup of apple cider for about 10 minutes until it is reduced to 2 tablespoons, then mix it with 2 tablespoons cider vinegar, 1 minced small shallot, 3/4 teaspoon Dijon mustard, and 1 tablespoon or more vegetable oil. Season the dressing to taste with salt and pepper, then prepare for a taste of autumn.

Nutrition Info

1 PORTION PROVIDES:

Vitamin C: 1 1/2 servings

Green leafy and yellow vegetables and
  fruits: 1 serving

Other fruits and vegetables: 1 serving

Mucho Mango Salad

Few fruits—or even vegetables—bring as many vitamins to the table as the sweet mango. This salad doubles the mango, and the nutrients, by using it in the dressing, too.

1½ large ripe mangoes, peeled
   and cubed
2 tablespoons whole-milk yogurt
1 tablespoon fresh lime juice
1 tablespoon orange juice
1 tablespoon orange juice
   concentrate or pineapple
   juice concentrate
2 teaspoons grated peeled fresh ginger
   (optional)
½ teaspoon ground coriander
Salt and black pepper
½ cup cubed kiwi
½ cup blueberries
2 cups mild baby greens,
   thick stems removed
2 tablespoons chopped
   macadamia nuts
Lime wedges, for serving

1. Place about one third of the mango cubes, along with the yogurt, lime juice, orange juice, orange juice concentrate, ginger, if using, and coriander in a food processor and process until smooth. Season the dressing with salt and pepper to taste.

2. Place the remaining mango cubes, kiwi, and blueberries in a large salad bowl, pour the dressing on top, and toss to coat evenly. Divide the greens between 2 salad plates, top each with half of the mango salad, then sprinkle the macadamia nuts on top. Serve with lime wedges.

SERVES 2

Nutrition Info
1 PORTION PROVIDES:

Vitamin C: 3½ servings

Green leafy and yellow vegetables and fruits: 2 servings

Fig and Arugula Salad with Parmesan Shavings

Fresh figs make this a very sensuous salad—serve it, and romance is sure to be on the menu.

1 large shallot, minced
2 tablespoons balsamic vinegar
1 to 2 tablespoons extra-virgin olive oil
1 teaspoon whole-grain mustard
Salt
8 fresh figs, cut in half
4 cups (packed) arugula, rinsed,
   thick stems removed
Black pepper
½ cup Parmesan cheese shavings
   (about 2 ounces; see box on
   page 317)

1. Place the shallot, balsamic vinegar, olive oil, mustard, and a pinch of salt in a large salad bowl and whisk to mix. Add the figs, toss to coat them evenly, and let stand, covered with plastic wrap, for 20 minutes.

2. Add the arugula to the figs and toss to mix. Season with salt and pepper to taste, then toss well. Divide the fig salad between 2 smaller salad bowls and top with the Parmesan shavings.

SERVES 2

Nutrition Info
1 PORTION PROVIDES:

Calcium: 1 serving

Vitamin C: ½ serving

Green leafy and yellow vegetables and fruits: 2 servings

Fat: ½ serving if made with 1 tablespoon oil; 1 serving if made with 2

Arugula with Shaved Fennel and Roasted Pepper Salad

For a very nutritious taste of Italy, serve this salad alongside grilled or broiled chicken or fish, or as a first stop on the way to a pasta dinner. If you prefer, substitute baby spinach or mixed baby greens for the arugula.

4 cups (packed) arugula, thick stems removed

2 tablespoons chopped fresh flat-leaf parsley

1 small fennel bulb, trimmed, halved, and very thinly sliced crosswise

2 to 4 tablespoons Lemon Vinaigrette (recipe follows)

1 roasted red bell pepper (leftover or from a jar), sliced into strips

½ cup Parmesan cheese shavings (about 2 ounces; see box on page 317)

1. Place the arugula, parsley, and fennel in a salad bowl and toss to mix. Toss with enough Lemon Vinaigrette to coat the salad evenly.

2. Divide the salad between 2 salad plates, then top it with the roasted peppers and Parmesan shavings.

SERVES 2

Nutrition Info
1 PORTION (WITHOUT DRESSING) PROVIDES:

Protein: 1 serving

Calcium: 1 serving

Vitamin C: 2½ servings

Green leafy and yellow vegetables and fruits: 3 servings

Lemon Vinaigrette

Simple yet versatile, this dressing can zest up almost any salad or vegetable. If the proportions in the recipe make the dressing a little too tart for your taste, increase the amount of olive oil.

5 tablespoons fresh lemon juice

3 to 5 tablespoons olive oil

Zest of 1 lemon

1 clove garlic (if raw garlic bothers you, see page 331), minced

Salt and black pepper

Place the lemon juice, olive oil, lemon zest, and garlic in a small bowl and whisk to mix. Season the vinaigrette with salt and pepper to taste. The dressing can be stored in an airtight container or jar for up to 1 week.

MAKES ABOUT ½ CUP

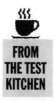

FROM THE TEST KITCHEN

CHEESE UP THE LEMON Vinaigrette by adding ¼ cup of grated Parmesan cheese. Add extra Italian flavor with a sprinkling of dried oregano.

Nutrition Info
1 PORTION (2 TABLESPOONS) PROVIDES:

Vitamin C: ½ serving

Fat: 1 serving if using 4 tablespoons oil

Broccoli, Tomato, and Mozzarella Salad

When broccoli takes on that favorite Italian salad, tomato and mozzarella, the result is both yummy and healthy. Just make sure you choose a pasteurized (not a raw) mozzarella. Domestic varieties are always a safe bet.

1¹⁄₂ cups small broccoli florets
2 ripe plum tomatoes, seeded and
   coarsely chopped
¹⁄₂ cup cubed pasteurized part-skim
   mozzarella (about 2 ounces)
3 tablespoons sliced fresh basil
2 tablespoons balsamic vinegar
1 to 2 tablespoons olive oil
¹⁄₂ medium-size lemon
Salt and black pepper
2 tablespoons toasted pine nuts
   (see page 272)

1. Steam the broccoli following the instructions on page 391 until crisp-tender, 5 to 6 minutes. Set the broccoli aside in a large salad bowl and let it cool completely, then add the tomatoes, mozzarella, and basil and toss to mix.

2. Place the balsamic vinegar and olive oil in a small bowl and whisk to mix. Pour the dressing over the salad and toss well to coat evenly. Squeeze a little lemon juice on top, season the salad with salt and pepper to taste, and toss again. Divide the broccoli salad between 2 smaller salad bowls, then sprinkle the pine nuts on top.

SERVES 2

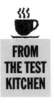

FROM THE TEST KITCHEN

NOT FEELING THE LOVE for broccoli? Leave it out, and substitute 2 sliced medium-size tomatoes.

Nutrition Info

1 PORTION PROVIDES:

Calcium: 1 serving

Vitamin C: 2 servings

Green leafy and yellow vegetables and fruits: 1¹⁄₂ servings

Fat: ¹⁄₂ serving if made with 1 tablespoon oil; 1 serving if made with 2 tablespoons

It's Mediterranean to Me Salad

This salad combines the best of Greece and Italy for a delicious Mediterranean hybrid. Here's a time-saving hint: Chop everything except the avocado early in the day; store the ingredients separately in the fridge, then toss the salad right before serving. You can beef it up by adding cubes of cooked chicken or turkey or chilled grilled shrimp.

2 cups chopped romaine lettuce
1/2 small red bell pepper, diced
1/2 medium-size avocado, preferably
    Hass, diced
1/4 hothouse (seedless English)
    cucumber, peeled and diced
1/4 medium-size red onion, chopped
2 plum tomatoes, seeded and diced
1/2 cup cubed sharp provolone cheese
    or other sharp Italian cheese
1/3 cup drained canned chickpeas
    (garbanzo beans)
1 tablespoon chopped fresh parsley
1 teaspoon chopped fresh oregano
    leaves, or 1/4 teaspoon dried oregano
1 teaspoon chopped fresh mint, or
    1/4 teaspoon dried mint (optional)
1/4 cup sliced pitted kalamata olives
    (optional)
2 tablespoons balsamic vinegar
1 to 2 tablespoons olive oil
1 1/2 teaspoons fresh lemon juice,
    or more to taste
1 small clove garlic (optional; if raw garlic
    bothers you, see page 331), minced
Salt and black pepper

1. Place the romaine, bell pepper, avocado, cucumber, onion, tomatoes, cheese, chickpeas, parsley, oregano, and mint and olives, if using, in a large salad bowl and stir to mix.

2. Place the balsamic vinegar, olive oil, lemon juice, and garlic, if using, in a small bowl and whisk to mix. Season the dressing with salt and black pepper to taste. Toss the salad with enough dressing to coat evenly. Taste for seasoning, adding more lemon juice, salt, and/or black pepper if desired. Divide the salad between 2 smaller salad bowls and serve.

SERVES 2

Nutrition Info
1 PORTION PROVIDES:

Calcium: 1 serving

Vitamin C: 1 1/2 servings

Green leafy and yellow vegetables and fruits: 1 1/2 servings

Other fruits and vegetables: 1 serving

Iron from the chickpeas

Fat: 1/2 serving if made with 1 tablespoon oil; 1 serving if made with 2

Asian Slaw

Move over, deli coleslaw. There's no room on the plate for the bland likes of you when this tangy slaw's in town. Rice vinegar, sesame oil, ginger, a hint of red pepper flakes, and cilantro give the dressing an Asian flair. Buy preshredded cabbage and carrots to save time.

1 cup coleslaw mixture
¹/₂ medium-size red bell pepper,
    thinly sliced
1 cup shredded carrots
3 tablespoons seasoned rice vinegar
1 tablespoon fresh lime juice
1 tablespoon sesame oil
1 tablespoon olive oil (optional)
1 tablespoon grated peeled fresh ginger
1 tablespoon white grape juice
    concentrate, Splenda, honey, brown
    sugar, or another sweetener, to taste
Pinch of crushed red pepper flakes
3 tablespoons chopped fresh cilantro
1 tablespoon toasted sesame seeds
    (see page 272)

1. Place the coleslaw mixture, bell pepper, and carrots in a large salad bowl and toss to mix.

2. Place the rice vinegar, lime juice, sesame oil, olive oil, if using, ginger, grape juice concentrate, pepper flakes, and cilantro in a small bowl and whisk to mix.

3. Just before serving, pour the dressing over the slaw mixture and toss to coat evenly. Sprinkle with sesame seeds and serve.

SERVES 2

FROM THE TEST KITCHEN

FOR A CRUNCHY and extra nutritious slaw, substitute 1 cup broccoli slaw (available prepacked at the supermarket) for the coleslaw mixture.

Nutrition Info
1 PORTION PROVIDES:

Vitamin C: 2 servings

Green leafy and yellow vegetables
and fruits: 3¹/₂ servings

Fat: ¹/₂ serving without olive oil;
    1 serving with it

CARROTS ONLY

▼ ▼ ▼

Can't stomach cabbage? Try a vitamin-packed all-carrot slaw instead. Drain 1 cup of canned crushed pineapple in juice, then mix it with 2 cups shredded carrots, 1½ cups raisins, and ½ cup plain low-fat yogurt. Add 2 teaspoons lemon juice; juice concentrate, honey, or Splenda to taste; a pinch of cinnamon; and 1 teaspoon grated peeled fresh ginger or ¼ teaspoon ground ginger. Chill the carrot slaw, then just before serving, stir in 2 tablespoons chopped toasted walnuts (you'll find toasting instructions on page 272). You'll have about 3 cups of slaw; it can be refrigerated for up to three days.

Dinner Salads

Looking for a light and easy way to end a long day? Turn off the oven, and chill out with a dinner salad. Pretty much any salad (from Caesar to Greek) can be turned into a meal when you top it with your choice of protein (fish, seafood, beef, poultry, or cheese). To keep things really cool, use last night's leftovers for your salad topper—you'll also save yourself time and effort. Serve dinner salads with crusty whole-grain bread or rolls.

◆◆◆◆◆

Curried Chicken Salad

Have some chicken left over from last night's dinner? Chop it up to make this yummy salad. Or, simply simmer a couple of chicken breasts in broth, let them cool, and you're ready to start. Serve the salad on top of greens or in a cantaloupe half (don't forget to count either in your Daily Dozen). Whatever chicken salad you have left over will make a great sandwich for tomorrow. Just pile it into a pita, and you're good to go.

1/2 cup plain yogurt

2 tablespoons mayonnaise

2 to 3 teaspoons curry powder

1 tablespoon fresh lime juice

2 teaspoons fresh peeled, grated ginger

2 tablespoons pineapple juice concentrate, Splenda, honey, or brown sugar

Salt and black pepper

1 pound cooked skinless, boneless chicken breasts or turkey breasts, cut into 1/2-inch pieces

4 scallions, both white and light green parts, trimmed and sliced

1 firm but ripe mango, chopped

1/2 cup chopped Granny Smith apple

1/2 red bell pepper, minced

1/3 cup toasted cashews (see page 272), coarsely chopped

Place the yogurt, mayonnaise, curry powder, lime juice, ginger, and pineapple juice concentrate in a large salad bowl and stir to mix. Add salt and pepper to taste. Add the chicken, scallions, mango, apple, bell pepper, and cashews and toss gently to combine. The salad can be refrigerated, covered, for up to 3 days.

SERVES 4

Nutrition Info

1 PORTION PROVIDES:

Protein: 1 serving

Vitamin C: 1 serving

Green leafy and yellow vegetables and fruits: 1/2 serving

Fat: 1/2 serving

Taco in a Salad

Unlike most taco salads, which tend to be astronomically high in fat and calories, this one's extra lean. Luckily, like those high-fat versions, this one is tasty, too—without all the calories.

1 tablespoon olive oil
2 cloves garlic, minced
1 medium red bell pepper, chopped
1/2 medium yellow bell pepper, chopped
1/2 small onion, chopped
8 ounces lean ground beef, buffalo,
   or ground turkey breast
2 teaspoons chili powder
1 teaspoon ground cumin
1/2 cup well-drained canned pinto
   or kidney beans, rinsed
1 1/2 cups prepared tomato salsa
2 tablespoons chopped fresh cilantro
   (optional)
Tabasco sauce (optional)
4 cups shredded romaine lettuce
2 large plum tomatoes, seeded
   and chopped
1/2 cup shredded cheddar cheese
   or Monterey Jack cheese
1/2 cup slightly crumbled baked
   taco chips

1. Heat the olive oil in a large skillet over medium heat. Add the garlic, bell peppers, and onion, and cook until softened, about 5 minutes.

2. Add the beef, chili powder, and cumin and cook, stirring frequently, until the meat is crumbly and cooked through, 3 to 4 minutes. Add the beans and salsa, bring to a boil, reduce the heat, and let simmer until the beans are heated through and the flavors are blended, about 2 minutes. Add the cilantro and Tabasco, if using.

3. Divide the lettuce between 2 large plates or bowls, then top each bed of lettuce with half of the meat mixture. Scatter half of the chopped tomato and cheese and 1/4 cup of the taco chips over each salad and serve immediately.

SERVES 2

Nutrition Info

1 PORTION PROVIDES:

Protein: 1 1/2 servings

Calcium: 1 serving

Vitamin C: 4 servings

Green leafy and yellow vegetables and fruits: 3 servings

Whole grains and legumes: 1/2 serving

Iron: if made with ground beef or buffalo

Fat: 1/2 serving

Steak Salad

No need to trek over to your local steakhouse. Here's steak and a salad, all on the same plate. You can substitute grilled or roasted portobello mushrooms for the sliced raw mushrooms.

Salt and cracked black pepper
1 strip steak or sirloin steak
   (about 1¼ inch thick and
   12 ounces), trimmed of fat
1 teaspoon finely grated lemon zest
2 tablespoons fresh lemon juice
1 to 2 tablespoons mayonnaise
Black pepper
1 medium-size red onion, cut into ¼-inch
   thick slices
4 cups (packed) arugula, or other tender
   greens, thick stems removed
1 cup thinly sliced button mushrooms
1 roasted red bell pepper (leftover or
   from a jar), thinly sliced
½ cup Parmesan cheese shavings
   (about 2 ounces; see box on page 317)

1. Preheat the broiler or set up the grill and preheat it to high.

2. Season the steak all over with salt and cracked pepper. Broil or grill the steak until the internal temperature taken with an instant-read meat thermometer is 160°F, 3 to 5 minutes per side.

3. Meanwhile, place the lemon zest, lemon juice, and mayonnaise in a small bowl and whisk to mix. Season with salt and pepper to taste. (If it's too tart for your taste, add an additional tablespoon of mayonnaise.) Set the dressing aside.

4. Transfer the steak to a cutting board, leaving the broiler on or the grill lit. Let the steak rest for 5 minutes, then slice it into ¼-inch strips. Reserve the meat juices.

5. Broil or grill the onion until cooked through and slightly charred, about 3 minutes per side. Place the cooked onions and the arugula, mushrooms, and bell pepper in a salad bowl and stir to mix. Add the dressing to the arugula mixture and toss to coat evenly.

6. Divide the arugula mixture between 2 plates. Arrange the steak slices on top of the salad and drizzle any meat juice over them. Sprinkle the Parmesan cheese over the salads and serve.

SERVES 2

Nutrition Info
1 PORTION PROVIDES:

Protein: 1½ servings

Calcium: 1 serving

Vitamin C: 2½ servings

Green leafy and yellow vegetables and fruits: 3 servings

Other fruits and vegetables: 2 servings

Fat: ½ serving if made with 1 tablespoon mayonnaise; 1 serving if made with 2

Salmon Salad Niçoise

Have leftovers from last night's grilled salmon fest? Use them to top this delicious dinner salad. Have leftover cooked green beans, too? Toss those in as well.

12 asparagus stalks, cut into 3-inch
    pieces
4 cups shredded romaine lettuce
2 cooked skinless salmon fillets
    (each about 4 ounces)
4 small cooked red potatoes
    (see box on page 253),
    quartered
2 plum tomatoes, quartered
2 large hard-cooked eggs, quartered
¼ cup sliced pitted kalamata olives
    (optional)
2 scallions, both white and light
    green parts, trimmed and
    thinly sliced
2 teaspoons drained capers
    (optional)
3 tablespoons fresh lemon juice
2 or 3 tablespoons olive oil
2 teaspoons Dijon mustard
1 clove garlic (optional; if raw garlic
    bothers you, see page 331),
    minced
1½ teaspoons fresh tarragon leaves,
    chopped, or ½ teaspoon dried
    tarragon
Salt and black pepper

1. Steam the asparagus following the instructions on page 391 until crisp-tender, 4 to 6 minutes, depending on the thickness. Pat dry with paper towels.

2. Divide the lettuce leaves between 2 plates and place a salmon fillet on top of each. Surround the salmon with the steamed asparagus and the potatoes, tomatoes, eggs, and olives, if using, dividing them equally between the 2 plates. Top the salmon with the scallions and capers, if using, dividing them equally.

3. Place the lemon juice, olive oil, mustard, garlic, if using, and tarragon in a small bowl and whisk to mix. Season with salt and pepper to taste. Spoon the dressing over the salads.

SERVES 2

Nutrition Info
1 PORTION PROVIDES:

Protein: 1 serving plus

Vitamin C: 2 servings

Green leafy and yellow vegetables and fruits: 2 servings

Fat: 1 serving if made with 1 tablespoon oil; 1½ if made with 2 tablespoons

Shrimp Caesar Salad

Perhaps you think grilled chicken as the standard topper for a Caesar, but you'll hail Caesar when it hosts a favorite friend from the sea.

12 large shrimp, shelled and
    deveined
Olive oil cooking spray
Black pepper
4 cups shredded romaine lettuce
1 medium-size red bell pepper,
    thinly sliced
1 cup small cherry or grape tomatoes
3 tablespoons Caesar Dressing
    (recipe follows) or Creamy Caesar
    Dressing (page 332)
1/2 cup grated Parmesan cheese,
    or more to taste
2 lemon wedges, for serving

1. Season the shrimp with black pepper.

2. Coat a skillet with olive oil cooking spray and heat it over high heat. Add the shrimp and cook it until cooked through, about 4 minutes. Set the shrimp aside.

3. Place the lettuce, bell pepper, tomatoes, salad dressing, and Parmesan cheese in a small bowl and toss to mix.

4. Divide the salad between 2 salad plates and top each with 8 shrimp. Serve with lemon wedges and more Parmesan, if desired.

SERVES 2

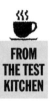

FROM THE TEST KITCHEN

THERE'S ALWAYS ROOM ON top of a Caesar for the old standard—grilled chicken breast. Grilled salmon's another tasty possibility.

Nutrition Info

1 PORTION (WITHOUT DRESSING) PROVIDES:

Protein: 1 serving

Calcium: 1 serving

Vitamin C: 4 servings

Green leafy and yellow vegetables and fruits: 3 servings

Caesar Dressing

A traditional Caesar dressing is made with raw or practically uncooked egg. This eggless version is better suited for the pregnant gourmet who wants all the taste of a great Caesar salad without any questionable ingredients.

1 teaspoon chopped garlic
   (from 2 large cloves; if raw garlic
   bothers you, see box)
4 tablespoons fresh lemon juice
3 tablespoons olive oil, or more
   to taste
2 anchovy fillets (optional),
   drained and coarsely chopped
1/4 cup grated Parmesan cheese,
   or more to taste
Salt and cracked black pepper

Place the garlic, lemon juice, olive oil, anchovies, if using, and Parmesan cheese in a blender or food processor and purée to form a smooth dressing. Season with salt and cracked pepper to taste, adding more olive oil and/or cheese, if desired.

MAKES ABOUT 1/2 CUP

THE HEART OF THE MATTER

▼ ▼ ▼

Love a good Caesar salad, but aren't so crazy about your post-Caesar breath? Removing the center core of the garlic before using it raw makes it easier on your breath—and your digestion.

Nutrition Info

1 PORTION (1/4 CUP) PROVIDES:

Calcium: 1/2 serving

Vitamin C: 1/2 serving

Fat: 11/2 servings

MOVE OVER, CROUTONS

▽ ▽ ▽

Here are two superfast and supernutritious ways to add crunch to a salad.

PARMESAN CRISPS: Preheat the oven to 325°F. Mound heaping tablespoons of freshly grated Parmesan cheese on a baking sheet that has been coated with olive oil cooking spray. Using the back of a spoon, pat each mound into a 3-inch circle. Bake until the cheese is bubbling, 6 to 8 minutes. Let the crisps cool slightly, then use a spatula to transfer them to paper towels to finish cooling and crisping. Serve on top of any cheese-friendly salad. Or just snack on them.

CRUNCHY CHICKPEAS: Preheat the oven to 375°F. Drain a can of chickpeas (garbanzo beans) and pat them dry thoroughly with paper towels. Spread the chickpeas out on a rimmed baking sheet, spray them with olive oil cooking spray, and sprinkle them with grated Parmesan cheese. Bake the chickpeas until crunchy, about 30 minutes. Use the chickpeas as a crouton substitute or enjoy them by the handful.

Creamy Caesar Dressing

Here's a dressing that's full of flavor but not full of fat.

¼ cup buttermilk
¼ cup plain whole-milk yogurt
¼ cup grated Parmesan cheese,
    or more to taste
2 tablespoons fresh lemon juice,
    or more to taste
2 tablespoons mayonnaise or olive oil
1 clove garlic (if raw garlic bothers you,
    see page 331), minced
1 shallot, chopped
2 anchovy fillets (optional), drained
    and chopped
½ teaspoon Worcestershire sauce,
    or more to taste
Salt and black pepper

Place the buttermilk, yogurt, Parmesan cheese, lemon juice, mayonnaise or oil, garlic, shallot, anchovies, if using, and Worcestershire sauce in a blender or food processor and pulse until they are combined. Taste for seasoning, adding more Parmesan, lemon juice, mayonnaise, and/or Worcestershire sauce as necessary, and salt and pepper to taste. If you prefer, you can toss more Parmesan with the salad rather than add it to the dressing.

MAKES ABOUT 1 CUP

Nutrition Info

1 PORTION (¼ CUP) PROVIDES:

Calcium: almost 1 serving

Fat: ½ serving

Shrimp and Mango Salad with Sesame Ginger Vinaigrette

Do the dog days of summer have you panting for something refreshing? Chill out with this salad—super-simple if you buy your shrimp cleaned and cooked. It's equally yummy with cubes of cooked chicken or turkey.

12 large shrimp, shelled and deveined
4 cups (packed) mesclun or other
    tender greens
1 Kirby (pickling) cucumber,
    peeled and thinly sliced

Sesame Ginger Vinaigrette
    (recipe follows)
1 ripe mango, thinly sliced
1 medium-size red bell pepper,
    thinly sliced

1. Steam the shrimp following the instructions on page 391 until they are cooked through and turn opaque, about 5 minutes.

2. Place the mesclun and cucumber in a salad bowl. Add ¼ cup of the Sesame Ginger Vinaigrette and toss to mix. Divide the greens between 2 salad plates.

3. Place the shrimp, mango, and bell pepper in the salad bowl. Toss with enough of the remaining Sesame Ginger Vinaigrette to coat evenly. Top the greens with the shrimp mixture.

SERVES 2

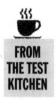

FROM THE TEST KITCHEN

OPEN, SESAME: If you have sesame seeds handy (preferably toasted), toss a couple of tablespoons in with the greens for a nutty crunch.

Nutrition Info

1 PORTION (WITHOUT DRESSING) PROVIDES:

Protein: 1 serving

Vitamin C: 3 servings

Green leafy and yellow vegetables and fruits: 3 servings

Other fruits and vegetables: 1/2 serving

Sesame Ginger Vinaigrette

The sweet and tangy punch of this Asian-inspired dressing comes from seasoned rice vinegar. If you substitute plain rice vinegar, you'll need to sweeten it to taste with your sweetener of choice.

2 scallions, both white and
    light green parts, trimmed
    and thinly sliced
1 tablespoon grated peeled
    fresh ginger
1 tablespoon chopped fresh cilantro
¼ teaspoon chopped garlic
    (if raw garlic bothers you,
    see page 331)
⅓ cup seasoned rice vinegar
1 tablespoon extra-virgin olive oil, or
    more to taste
1 tablespoon low-sodium soy sauce
1 tablespoon sesame oil
Black pepper

Place the scallions, ginger, cilantro, garlic, rice vinegar, olive oil, soy sauce, and sesame oil in a small bowl and whisk to mix. Add black pepper to taste.

MAKES ABOUT ½ CUP

Nutrition Info

1 PORTION (¼ CUP) PROVIDES:

Fat: 1 serving

Southwest Russian Dressing

Pair a pregnancy version of a Cobb salad (chopped chicken or turkey, avocado, pasteurized blue cheese, chopped hard-cooked egg, chopped tomato, chopped romaine lettuce) with this great Russian dressing, which has a zippy taste of the Southwest. It's also good with a simple chopped lettuce and tomato salad. Use any leftovers as a dip for veggies or as a spread on sandwiches.

½ cup buttermilk
¼ cup store-bought mild salsa
  (preferably a chunky tomato one)
2 tablespoons mayonnaise
1 tablespoon chopped fresh parsley
2 teaspoons fresh lemon juice
¼ teaspoon dry mustard
1 tablespoon sweet pickle relish
Salt and black pepper

Place the buttermilk, salsa, mayonnaise, parsley, lemon juice, and mustard in a blender and blend at low speed until a smooth paste forms. Transfer the dressing to a bowl and stir in the pickle relish. Season the dressing with salt and pepper to taste. The dressing can be stored in the refrigerator, covered, for 2 days.

MAKES ABOUT 1 CUP

FROM THE TEST KITCHEN

LIKE YOUR RUSSIAN SWEET?
Add white grape juice concentrate, Splenda, honey, or another sweetener to taste. Like it spicy? Spike it with hot sauce.

Nutrition Info
1 PORTION (¼ CUP) PROVIDES:

Fat: ½ serving

Meat

Has red meat always been your guilty pleasure? Well, lose the guilt—and bring on the pleasure. Red meat gets a green light when you're expecting, for a couple of reasons. First, cholesterol's not a concern for the pregnant set. Second, red meat is among the best sources of dietary iron, plus it packs plenty of protein and other pregnancy-friendly nutrients (like the B vitamins) into every bite (omega-3's, too, if you use grass-fed beef or buffalo). Whether you're looking for a taste of nostalgia (in good old-fashioned dishes like Tomato-Layered Mini Meat Loaves and Here's the Beef Stew), or you're craving contemporary (like Pork Medallions with Arugula and Tomatoes or Beef Kebabs with Cumin Marinade), or you'd like to put an international spin on supper (with Ginger Beef Stir-Fry or Mexican Lasagna), there's a meat recipe for everyone in this section. So dig in like the carnivore you've always wanted to be.

Here's the Beef Stew

Nothing warms up a cold winter's night like a hot stew. This hearty and healthy one combines tender beef and carrots, potatoes, mushrooms, onion, and sugar snap peas in a rich tomato sauce. It'll taste even better a day or two later, so don't forget to eat the leftovers.

1¼ pounds lean beef stew meat,
    well trimmed
Salt and black pepper
Cooking oil spray
1½ teaspoons olive oil
1 small onion, chopped
3 cloves garlic, minced
2½ cups low-sodium beef broth
1 can (about 14 ounces) diced
    tomatoes, drained
1 tablespoon tomato paste
1 tablespoon balsamic vinegar
2 tablespoons fresh thyme leaves,
    or 2 teaspoons dried thyme
1 tablespoon minced fresh rosemary,
    or 1 teaspoon dried rosemary
2 cups baby carrots
3 small Yukon Gold potatoes,
    peeled and cut into 1-inch cubes
½ pound white button mushrooms,
    wiped clean and cut into quarters
1 cup sugar snap peas
¼ tablespoon minced fresh parsley

WANT TO BEEF UP?

▼ ▼ ▼

Most of the recipes in this section call for 4 ounces of meat per serving, not only because that's all you need to net a protein serving, but because smaller portions are easier to handle when digestion is as slow-going as it is during pregnancy. But if you've got the appetite for a bigger slab, knock yourself out with it—eat a 6-ounce portion and tally up 1½ protein servings . . . or on a really hungry day, tackle an 8-ouncer, and count out 2 servings.

1. Season the beef with salt and pepper. Coat a large saucepan with cooking oil spray. Add the olive oil and place over medium-high heat. Add the beef and cook, stirring occasionally, until browned all over, 5 to 7 minutes. Remove the beef and set aside.

2. Add the onion and garlic to the saucepan and cook until the onion is very soft, about 10 minutes.

3. Return the beef and any juices to the pan. Add the beef broth, tomatoes, tomato paste, vinegar, 1 tablespoon of the thyme, and the rosemary. Let come to a boil. Reduce the heat to medium-low, cover the pan, and let simmer until the beef is almost tender, about 1 hour.

4. Add the carrots, potatoes, and mushrooms to the pan. Let simmer, uncovered, until the meat is very tender and the stew is slightly thickened, about 45 minutes.

5. Add the sugar snap peas, the remaining tablespoon of thyme, and the parsley. Cover and let simmer until the sugar snap peas are heated through, about 5 minutes. The stew can be refrigerated, covered, for up to 3 days.

SERVES 4

Nutrition Info
1 PORTION PROVIDES:

Protein: 1 serving

Vitamin C: 1 serving

Green leafy and yellow vegetables and fruits: 2 servings

Other fruits and vegetables: 1 serving

Iron: from the beef

Braised Roast Beef in Tomato Sauce

In less than five minutes, this hearty roast is ready to pop into the oven. Of course, you'll have to wait for it to slowly cook before you get to dig in—while you sit back, relax, and breathe in those tantalizing smells. If you're making this for two, you'll have plenty of leftovers to look forward to.

1 teaspoon canola oil
1 boneless beef chuck roast or bottom round roast (about 3 pounds), trimmed
Salt and black pepper
2 medium-size onions, chopped
2 tablespoons low-sodium beef broth
1 can (28 ounces) crushed tomatoes, with their juices
1 tablespoon fresh thyme leaves, or 1 teaspoon dried thyme
1 tablespoon chopped fresh oregano, or 1 teaspoon dried oregano

1 tablespoon chopped fresh rosemary, or 1 teaspoon dried rosemary
2 tablespoons Worcestershire sauce (optional)
5 cloves garlic, peeled
½ cup sliced carrots

1. Preheat the oven to 300°F.

2. Heat the oil in a large heavy saucepan over high heat. Season the roast with salt and pepper and place it in the pan. Sear the meat on all sides until dark brown. Remove the roast from the saucepan.

3. Add the onions to the saucepan and cook until browned, about 7 minutes. Pour the broth into the saucepan, let come to a boil, then boil until the liquid is nearly gone, scraping up any brown bits from the bottom of the pan.

4. Place the roast in a 4- to 5-quart casserole. Place the onion mixture and the tomatoes, thyme, oregano, rosemary, and Worcestershire sauce, if using, on top of the roast. Scatter the garlic and carrots around it.

5. Cover the casserole and bake it until the roast is very tender, 3 to 4 hours. The roast can be refrigerated, covered, for up to 2 days.

SERVES 6

Nutrition Info
1 PORTION PROVIDES:

Protein: 2 servings

Vitamin C: 1/2 serving

Green leafy and yellow vegetables and fruits: 1 serving

Iron: from the beef

Many Peppers Steak

While standard recipes stop at green, this Many Peppers Steak features red, yellow, and orange bell peppers. And as if that's not enough color and nutrients for one recipe, carrots and red onion show up, too. A sprinkling of crunchy cashews tops it off, making this dish a feast for the eyes—and the taste buds. It's also delicious with chicken or turkey strips.

2 tablespoons low-sodium soy sauce

1½ teaspoons cornstarch

1 tablespoon fresh lemon juice

1/3 cup plus 2 tablespoons low-sodium beef broth

1/2 pound boneless lean beef sirloin steak, thinly sliced

Salt, black pepper, and garlic powder

1½ tablespoons olive oil

1 medium-size red bell pepper, cut into 1/4-inch-thick strips

1 medium-size yellow bell pepper, cut into 1/4-inch-thick strips

1 medium-size orange bell pepper, cut into 1/4-inch-thick strips

1/2 cup shredded carrots

1/2 large red onion, thinly sliced

3 cloves garlic, chopped

1 teaspoon minced peeled fresh ginger

Crushed red pepper flakes (optional)

1/4 cup toasted cashews (see page 272)

1 cup cooked brown rice (optional), for serving

COOK IT ONCE, EAT IT ALL WEEK

▼ ▼ ▼

If you cook a pound of brown rice once a week, you can simply reheat smaller portions in the microwave. It will take only a minute or two to reheat ½ cup of rice.

1. Place the soy sauce, cornstarch, lemon juice, and ⅓ cup of the beef broth in a small bowl and whisk to mix.

2. Season the beef with salt, black pepper, and garlic powder.

3. Heat ½ tablespoon of the olive oil in a large skillet over medium-high heat. Add the meat and stir-fry until browned and cooked through, about 5 minutes. Transfer the beef to a plate.

4. Reduce the heat to medium-low. Add the remaining 1 tablespoon of olive oil to the skillet, then add the bell peppers, carrots, onion, chopped garlic, and ginger and stir-fry until the onion is golden, 6 to 7 minutes. Reduce the heat to low, stir in the remaining 2 tablespoons of broth, cover the skillet, and cook to soften the vegetables, 3 minutes.

5. Return the beef and any juices to the skillet. Stir in the cornstarch mixture. Season the stir-fry with crushed red pepper to taste, if desired. Let come to a boil and cook, stirring, until the meat is heated through, about 2 minutes. Stir in the cashews. Serve over brown rice, if desired.

SERVES 2

Nutrition Info

1 PORTION PROVIDES:

Protein: 1 serving

Vitamin C: 6 servings

Green leafy and yellow vegetables and fruits: 2 servings

Other fruits and vegetables: 1 serving

Whole grains and legumes: 1 serving if served with brown rice

Iron from the beef

Fat: ½ serving

Ginger Beef Stir-Fry

Probably quicker than take-out, with the help of a couple packages of broccoli florets, this stir-fry can be on your table in less than 20 minutes (without those leaky cardboard containers). A boldly sauced and delicious combination of beef sirloin, yellow or red bell pepper, carrots, and broccoli cooks up in no time flat—and packs in both protein and vitamins. A bonus: The ginger is great for queasy days. Sniff some while you cook. The stir-fry is just as tasty prepared with chicken, turkey, lean pork, firm tofu, or shrimp.

Cooking oil spray
1 tablespoon sesame oil
1/2 pound lean beef, such as
    boneless beef sirloin,
    thinly sliced
1 clove garlic, minced
1 medium-size yellow or
    red bell pepper, sliced
1 1/2 cups small broccoli florets
1/2 cup baby carrots
2 scallions, both white and
    light green parts, trimmed
    and thinly sliced
1/4 cup low-sodium beef broth
Ginger Sauce (recipe follows)
1 tablespoon chopped fresh cilantro
1 cup cooked brown rice (optional),
    for serving

1. Coat a large skillet with cooking oil spray. Add 1 teaspoon of the sesame oil and heat over medium-high heat. Add the beef and stir-fry until browned and cooked through, about 5 minutes. Set the beef aside.

2. Heat the remaining 2 teaspoons of sesame oil in the skillet over medium-high heat. Add the garlic and cook until the flavor releases, about 1 minute. Add the bell pepper, broccoli, carrots, and scallions and cook until slightly softened, about 2 minutes. Add the beef broth to the skillet. Turn the heat down to medium, cover and let cook, stirring occasionally, until the vegetables are tender but still slightly crunchy, about 3 minutes..

3. Return the beef to the skillet. Turn heat to high, add the Ginger Sauce, and cook, stirring frequently, until heated through, about 2 minutes. Sprinkle the cilantro over the stir-fry and serve over brown rice, if desired.

SERVES 2

Ginger Sauce

This assertive ginger-flavored sauce can be tossed with just about any stir-fry. If you're feeling the burn (heartburn, that is), you may want to omit the hot sauce.

1 tablespoon grated fresh ginger,
   or 1/2 teaspoon ground ginger
2 tablespoons rice vinegar
1 tablespoon low-sodium beef broth
1 tablespoon white grape juice
   concentrate, Splenda, honey,
   or brown sugar
2 tablespoons low-sodium soy sauce
2 teaspoons sesame oil
Hot sauce, to taste

Place the ginger, rice vinegar, beef broth, juice concentrate, soy sauce, sesame oil, and hot sauce in a small bowl and whisk to mix.

MAKES ABOUT 1/3 CUP

Nutrition Info
1 PORTION PROVIDES:

Protein: 1 serving

Vitamin C: 3 1/2 servings

Green leafy and yellow vegetables and fruits: 2 1/2 servings if made with yellow bell pepper; 3 1/2 if made with red bell pepper

Whole grains and legumes: 1 serving if served with brown rice

Iron: from the beef

Fat: 1/2 serving

STIR-FRY MADE EVEN EASIER

Stir-frying is probably one of the quickest ways to get dinner on the table. The only time-consuming part is the chopping, grating, and slicing involved in prepping the ingredients for the wok or skillet. Fortunately for the perpetually time challenged there's good news on that front: Almost everything you'd want to toss into a stir-fry can be bought pan-ready. Check your supermarket's meat case for pre-sliced beef, chicken, or turkey. Scour the produce section for chopped, sliced, shredded, or peeled fresh onions, garlic, broccoli, cauliflower, cabbage, carrots, and bell peppers. If the store has a salad bar, you can round up vegetables not usually found prepped and packaged. And if the produce section is running on empty, head to the frozen food aisle for some ready-to-use veggies.

Beef Kebabs with Cumin Marinade

Here's a meal on a stick—once you've placed the stick over some cous-cous, quinoa, brown rice, or another grain. You'll need to plan ahead a bit; the beef marinates for at least three hours (marinate in the morning; enjoy at night). Serving two is easy—just cut the recipe in half. If you are using wooden skewers, be sure to soak them in water first for half an hour.

½ pound lean beef, such as top sirloin, well trimmed and cut into 1-inch pieces

2 tablespoons low-sodium soy sauce

2 tablespoons fresh lemon juice

1 tablespoon olive oil

1 teaspoon ground cumin

1 medium-size red bell pepper, cut into 2-inch pieces

½ medium-size red onion, cut into 2-inch pieces

12 white button mushrooms, caps only, wiped clean

12 cherry or grape tomatoes

1. Place the beef, soy sauce, lemon juice, olive oil, and cumin in a bowl and stir to coat the beef evenly with the marinade. Cover the bowl with plastic wrap and refrigerate for at least 3 hours or as long as overnight.

2. Preheat the broiler or set up the grill and preheat it to high.

3. Remove the beef from the marinade and thread it onto 8 skewers, alternating pieces of bell pepper, onion, mushrooms, and tomatoes between the pieces of meat.

4. Broil or grill the kebabs until the beef is tender, turning occasionally, 8 to 10 minutes.

SERVES 4

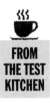

FROM THE TEST KITCHEN **IF YOU WANT SWEET BEEF** kebabs instead, substitute 2 tablespoons of pineapple juice concentrate for the 2 tablespoons of lemon juice. And use pineapple and mango chunks instead of the mushroom caps and tomatoes.

Nutrition Info

1 PORTION PROVIDES:

Protein: 1 serving

Vitamin C: 2½ servings

Green leafy and yellow vegetables and fruits: 1 serving

Other fruits and vegetables: 1½ servings

Iron: from the beef

Tomato-Layered Mini Meat Loaves

Your favorite comfort food—just like the meat loaf mother used to make, except smaller. Leftovers can be easily rewarmed one mini loaf at a time or sliced for a cold meat loaf sandwich.

2 pounds lean ground beef

1 cup shredded cheddar cheese

2 tablespoons ketchup

1 large egg, lightly beaten

3 tablespoons old-fashioned rolled oats

1½ teaspoons chopped fresh oregano, or ½ teaspoon dried oregano

¾ teaspoon chopped fresh dill, or ¼ teaspoon dried dill

¼ teaspoon garlic powder

¼ teaspoon salt

¼ teaspoon black pepper

2 medium-size ripe tomatoes, thinly sliced

1. Preheat the oven to 375°F.

2. Place the beef, cheddar cheese, ketchup, egg, oats, oregano, dill, garlic powder, salt, and pepper in a large bowl and mix them together with a fork. Press half of the beef mixture into 6 cups of a muffin tin, dividing it evenly among them. Top each meat loaf with a slice of tomato, then press the remaining beef mixture into the muffin cups.

3. Bake the meat loaves until cooked through, about 20 minutes.

4. Remove the meat loaves from the muffin tin immediately and serve. Wrap any leftover meat loaves in aluminum foil and refrigerate them. To reheat, pop the meat loaves (covered with foil) in a preheated 350°F oven for 10 minutes or in the microwave (remove the foil first) for 1 minute on high power. The baked meat loaves can be refrigerated for 2 days; they can be frozen for 2 weeks. The meat loaves can also be frozen uncooked, wrapped in plastic wrap, for 1 month. To thaw, leave the meat loaves in the refrigerator overnight.

SERVES 6

FROM THE TEST KITCHEN

NOT IN THE MOOD for beef? Make the meat loaves with 2 pounds of ground breast of turkey or lean ground pork instead. Want to A-List your meat loaf? Stir in finely grated carrot.

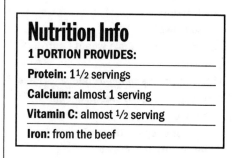

Nutrition Info

1 PORTION PROVIDES:

Protein: 1½ servings

Calcium: almost 1 serving

Vitamin C: almost ½ serving

Iron: from the beef

Mexican Lasagna

Who says Italy has a corner on the lasagna market? This decidedly different and delicious take on the traditional Italian favorite begs to differ. Red bell pepper, carrot, and corn add color, flavor, and unexpected nutrients; enchilada sauce and a Mexican-style tomato sauce add a kick. And tasty and nutritious tortillas stand in for the traditional pasta.

2 teaspoons olive oil
1 medium-size onion, chopped
1 medium-size red bell pepper, chopped
2 cloves garlic, minced
1 pound extra-lean ground beef
¾ cup grated carrots
1 tablespoon chili powder
1½ teaspoons ground cumin
1 tablespoon chopped fresh oregano, or 1 teaspoon dried oregano
1 cup fresh or frozen yellow corn kernels
1 cup prepared enchilada sauce
1 can (15 ounces) tomato sauce (preferably Mexican-style)
1 container (16 ounces) low-fat cottage cheese
2 large eggs, lightly beaten
¼ cup grated Parmesan cheese
Black pepper
Cooking oil spray
12 small corn or whole wheat flour tortillas
1½ cups finely shredded cheddar cheese
Plain yogurt or sour cream, chopped fresh cilantro, chopped fresh tomato, and/or chopped black olives (optional), for serving

1. Preheat the oven to 375°F.

2. Heat the olive oil in a large nonstick skillet over medium heat. Add the onion, bell pepper, and garlic and cook until softened, about 5 minutes. Add the beef, carrots, chili powder, cumin, and oregano and cook, chopping up the meat with a spoon, until the meat cooks through, about 10 minutes. Stir in the corn, enchilada sauce, and tomato sauce and let simmer, stirring frequently, until the flavors blend, about 5 minutes.

3. Place the cottage cheese, eggs, and Parmesan cheese in a bowl and stir to mix. Season lightly with black pepper, then set aside.

4. Coat a 13-by-9-inch baking dish with cooking oil spray. Place 6 of the tortillas on the bottom (they'll overlap slightly). Spread half of the meat mixture over the tortillas. Spread the cottage cheese mixture over the meat mixture. Arrange the remaining 6 tortillas on top of the cottage cheese mixture. Top the tortillas with the remaining meat mixture.

5. Bake the lasagna for 20 minutes. Remove it from the oven and sprinkle the cheddar cheese evenly over the top. Return the lasagna to the oven and bake until the cheese is melted, about 10 minutes longer.

6. Let the lasagna stand for 10 minutes before serving. Top with yogurt, cilantro, tomato, and/or olives, if desired. The lasagna can be refrigerated, covered, for 3 days. Reheat leftovers in the microwave.

SERVES 6

Nutrition Info

1 PORTION PROVIDES:

Protein: 1½ servings

Calcium: 1 serving

Vitamin C: 1 serving

Green leafy and yellow vegetables and fruits: 1 serving

Other fruits and vegetables: 1 serving

Whole grains and legumes: 2 servings

Pork Medallions with Arugula and Tomatoes

Here's a very quick dish that's elegant enough for company but easy enough for the most harried weekday. Sauté extra tenderloin while you're at it—it would make a delicious sandwich with fresh arugula and tomatoes.

Olive oil cooking spray
1 tablespoon olive oil
2 cloves garlic, minced
½ pound pork tenderloin,
    cut into 1-inch-thick slices
Salt and black pepper
2 tablespoons balsamic vinegar

4 ripe plum tomatoes, seeded and
    chopped
1 package (5 or 6 ounces) arugula
    or baby spinach
¼ cup coarsely grated Parmesan
    cheese

1. Coat a large nonstick skillet with olive oil cooking spray. Add 2 teaspoons of olive oil and heat over medium heat. Add the garlic and cook, stirring, until golden, about 4 minutes. Remove the garlic and set aside.

2. Season the pork slices with salt and pepper and add them to the skillet. Increase the heat to medium-high and cook until the pork is well browned and cooked through, about 5 minutes per side. Transfer the pork to a plate and cover it with aluminum foil to keep warm.

3. Let the skillet cool for a minute off the heat. Then heat the skillet over low heat and add the remaining 1 teaspoon of oil and the balsamic vinegar, stirring to scrape up any brown bits. Add the tomatoes and the cooked garlic and stir for 1 minute. Add the arugula and toss until wilted. Season with salt and pepper to taste.

4. Spoon the arugula and tomato mixture over the pork, sprinkle the Parmesan cheese on top and serve immediately.

SERVES 2

Nutrition Info
1 PORTION PROVIDES:

Protein: 1 serving

Calcium: 1/2 serving

Vitamin C: 2 servings

Green leafy and yellow vegetables and fruits: 3 servings

Iron: from the spinach, if using

Fat: 1/2 serving

Pork Quesadillas

Another great taste of Mexico, this time starring pork. Besides packing loads of flavor in every bite, these quesadillas have loads of nutrients—vitamins from the red bell peppers, protein from the pork and Monterey Jack cheese, and the right kind of carbs from the whole wheat tortillas. Just two for dinner? Use half the pork tonight, and the rest in tomorrow's sandwiches.

FOR THE MARINADE AND PORK

3 tablespoons fresh lime juice
1 tablespoon olive oil
2 tablespoons chopped fresh cilantro
1 teaspoon white grape juice
   concentrate, Splenda, honey,
   or brown sugar
1 teaspoon ground cumin
1 teaspoon chili powder
1 pound lean pork tenderloin,
   cut into ¼-inch-thick slices
Olive oil cooking spray

FOR THE QUESADILLAS

6 scallions, both white and light green
   parts, trimmed and thinly sliced
2 medium-size red bell peppers,
   thinly sliced
4 whole wheat tortillas
   (each 12 inches in diameter)
1 cup shredded Monterey Jack cheese
1 medium-size avocado (optional),
   preferably Hass, diced
1 large ripe tomato (optional),
   chopped

1. Make the marinade: Place the lime juice, olive oil, cilantro, grape juice concentrate, cumin, and chili powder in a large mixing bowl and stir to mix. Add the pork slices and toss to coat evenly with the marinade. Refrigerate, covered, for at least 15 minutes or as long as overnight.

2. Coat a skillet with olive oil cooking spray, then heat it over medium-high heat. Remove the pork from the marinade and add the pork to the skillet. Cook the pork until cooked through, turning once, about 6 minutes. Remove the pork and set aside.

3. Make the quesadillas: Add the scallions and bell peppers to the skillet and cook until beginning to soften, about 2 minutes. Add the pork, cook until heated through, then reduce the heat to keep warm.

4. Coat another skillet with cooking oil spray, then heat it over medium heat. Working with 1 tortilla at a time, heat it until warmed through, about 30 seconds per side.

5. Place the tortillas on a work surface. Spoon the pork mixture over half of each tortilla, dividing it evenly among them. Sprinkle ¼ cup of the Monterey Jack cheese over the pork on each tortilla. Fold the bare half of the tortilla over the filling.

6. Place the filled tortillas in a skillet over medium heat and cook for 2 minutes. Turn the quesadillas over and cook until the cheese has melted, about 2 minutes. Cut each quesadilla into wedges and serve with the avocado and tomato, if desired.

SERVES 4

Nutrition Info

1 PORTION PROVIDES:

Protein: 1 serving

Calcium: 1 serving

Vitamin C: 2 servings

Green leafy and yellow vegetables and fruits: 1 serving

Other fruits and vegetables: ½ serving if made with avocado

Whole grains and legumes: 2 servings

Pacific Rim Pork Kebabs

Looking for a super-easy dish with a nice Hawaiian punch? These sweet and tangy pork kebabs are heady with grated ginger and could be particularly appealing during those queasy months. If you're using wooden skewers, soak them in water first for half an hour. And try chicken or shrimp.

1 pound lean pork tenderloin,
   cut into 1-inch cubes
2 medium-size red bell peppers,
   cut into 1-inch pieces
1 can (20 ounces) pineapple
   chunks in juice, drained
¼ cup pineapple juice concentrate
2 tablespoons fresh lime juice
2 teaspoons canola oil
2 teaspoons grated peeled fresh ginger
1 teaspoon curry powder
1 teaspoon minced garlic (optional)
2 cups cooked brown rice or quinoa,
   for serving

1. Thread the pork, bell peppers, and pineapple onto 8 skewers, alternating pieces of each. Set the kebabs aside.

2. Place the pineapple juice concentrate, lime juice, oil, ginger, curry powder, and garlic, if using, in a large resealable plastic bag and squeeze the bag to blend the marinade. Add the kebabs, seal the bag, and gently shake and turn the bag to coat the kebabs evenly. Let the kebabs marinate for about 30 minutes.

3. Preheat the broiler or set up the grill and preheat it to high.

4. Remove the kebabs from the marinade and broil or grill until the pork is cooked through, turning occasionally, about 10 minutes. Unskewer the kebabs and serve on top of the brown rice.

SERVES 4

Nutrition Info

1 PORTION PROVIDES:

Protein: 1 serving

Vitamin C: 3 servings

Green leafy and yellow vegetables and fruits: 1 serving

Whole grains and legumes: 1 serving

Poultry

Tired of the same old chicken that tastes, well, like chicken? Here's a flock of recipes that'll shake (and bake and sauté and grill) the way you feel about America's ubiquitous bird. They're easy, they're quick, and best of all, they fill your nutritional requirements deliciously. Looking for some excitement? Look no further than Chicken with Pomegranate Glaze. Want to fill your bucket with something healthy and crunchy? Try Oven-Fried Chicken Breasts. Take your bird on a round-the-world tour with Basque Chicken, Tandoori Chicken Breasts with Mango and Orange Salad, and Thai Chicken Curry. Or play it safe—and soothing—with Apricot Ginger Glazed Chicken. Talking turkey? You will be once you try Grilled Turkey Breast with Corn and Edamame Salsa and Turkey Cutlets in Mushroom Sauce. What's more, since most of these recipes serve four, you can get two meals for the cooking effort of one. Pack a leftover cold chicken cutlet sandwiched in a whole-grain roll for lunch.

Rosemary Lemon Chicken

A simple vinaigrette of fragrant fresh rosemary and tangy lemon brightens this super-simple chicken dish, making it perfect for a quick meal or leisurely dinner. Serve it hot the first night, and serve the leftovers (if there are any) cold the next night, perhaps sliced over a salad. Or, make a tasty sandwich for lunch.

1 tablespoon chopped fresh rosemary
1 tablespoon drained capers
1 teaspoon chopped garlic (optional)
1 teaspoon olive oil
Juice of 1 medium-size lemon, plus
   1 lemon, very thinly sliced
1 tablespoon pine nuts
4 skinless, boneless chicken breast
   halves (each 4 ounces)
Salt and black pepper

1. Preheat the oven to 350°F.

2. Place the rosemary, capers, garlic, if using, olive oil, lemon juice, and pine nuts in a small bowl and stir to mix. Set aside.

3. Place the lemon slices in a single layer in a baking dish large enough to hold the chicken breasts in a single layer. Season the chicken breasts with a pinch each of salt and pepper, then place them on top of the lemon slices. Spoon about a tablespoon of the rosemary mixture over each chicken breast. Bake the chicken until it is cooked through (there should be no pink), 20 to 25 minutes.

SERVES 4

BIGGER BREASTS?

▼ ▼ ▼

The recipes in this section call for 4 ounces of chicken or turkey per person—because that's all you need for 1 portion. Plus, petite portions are easier on pregnant-sluggish digestion. But if you've got the appetite and larger breasts in your refrigerator, go right ahead and enjoy them. If you use 6-ouncers, count yourself in for 1½ protein servings. If you're really running on empty, go for a full 8 ounces and score 2 full servings.

Nutrition Info
1 PORTION PROVIDES:

Protein: 1 serving

Oven-Fried Chicken Breasts

Who needs to send out for a bucket? These chicken breasts are crunchy on the outside, moist on the inside, completely greaseless—and still, finger-licking good.

1/2 cup whole wheat bread crumbs
1/4 cup grated Parmesan cheese
1 teaspoon paprika
1/2 teaspoon garlic powder
Salt and black pepper
1/3 cup buttermilk
1 tablespoon Dijon mustard (optional)
1 tablespoon mayonnaise
2 skinless, boneless chicken breast
   halves (each 4 ounces)
Olive oil cooking spray

1. Preheat the oven to 400°F.

2. Place the bread crumbs, Parmesan cheese, paprika, and garlic powder in a large shallow bowl and stir to mix. Season with salt and pepper to taste.

3. Place the buttermilk, mustard, if using, and mayonnaise in another shallow bowl and stir to mix.

4. Dip the chicken breasts in the buttermilk mixture, then dredge them in the bread crumb mixture. Place the breasts on a baking sheet coated with olive oil cooking spray. Spray the breasts with a little olive oil, too. Bake the chicken until cooked through (there should be no pink), about 25 minutes.

SERVES 2

Nutrition Info
1 PORTION PROVIDES:

Protein: 1 serving

Calcium: 1/2 serving

Whole grains and legumes:
  1 serving

Fat: 1/2 serving

Chunky Tomato Chicken Parmesan

Mama mia! Baby's going to love this dish because it's nutritious, but you're going to love it for its taste. Vitamin-packed roasted red peppers, rich tomato sauce, freshly chopped tomatoes, and a blanket of provolone top chicken breasts in a wholesome remake of an old Italian favorite. Serve the chicken on whole-grain or soy pasta.

¼ cup whole wheat bread crumbs

2 tablespoons grated Parmesan cheese

2 skinless, boneless chicken breast halves (each 4 ounces)

Salt and cracked black pepper

½ teaspoon dried oregano

½ roasted red bell pepper (leftover or from a jar), cut into 8 strips

½ cup good-quality commercial tomato sauce

½ cup seeded chopped ripe tomatoes

2 slices provolone cheese (about 2 ounces total)

1. Preheat the oven to 350°F.

2. Place the bread crumbs and Parmesan cheese in a small bowl and stir to mix, then set aside.

3. Season the chicken breasts lightly with salt and pepper and the oregano. Sprinkle the bread crumb mixture evenly over the chicken breasts, then place them in a baking dish. Top each chicken breast half with 2 strips of roasted pepper, half of the tomato sauce, and half of the tomatoes. Place a slice of provolone cheese on top of each breast half. Bake the chicken until it is cooked through (there should be no pink), about 25 minutes.

SERVES 2

Nutrition Info

1 PORTION PROVIDES:

Protein: 1 serving

Calcium: 1 serving

Vitamin C: 1½ servings

Green leafy and yellow vegetables and fruits: ½ serving

Whole grains and legumes: ½ serving

Apricot Ginger Glazed Chicken

Craving something sweet but in the market for dinner, not dessert? Here's the ticket. An added bonus for queasy moms: The ginger is sure to soothe. Serve the chicken with a wild rice or quinoa pilaf tossed with dried apricots and toasted sliced almonds.

1 tablespoon all-fruit apricot
   preserves
½ tablespoon low-sodium
   soy sauce
½ teaspoon ground ginger
2 skinless, boneless chicken breast
   halves (each 4 ounces)
Salt and black pepper (optional)

1. Place the apricot preserves, soy sauce, and ginger in a small bowl and stir to mix. Divide the apricot and ginger glaze in half and set aside.

2. Preheat the broiler or set up the grill and preheat it to high.

3. Lightly season the chicken breast halves with salt and pepper, if desired, then brush one side of each with half of the glaze. Broil or grill the chicken glazed-side up until cooked through (there should be no pink), 5 to 6 minutes per side. Brush the second side of the breast halves with the remaining glaze after you turn them over.

SERVES 2

Nutrition Info
1 PORTION PROVIDES:

Protein: 1 serving

Chicken with Pomegranate Glaze

Make a double batch of this tasty pomegranate glaze; use it tonight on chicken breasts, tomorrow night on pork or lamb chops.

½ cup pomegranate juice
2 tablespoons cider vinegar
1 tablespoon white grape juice
  concentrate, Splenda, honey,
  brown sugar, or another sweetener,
  or more to taste
4 skinless, boneless chicken breast
  halves (each 4 ounces)
Salt and black pepper
2 tablespoons chopped fresh
  flat-leaf parsley

1. Pour the pomegranate juice, cider vinegar, and grape juice concentrate in a small saucepan, whisk to mix, and let come to a boil over medium heat. Reduce the heat to medium-low and cook the juice mixture until it is reduced to about ¼ cup. Set the glaze aside.

2. Season the chicken with a pinch each of salt and pepper.

3. Preheat the broiler or set up the grill and preheat it to high.

4. When ready to cook, set aside 2 table-spoons of the pomegranate glaze to use when serving, then brush the chicken with the remaining glaze. Broil or grill the chicken until cooked through (there should be no pink), 5 to 6 minutes per side.

5. Brush the cooked chicken with the remaining pomegranate glaze, then sprinkle the parsley over it. The chicken can be served hot or at room temperature.

SERVES 4

FROM THE TEST KITCHEN POMEGRANATE JUICE is fast becoming a staple in supermarkets; look for it in the refrigerated juice section or with the fresh produce. Can't find it? You can easily substitute cranberry juice—just omit the cider vinegar. Serving just two tonight? Cut the recipe in half, or save the extra breasts for a salad or sandwich.

Nutrition Info
1 PORTION PROVIDES:

Protein: 1 serving

Teriyaki Chicken

Just about anything you're cooking—from turkey cutlets, to steak, to pork, to salmon, to portobello mushrooms—tastes better prepared teriyaki style. Serve the chicken with brown rice and a veggie stir-fry.

2 tablespoons low-sodium
  soy sauce
1 tablespoon white grape juice
  concentrate, Splenda, honey,
  or brown sugar
1½ teaspoons grated peeled
  fresh ginger, or ½ teaspoon
  ground ginger
1 teaspoon sesame oil
1 tablespoon chopped fresh
  cilantro, or ½ teaspoon
  ground coriander
2 skinless, boneless chicken breast
  halves (each 4 ounces)

1. Place the soy sauce, grape juice concentrate, ginger, sesame oil, and cilantro in a small bowl and whisk to mix.

2. Place the chicken in a baking dish and pour the teriyaki marinade over it, turning the breasts to coat them evenly. The chicken can marinate, covered, in the refrigerator for up to 8 hours.

3. Preheat the broiler or set up the grill and preheat it to high.

4. Broil or grill the chicken until cooked through (there should be no pink), 5 to 6 minutes per side.

SERVES 2

Nutrition Info
1 PORTION PROVIDES:

Protein: 1 serving

Tandoori Chicken Breasts with Mango and Orange Salad

Tired of dried-out chicken breasts? The yogurt keeps these moist, moist, moist—and the spices make them intriguingly tasty but not too hot. Leftover breasts (if you're cooking for two) will make a yummy salad or sandwich.

¾ cup plain low-fat yogurt
Juice of 1 lime
2 tablespoons grated peeled
 fresh ginger
½ teaspoon chopped garlic,
 or 1 clove garlic, minced
1½ teaspoons ground cumin
1½ teaspoons ground coriander
1½ teaspoons ground turmeric
1½ teaspoons paprika
½ teaspoon crushed red pepper
 flakes (optional)
Pinch of salt
4 skinless, boneless chicken breast
 halves (each 4 ounces)
Mango and Orange Salad
 (recipe follows)

1. Place the yogurt, lime juice, ginger, garlic, cumin, coriander, turmeric, paprika, red pepper flakes, if using, and salt in a large bowl and stir to mix.

2. Add the chicken breast halves to the yogurt mix and turn to coat evenly. The chicken can marinate in the refrigerator, covered, for up to 24 hours. Turn it a few times so that it marinates evenly.

3. Preheat the broiler or set up the grill and preheat it to high.

4. Broil or grill the chicken until cooked through (there should be no pink), 5 to 6 minutes per side. Serve the chicken with the Mango and Orange Salad.

SERVES 4

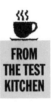

PLANNING to serve Tandoori Chicken Breasts tomorrow night? You're in luck—the longer the chicken marinates in the yogurt mixture, the moister it will be.

FROM THE TEST KITCHEN

Nutrition Info

1 PORTION (WITHOUT SALAD)
PROVIDES:

Protein: 1 servings

Mango and Orange Salad

Mango, orange, and mint mingle with a balsamic vinegar dressing in a refreshing salad that's just about bursting with flavor. It's pleasing to the eye and the palate.

2 ripe mangoes, peeled and pitted
2 medium seedless oranges,
   peeled and white pith removed
2 tablespoons balsamic vinegar
2 teaspoons chopped fresh mint

Cut the mangoes into thin slices and place in a bowl. Segment the oranges and add to the bowl. Add the balsamic vinegar and mint and toss to mix.

SERVES 4

Nutrition Info

1 PORTION PROVIDES:

Vitamin C: 2 servings

Green leafy and yellow vegetables and fruits: 1 serving

Thai Chicken Curry

Here's a curry of a different flavor—milder and creamier, thanks to unsweetened coconut milk. Serve it on brown rice or udon noodles to soak up all the broth, and you've got a meal in one. Or two meals in one, if you've thought ahead and doubled the recipe.

1 tablespoon canola oil
1 small red onion, chopped
2 cloves garlic, minced
1 medium red bell pepper,
     cut into 1/2-inch chunks
2 teaspoons minced peeled
     fresh ginger
1 teaspoon ground coriander
1 teaspoon ground cumin
1 teaspoon curry powder
1 teaspoon ground turmeric
2 teaspoons white grape juice
     concentrate, Splenda, honey,
     or brown sugar
1 can (141/2 ounces) diced tomatoes
     in juice, with their juice
1 cup unsweetened low-fat
     coconut milk
1 tablespoon low-sodium soy sauce
1/2 pound skinless, boneless chicken
     breasts, cut into 1-inch cubes
1 cup cauliflower florets
1/2 cup frozen peas
Juice of 1/2 lime, or more to taste
Chopped fresh cilantro (optional),
     for serving
Chopped toasted cashews
     (optional; see page 272),
     for serving

1. Heat the oil in a large nonstick skillet over medium heat. Add the onion and garlic and cook, stirring frequently, until softened, about 5 minutes.

2. Reduce the heat to medium-low. Add the bell pepper, ginger, coriander, cumin, curry powder, turmeric, and grape juice concentrate and stir to mix. Cook, stirring frequently, for 1 minute.

3. Stir in the tomatoes, coconut milk, and soy sauce. Raise the heat to medium and let come to a boil. Reduce the heat to low and let simmer until the flavors blend, about 15 minutes. Add the chicken and cauliflower, raise the heat to medium, and let come to a boil again. Reduce the heat to low and let simmer, stirring frequently, until the chicken is cooked through (there should be no pink) and the cauliflower is crisp-tender, about 8 minutes.

4. Add the peas and let simmer until they are heated through, about 2 minutes. Sprinkle the lime juice over the curry and garnish it with cilantro and/or cashews, if desired.

SERVES 2

FROM THE TEST KITCHEN

THIS CURRY IS just as tasty made with different ingredients. Try it with turkey, shrimp or another seafood, and with any vegetable or fruit that strikes your fancy—sliced carrots and pineapple, for instance. You can also stir in some baby spinach at the end. Like things spicier? Add some chili garlic sauce (you'll find it in the Asian section of the supermarket).

Nutrition Info

1 PORTION PROVIDES:

Protein: 1 serving

Vitamin C: 4 servings

Green leafy and yellow vegetables and fruits: 1 serving

Other fruits and vegetables: 1 serving

Fat: 1/2 serving

COOKING IN A PACKET

▼ ▼ ▼

Do you like a home-cooked meal but hate the cleanup that comes after? Skip the pots and pans, and cook your dinner in a packet! Most any combination of poultry, meat, or fish, vegetables, and seasonings can be adapted to pouch cooking. All you need is a lot of aluminum foil and a little imagination. Here are some tips:

■ Choose ingredients that cook quickly—boneless chicken breasts instead of legs; shredded carrots not chunks; and summer rather than winter squash.

■ Tear off a square of heavy-duty aluminum foil large enough to completely enclose one portion of meat or fish and veggies and place it on a work surface.

■ Layer the ingredients you want to cook on the foil, starting with the heaviest, such as sliced onions and strips of beef and ending with the lightest ones, like mushrooms. Top everything with herbs and other seasonings.

■ Season aggressively, using generous amounts of spices and fresh herbs—more than you would ordinarily. They'll have to stand up to the steam created in the packet.

■ If the ingredients aren't likely to form a sauce (tomatoes will, cabbage won't), pour a couple of tablespoons of broth, a little soy sauce, or a few squeezes of lemon, lime, or orange juice over everything. Citrus slices make an ideal addition to many fish and poultry packets.

■ Fold the foil over the ingredients and crimp the edges all around to seal the packet very tightly. This will seal in the steam and those very intense flavors and aromas.

■ Bake the packet on a rimmed baking sheet in a hot oven, 400°F. Cooking times will vary depending on the ingredients you use but will usually be between 15 and 25 minutes.

■ For a dramatic and aromatic presentation, open the foil packet at the table, but do it carefully. The escaping steam is very hot, so keep your face and hands out of harm's way.

Chicken Enchiladas

In this case, the whole enchilada offers a whole lot of nutrition—and flavor—but very little fat. Plus, leftovers reheat deliciously.

1 pound skinless, boneless chicken breasts, cut into 1/2-inch cubes
1 medium-size red bell pepper, cut into small dice
2 teaspoons chili powder
1/2 teaspoon dried oregano
Pinch of salt
1 tablespoon plus 2 teaspoons olive oil
1 can (14 1/2 ounces) diced tomatoes with mild green chiles, with their juices
1 can (about 15 ounces) black beans, rinsed and drained
1 can (10 ounces) enchilada sauce
4 large corn tortillas (each about 10 inches in diameter)
1 cup shredded cheddar cheese

1. Preheat the oven to 300°F.

2. Place the chicken, bell pepper, chili powder, oregano, salt, and 1 tablespoon of olive oil in a large bowl and toss to mix.

3. Heat the remaining 2 teaspoons of olive oil in a large nonstick skillet over medium heat. Add the chicken and bell pepper mixture and cook until the chicken is cooked through (there should be no pink), 5 to 7 minutes. Add the tomatoes and black beans and cook until heated through, about 3 minutes.

4. Place the enchilada sauce in a small saucepan over medium heat and cook until heated through, 3 to 5 minutes.

5. Brush each of the tortillas with a little of the enchilada sauce. Spoon some of the chicken and bean mixture into the center of a tortilla and roll it up. Place the filled tortilla in a 9-by-13-inch baking dish, seam side down. Repeat with the remaining tortillas and chicken mixture. Pour the remaining enchilada sauce over the filled tortillas and sprinkle the cheddar cheese on top.

6. Bake the enchiladas until the cheese melts, 15 to 20 minutes. If you are not ready to serve the enchiladas immediately, reduce the oven temperature to 200°F; the enchiladas will keep warm until ready to serve.

SERVES 4

Nutrition Info
1 PORTION PROVIDES:

Protein: 1 1/2 servings

Calcium: 1 serving

Vitamin C: 2 servings

Green leafy and yellow vegetables and fruits: 1 serving

Whole grains and legumes: 2 servings

Iron: from the beans

Fat: 1/2 serving

Basque Chicken

In this rustic dish, the combination of tomatoes, kalamata olives, and bell peppers that have practically melted through slow cooking gives chicken a distinctively Mediterranean flavor. Serve it over a bed of rice or quinoa.

2 teaspoons olive oil
½ pound skinless, boneless chicken
  breasts, sliced into 1-inch-long strips
½ medium-size Spanish onion, thinly sliced
2 cloves garlic, thinly sliced
1 small red bell pepper, cut into
  julienne strips
1 small green bell pepper, cut into
  julienne strips
1 small yellow or orange bell pepper,
  cut into julienne strips
4 ripe plum tomatoes, seeded and
  finely chopped, or 1 cup drained
  canned diced tomatoes
¼ cup pitted kalamata olives, halved
2 teaspoons fresh thyme leaves
1 teaspoon hot paprika, or 1 teaspoon
  sweet paprika and a pinch of crushed
  red pepper flakes, or more to taste
¼ cup chopped fresh flat-leaf parsley
Salt and black pepper

1. Heat 1 teaspoon of the olive oil in a large nonstick skillet over medium heat. Add the chicken and sauté until it's just cooked through (there should be no pink), 5 to 7 minutes. Remove the chicken from the skillet and set aside.

2. Add the remaining teaspoon of olive oil to the skillet along with the onion, garlic, and bell peppers, reduce the heat to medium-low, and cook until softened,

about 8 minutes. Stir in the tomatoes, olives, thyme, paprika, and 2 tablespoons of the parsley. Cook, stirring frequently, until the flavors blend, about 5 minutes. Season with salt, pepper, and additional paprika to taste. Add the cooked chicken, toss to coat with the sauce, and cook until heated through. Sprinkle the remaining 2 tablespoons of parsley over the top.

SERVES 2

FROM THE TEST KITCHEN

IN BASQUE COUNTRY, the chicken might be served topped with a sheep's milk cheese—probably an unpasteurized one. For your pregnant purposes, some crumbled pasteurized feta can safely, and deliciously, stand in.

Nutrition Info
1 PORTION PROVIDES:

Protein: 1 serving

Vitamin C: 5 servings

Green leafy and yellow vegetables and
  fruits: 1½ servings

Other fruits and vegetables: 1 serving

Fat: ½ serving

Chicken Pot Shepherd's Pie

Here's the best of both worlds—a nutritious cross between a chicken pot pie and a shepherd's pie. It has a delicious cheesy mashed potato crust—the ultimate (low-fat) comfort food. Though this recipe takes a little longer to prepare, your efforts will be rewarded once you take a taste. To save prep time, consider making the filling the day before. Serving only two? Save the other half for tomorrow.

FOR THE FILLING:

2 cups low-sodium chicken broth,
   or more if necessary
1 pound skinless, boneless chicken
   breast halves, cut into 1-inch cubes
3 carrots, cut into $1/2$-inch-thick
   chunks
2 ribs celery, cut into $1/2$-inch-thick
   chunks
1 tablespoon plus 2 teaspoons butter
   or olive oil
$1/2$ pound button mushrooms,
   wiped clean and quartered
1 cup frozen peas
1 small onion, finely chopped
1 bay leaf
2 teaspoons fresh thyme leaves
1 teaspoon fresh tarragon leaves
$1/2$ teaspoon dried marjoram
$1/4$ cup whole wheat flour
Pinch of ground nutmeg
Salt and black pepper

FOR THE TOPPING:

4 small Yukon Gold potatoes,
   peeled and cubed
$1/3$ cup buttermilk, or more
   if necessary

$1/2$ cup shredded sharp cheddar
   cheese
$1/4$ cup grated Parmesan cheese
2 tablespoons minced fresh chives
Salt and black pepper

1. Make the filling: Place the chicken broth in a large saucepan and let come to a boil over medium-high heat. Add the chicken, carrots, and celery (add additional chicken broth to cover if necessary), reduce the heat to low, and let simmer until the chicken is cooked through (there should be no pink) and the carrots are just tender, about 10 minutes. Remove the chicken and vegetables from the broth, place them in a large bowl and set aside. Set aside the broth.

2. Melt 2 teaspoons of the butter in a large nonstick skillet over medium heat. Add the mushrooms and cook, stirring frequently, until softened and golden brown and any liquid evaporates, about 5 minutes. Remove the mushrooms from the skillet and add them to the chicken mixture.

3. Add the remaining 1 tablespoon of butter to the skillet, reduce the heat to low, and add the peas, onion, bay leaf, thyme, tarragon, and marjoram. Cook, stirring, until the onion is softened, about 5 minutes. Stir in the flour and cook, stirring, 3 minutes longer. Gradually whisk in 1½ cups of the reserved chicken broth. Add the nutmeg and season with salt and pepper to taste. Let simmer, stirring frequently, for 5 minutes.

4. Remove and discard the bay leaf, then add the broth mixture to the chicken and vegetables. Toss well to combine. The filling can be made a day ahead and refrigerated, covered. Let come to room temperature before proceeding with the recipe.

5. Preheat the oven to 425°F.

6. Make the topping: Place the potatoes in a medium-size saucepan and cover them with water. Let come to a boil over high heat, then reduce the heat to low and let simmer until very tender, about 15 minutes. Drain the potatoes and place them in a bowl with the buttermilk and the cheddar and Parmesan cheeses. Mash the potatoes until very smooth, stir in the chives, then season with salt and pepper. Add more buttermilk if necessary, but keep the potatoes fairly dry.

7. Pour the chicken mixture into a 2-quart baking dish. Spread the mashed potatoes evenly over the top and bake until golden and bubbling, about 25 minutes.

SERVES 4

Nutrition Info

1 PORTION PROVIDES:

Protein: 1 serving

Calcium: 1 serving

Vitamin C: ½ serving

Green leafy and yellow vegetables and fruits: 1½ servings

Other fruits and vegetables: 2 servings

Fat: ½ serving

Turkey Cutlets in Mushroom Sauce

Love mushrooms? You're in for a treat, in just minutes. This colorful and flavorful one-pot dish teams turkey with lots of mushrooms (use wild for even more flavor), peas, carrots, and fresh herbs. Complement this earthy entrée by serving it on a bed of noodles.

Whole wheat flour
2 turkey cutlets (each 6 ounces and
   1/2-inch thick, see Note)
Salt and black pepper
Olive oil cooking spray
1 teaspoon olive oil
2 teaspoons butter
2 shallots, finely minced
1/2 pound sliced wild or cultivated
   mushrooms (about 3 cups)
1 cup shredded (not grated) carrots,
   or 1 cup carrots cut into matchstick
   strips
1/2 cup frozen peas
1 teaspoon fresh tarragon leaves,
   minced
2 tablespoons chopped fresh flat-leaf
   parsley, plus more for garnish
2 tablespoons snipped fresh chives,
   plus more for garnish
3/4 cup low-sodium chicken or
   mushroom broth

1. Place some flour in a shallow bowl. Season the turkey cutlets with salt and pepper, then lightly dredge both sides of each cutlet with flour.

2. Coat a large, heavy nonstick skillet with olive oil spray. Place 1 teaspoon of the olive oil in the skillet and heat over medium heat. Cook the cutlets until browned but not cooked through, about 2 minutes per side. Remove the cutlets from the skillet and set aside.

3. Coat the skillet again with olive oil spray and melt the butter in it over medium-low heat. Add the shallots and cook until slightly softened, about 2 minutes. Increase the heat to medium-high, add the mushrooms and cook for 2 minutes.

Nutrition Info

1 PORTION PROVIDES:

Protein: 1 1/2 servings

Green leafy and yellow vegetables and fruits: 2 servings

Other fruits and vegetables:
3 servings

4. Add the carrots, peas, tarragon, parsley, chives, and broth and let come to a boil, then lower the heat and let simmer for 2 minutes. Return the cutlets to the skillet. Let simmer, stirring frequently, until the sauce is slightly reduced and the turkey is cooked through (there should be no pink), about 2 minutes. Season with salt and pepper to taste, and garnish with more parsley and chives.

SERVES 2

NOTE: If your turkey cutlets are more than ½ inch thick, pound them with a heavy skillet or meat pounder until they are an even ½ inch in thickness.

Turkey Breast with Corn and Edamame Salsa

No need to wait until Thanksgiving for this turkey dish—and no need to wait hours for your bird to be ready. Make summer turkey season, too, with a tasty and quick-grilled turkey breast topped with a crisp, cool salsa. New to edamame ? This will be a delicious introduction to chewy, nutritious soybeans.

4 plum tomatoes, seeded and chopped
1 cup cooked corn kernels
1 cup cooked shelled edamame
    (soybeans)
1 teaspoon chili powder
2 tablespoons chopped fresh cilantro,
    or more to taste
2 tablespoons olive oil
2 tablespoons fresh lime juice

Salt and black pepper
1/2 pound piece boneless
    turkey breast
1/2 teaspoon ground cumin
Olive oil cooking spray
Garlic powder
1 medium-size avocado,
    preferably Hass, sliced
4 lime wedges, for serving

1. Place the tomatoes, corn, edamame, chili powder, 1 tablespoon of the cilantro, 1 tablespoon of the olive oil, and the lime juice in a bowl and stir to mix. Season with salt, pepper to taste and add additional cilantro, if desired. Set the salsa aside.

2. Using a very sharp knife, slice the turkey breast into ½-inch-thick medallions. Place the remaining tablespoon of olive oil and the cumin in a small bowl and stir to mix. Brush the cumin oil on the turkey and season it with salt, pepper, and garlic powder.

3. Coat a large skillet with olive oil cooking spray and heat over medium-high heat. Add the turkey and cook until completely cooked through (there should be no pink), 2 to 4 minutes per side.

4. To serve, place the turkey on top of the salsa. Sprinkle the remaining tablespoon of cilantro over the turkey, then garnish it with avocado slices and lime wedges.

SERVES 2

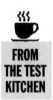

HERE'S A TIME-SAVING TIP: Grill a whole pound of turkey while you're at it, then have the leftovers on a salad tomorrow (or in Fruity Turkey Salad, page 278).

FROM THE TEST KITCHEN

Nutrition Info
1 PORTION PROVIDES:

Protein: 1½ servings

Vitamin C: ½ serving

Other fruits and vegetables:
1½ servings

Whole grains and legumes: 1 serving

Fat: 1 serving

Fish and Seafood

Maybe you're a fish fan from way back. Or maybe you feel lukewarm about seafood—you don't mind it, but you probably wouldn't make it your entrée of choice. Or maybe you know you *should* embrace the seafood side of life (for its high-protein, low-fat benefits), but fish is a taste you're still waiting to acquire. No matter how you feel about fish and seafood, these recipes will win you over.

Looking for something exotic? Try Sautéed Halibut with Watercress, Mango, and Avocado or Salmon Poached in Thai Carrot Broth. Seeking the simple and soothing? Opt for Flounder with Carrot, Fennel, and Leeks, or Salmon Fillets with Ginger and Lime. Going gourmet? How about Shrimp with Feta or Seared Scallops on White Beans and Kale. Fishing for a quick yet memorable meal? You'll find it here.

Sautéed Halibut with Watercress, Mango, and Avocado

Sautéed halibut sits on a vitamin-packed bed of wilted watercress, crowned by a sweet and tangy salsa of mango and avocado. It's a dish that's almost too pretty to eat—with a taste too luscious to resist.

½ large ripe mango, diced
½ medium-size avocado, preferably
  Hass, diced
1 tablespoon fresh lime juice
2 halibut fillets (each about 6 ounces)
Salt and black pepper
½ teaspoon thinly sliced fresh
  mint leaves
1 tablespoon whole wheat bread
  crumbs
1 tablespoon olive oil
2 cups (packed) watercress,
  thick stems removed

1. Place the mango, avocado, and lime juice in a small bowl and stir to mix. Set the mango and avocado salsa aside until ready to serve.

2. Lightly season the top of each halibut fillet with salt and pepper. Sprinkle ¼ teaspoon of mint and 1½ teaspoons of bread crumbs over each fillet.

3. Heat the olive oil in a large skillet over medium-high heat. Add the halibut fillets, seasoned side down, and cook until they are cooked through and flake easily

when pierced with a fork, about 3 minutes per side. Remove the fish from the skillet and cover loosely with aluminum foil to keep warm.

4. Reduce the heat to low, add the watercress, and cook just until it begins to wilt, about 1 minute.

5. Divide the wilted watercress between 2 serving plates and place a halibut fillet on top of each. Spoon the mango and avocado salsa over the fillets, dividing it equally between them.

SERVES 2

Nutrition Info
1 PORTION PROVIDES:

Protein: 1½ servings

Vitamin C: 1½ servings

Green leafy and yellow vegetables and
  fruits: 1½ servings

Other fruits and vegetables:
  1½ servings

Fat: ½ serving

Ginger Steamed Halibut

Aluminum foil packets enclose an intensely flavored meal-in-one, steaming not only the halibut but also couscous and a delicious mix of vegetables.

¼ cup uncooked couscous
½ large red bell pepper, thinly sliced
1 cup sugar snap peas
½ cup sliced shiitake mushrooms, or ½ cup chopped enoki mushrooms
1 cup (packed) baby spinach leaves
2 teaspoons grated peeled fresh ginger
Salt and black pepper
¼ cup vegetable broth or fish broth
2 halibut or salmon fillets (each about 6 ounces)
4 fresh basil leaves (optional)

1. Preheat the oven to 450°F.

2. Tear off 2 pieces of heavy-duty aluminum foil each 12 inches long. Place the pieces of foil on a work surface and put 2 tablespoons of couscous in the center of each.

3. Place the bell pepper, sugar snap peas, mushrooms, spinach, and ginger in a bowl and stir to mix. Season the vegetable mix lightly with salt and black pepper, then place half of it in the center of each piece of foil.

4. Fold up the edges of each piece of foil slightly, then spoon 2 tablespoons of broth into each.

FULL OF FISH?

▼ ▼ ▼

Most recipes in this chapter call for 6-ounce fish fillets—because that's the size that's most commonly encountered at fish markets. That means you'll be racking up 1½ protein servings in each portion. But if that's too much fish for you, scale it back to 4-ounce portions, and you'll cut your protein serving down to 1. On the other hand, if you can never get your fill of fish, you can occasionally feast on 8 ounces—a portion that will yield a full 2 protein servings.

5. Lightly season the fish fillets with salt and black pepper and place one on top of each mound of vegetables. Top each fish fillet with 2 basil leaves, if using.

6. Seal a packet by bringing together the two longest edges of the foil and double folding them, leaving room for heat circulation inside. Crimp the edges to make a tight seal. Double fold and crimp the remaining 2 edges to finish sealing the packet (there should be no gaps where juices can leak out). Repeat with the remaining piece of aluminum foil.

7. Transfer the foil packets to a rimmed baking sheet and bake them until the fish is cooked through, 12 to 15 minutes, depending upon the thickness of the fillets. To test for doneness, carefully open a packet; when the fish is cooked through

it will flake easily when pierced with a fork.

8. To serve, place the packets on serving plates and open them at the table, taking care to avoid the escaping hot steam.

SERVES 2

Nutrition Info
1 PORTION PROVIDES:

Protein: 1 1/2 servings

Vitamin C: 2 servings

Green leafy and yellow vegetables and fruits: 1 serving

Other fruits and vegetables: 1/2 serving

Whole grains and legumes: 1/2 serving

Iron: from the spinach

CUCUMBER SAUCE

▼ ▼ ▼

Any roasted, poached, or grilled fish tastes better with a sauce, but you'll feel better if you know the sauce isn't adding a lot of extra calories. Try this cucumber sauce on for size. It's enough for two servings.

1/2 cup plain yogurt (whole-milk yogurt will produce a richer flavor)
2 Kirby (pickling) cucumbers, peeled, cut in half, and seeded

1 tablespoon chopped fresh dill, or 1/2 teaspoon dried dill
1 ripe tomato, diced
Salt and black pepper

Place the yogurt, cucumbers, and dill in a food processor and process until just chunky. Fold in the tomato and season the sauce with salt and pepper to taste. Like a little bite? Add a teaspoon or two of well-drained prepared horseradish.

Flounder with Carrot, Fennel, and Leeks

Root vegetables, poached in cider, make a delicately flavored companion for delicate fish fillets. Plus, cleanup's a snap, thanks to the foil packets the fish is baked in.

½ cup apple cider

2 leeks, both white and pale green parts, trimmed, rinsed well, and thinly sliced

1 medium-size carrot, thinly sliced

1 small fennel bulb, outer layers removed and discarded, thinly sliced crosswise

1 teaspoon fresh thyme leaves, or ¼ teaspoon dried thyme

Olive oil cooking spray

2 flounder, sole, or halibut fillets (each about 6 ounces)

2 lime or lemon wedges

1. Preheat the oven to 450°F.

2. Place the apple cider in a small saucepan, and let come to a simmer over medium-low heat. Add the leeks, carrot, fennel, and thyme and cook just until the vegetables soften, about 3 minutes.

3. Tear off 2 pieces of heavy-duty aluminum foil, each 12 inches long. Place the pieces of foil on a work surface and coat them with olive oil spray.

4. Place a fish fillet in the center of each piece of foil. To hold in the cooking juices of the vegetables, fold up the edges of the foil slightly. Spoon half of the poached vegetables and their juices over each fillet.

5. Seal a packet by bringing together the two longest edges of foil and double folding them, leaving room for heat circulation inside. Crimp the edges to make a tight seal. Double fold and crimp the remaining 2 edges to finish sealing the packet (there should be no gaps where juices can leak out). Repeat with the remaining piece of aluminum foil.

6. Transfer the foil packets to a rimmed baking sheet and bake them until the fish is cooked through, about 12 to 15 minutes, depending upon the thickness of the fillets. To test for doneness, carefully open a packet; when the fish is cooked through it will flake easily when pierced with a fork.

7. To serve, place the packets on serving plates and open them at the table, taking care to avoid the escaping hot steam. Serve lime or lemon wedges alongside.

SERVES 2

Nutrition Info
1 PORTION PROVIDES:

Protein: 1¹/2 servings

Green leafy and yellow vegetables and fruits: 1 serving

Other vegetables and fruits: 1¹/2 servings

MINUTE MEALS

▼ ▼ ▼

For a fish dinner without any fuss (or unpleasant smells), turn to the microwave. Place a fish fillet in a microwave-safe baking dish; use a fillet that's no more than ¹/2 inch thick. Season the fish with a combination of any of the following: grated lemon or orange zest, a sprinkling of chopped fresh herbs (such as tarragon and dill), and a coating of equal parts grainy mustard and mayonnaise. Cover the baking dish with plastic wrap, folding back one corner to allow the steam to escape. Microwave the fish on high power until it's cooked through, 2 to 3 minutes. Presto! With a squeeze of lemon or lime juice, dinner is ready.

Red Snapper with Mango Salsa

Topping broiled red snapper with a snappy mango salsa gives the fish an authentic island kick. The mango salsa also goes well with turkey, beef, pork, or chicken and will keep nicely in the refrigerator for one or two days.

1 medium-size ripe mango,
    cut into small dice
1/2 medium-size red bell pepper,
    cut into small dice
2 scallions, both white and
    light green parts, trimmed
    and thinly sliced
1/2 teaspoon canned sliced jalapeño
    pepper (optional)
2 tablespoons fresh lime juice
2 tablespoons chopped fresh cilantro
1 tablespoon olive oil
2 red snapper fillets
    (each about 6 ounces)
Salt and black pepper

1. Preheat the broiler.

2. Place the mango, bell pepper, scallions, jalapeño, if using, lime juice, cilantro, and 1 teaspoon of the oil in a bowl and stir to mix. Set the mango salsa aside.

3. Brush the fish fillets with the remaining oil and season with salt and black pepper. Broil them until they are cooked through and flake easily when pierced with a fork, 4 to 5 minutes per side.

4. Serve the fish with large spoonfuls of the mango salsa.

SERVES 2

FROM THE TEST KITCHEN

HEARTBURN getting you down? Skip the heat—substitute a teaspoon of ground cumin for the jalapeño pepper.

Nutrition Info
1 PORTION PROVIDES:

Protein: 1 1/2 servings

Vitamin C: 2 servings

Green leafy and yellow vegetables and fruits: 1 1/2 servings

Fat: 1/2 serving

Greek Salad Snapper

Bake snapper with a delicious sauce that combines all of your favorite Greek salad ingredients—tomatoes, red pepper, capers, kalamata olives, oregano, and feta cheese. The results are mouthwatering.

1 tablespoon olive oil

2 scallions, both white and light green
parts, trimmed and thinly sliced

2 ripe plum tomatoes, cut into
1/2-inch pieces

1/2 large red bell pepper, cut into
1/2-inch pieces

1 teaspoon fresh oregano, or
1/2 teaspoon dried oregano

1 teaspoon drained capers, or more,
to taste

6 pitted kalamata olives, chopped

1/4 cup crumbled pasteurized feta cheese

2 tablespoons chopped fresh
flat-leaf parsley

Fresh lemon juice (about 1/2 lemon)

Olive oil cooking spray

2 red snapper fillets (each about 6 ounces)

1/2 teaspoon dried dill

Salt and black pepper

1. Preheat the oven to 400°F.

2. Heat the olive oil in a small skillet over medium-high heat. Add the scallions and cook until softened slightly, about 1 minute. Add the tomatoes, bell pepper, oregano, and capers and cook until the vegetables soften, about 4 minutes. Remove from the heat and add the olives and feta cheese, then sprinkle parsley on top and season with black pepper and lemon juice to taste.

3. Coat an 8-inch-square baking dish with olive oil spray. Place the fish fillets in the center of the baking dish, sprinkle the dill over them and season them with salt and black pepper. Spoon the tomato and feta mixture on top. Cover the baking dish with aluminum foil and bake until the fish is cooked through, and flakes easily when pierced with a fork, 8 to 10 minutes. Serve the fish with the tomato and feta mixture.

SERVES 2

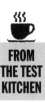

FROM THE TEST KITCHEN

NOT A RED SNAPPER FAN? You can substitute haddock, tilapia, orange roughy, bass, cod, or flounder for any recipe that calls for red snapper.

Nutrition Info

1 PORTION PROVIDES:

Protein: 1/2 serving

Calcium: 1 serving

Vitamin C: 1 1/2 servings

**Green leafy and yellow vegetables and
fruits:** 1/2 serving

Fat: 1/2 serving

Roasted Mediterranean Sea Bass with Red Pepper and White Beans

Here's a quick and easy way to bring the flavors of the Mediterranean to your table. White beans and red bell pepper pair up to provide a simple yet satisfying base for the bass.

4 scallions, both white and light green
   parts, trimmed and chopped
1/2 cup fresh-leaf parsley leaves
1/4 cup vegetable broth
1 tablespoon olive oil
1 medium-size red bell pepper,
   thinly sliced
1 can (14 ounces) Great Northern
   beans, rinsed and drained
2 sea bass, halibut, or salmon fillets
   (each about 6 ounces)
1 lemon, halved and seeded
   (1 half, thinly sliced)

1. Preheat the oven to 375°F.

2. Place the scallions, parsley, vegetable broth, and olive oil in a blender or food processor and purée them.

3. Place the bell pepper and beans in an 8-inch-square baking dish. Set aside 3 tablespoons of the scallion and parsley purée, then spoon the rest over the bell pepper and beans. Arrange the fish fillets on top and spoon the remaining scallion and parsley purée over the fish. Scatter the lemon slices on top.

4. Bake the fish until it is cooked through and flakes easily when pierced with a fork, about 15 minutes. Squeeze the remaining lemon half over the fish just before serving it.

SERVES 2

Nutrition Info

1 PORTION PROVIDES:

Protein: 2 servings

Calcium: 1/2 serving

Vitamin C: 2 servings

Green leafy and yellow vegetables and fruits: 2 servings

Whole grains and legumes: 21/2 servings

Iron: from the beans

Marinated Salmon Fillets with Ginger and Lime

Simple broiled or grilled salmon is easy to prepare but much tastier—and just as easy—in this Pacific Rim–inspired dish. The lime and ginger marinade makes it fragrant and flavorful. The recipe is easy to cut in half—or enjoy any leftovers the next day. It's good on shrimp, too.)

Zest and juice of 2 limes
2 teaspoons olive oil
2 teaspoons low-sodium soy sauce
1 teaspoon sesame oil
2 teaspoons grated peeled fresh
    ginger
4 skinless salmon fillets
    (each about 6 ounces)
3 scallions, both white and
    light green parts, trimmed
    and thinly sliced

1. Place the lime zest and juice, olive oil, soy sauce, sesame oil, and ginger in a small bowl and stir to mix.

2. Place the salmon in a 9-by-13-inch glass baking dish. Pour half of the lime and ginger mixture over the salmon; set the rest aside. Turn the salmon fillets to coat them evenly with the marinade.

3. Preheat the broiler or set up the grill and preheat it to high.

4. Broil or grill the salmon until it is cooked through and flakes easily when pierced with a fork, 3 to 5 minutes per side.

5. Place the salmon fillets on serving plates and spoon the reserved lime and ginger mixture over them. Top the fillets with the scallions.

SERVES 4

Nutrition Info

1 PORTION PROVIDES:

Protein: 1½ servings

Fat: ½ serving

Pan-Roasted Salmon with a Mild Mustard Crust

Salmon's rich taste stands up beautifully to this flavorful mustard coating. But don't shy away from trying this crust on a milder fish, like halibut. For that matter, try it on chicken breasts.

Olive oil cooking spray
2 skinless salmon fillets
   (each about 6 ounces)
Salt and black pepper
1½ tablespoons grainy mustard
2 teaspoons mayonnaise
2 teaspoons chopped fresh dill,
   or ½ teaspoon dried dill

1. Preheat the oven to 375°F.

2. Coat the bottom of an 8-inch-square baking dish with olive oil cooking spray. Place the salmon fillets in the baking dish and lightly season them with salt and pepper.

3. Place the mustard, mayonnaise, and dill in a small bowl and stir to mix.

4. Spread the mustard mixture on the salmon fillets.

5. Bake the salmon until it is cooked through and flakes easily when pierced with a fork, about 10 minutes.

SERVES 2

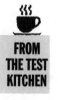

FROM THE TEST KITCHEN FOR A SWEET-AND-PUNGENT taste, skip the dill and add 2 teaspoons fruit-only apricot preserves to the mustard mixture in the crust.

Nutrition Info
1 PORTION PROVIDES:

Protein: 1½ servings

Roast Salmon on a Bed of Lentils

Earthy lentils provide a nutritious bed for roast salmon. The result is a hearty dish that's sure to satisfy.

2 skinless salmon fillets
  (each about 6 ounces)
2 teaspoons olive oil
2 teaspoons fresh thyme leaves
Pinch each of salt and black pepper
Warm Lentil Ragout (recipe follows)
1 tablespoon finely chopped fresh
  parsley

1. Preheat the oven to 450°F.

2. Place the salmon fillets in an 8-inch-square baking dish and rub the olive oil over them. Sprinkle the thyme, salt, and pepper on top of the salmon.

3. Bake the salmon until it is cooked through and flakes easily when pierced with a fork, 10 to 15 minutes.

4. Spoon a serving of the lentils onto each of 2 serving plates and place a salmon fillet on top. Sprinkle parsley over each fillet and serve.

SERVES 2

Nutrition Info
1 PORTION SALMON
(WITHOUT LENTILS) PROVIDES:

Protein: 1½ servings

Warm Lentil Ragout

This recipe makes twice as many lentils as you'll need for the Roast Salmon on a Bed of Lentils. So tomorrow you can serve chicken or beef over the leftovers.

2 teaspoons olive oil
1 medium-size onion, chopped
2 cloves garlic, minced
2 medium-size carrots, diced
1 cup green lentils
1 sprig fresh thyme
1 bay leaf
3 cups low-sodium chicken broth or
  vegetable broth
Salt and black pepper

1. Heat the olive oil in a medium-size saucepan over medium-low heat. Add the onion and garlic and cook until just beginning to soften, 3 minutes.

2. Add the carrots and cook, stirring frequently, until they soften slightly, about 3 minutes. Add the lentils, thyme, and bay leaf and cook, stirring to mix well, for about 1 minute.

3. Stir in the chicken broth, raise the heat to medium-high and bring to a boil. Reduce the heat, and let simmer until the lentils are tender, about 20 minutes. Season with salt and pepper to taste. Remove and discard the sprig of thyme and bay leaf before serving. The lentils can be refrigerated, covered, for up to 5 days.

SERVES 4

Nutrition Info

1 PORTION PROVIDES:

Protein: 1/2 serving

Green leafy and yellow vegetables and fruits: 1 serving

Other fruits and vegetables: 1/2 serving

Whole grains and legumes: 1 1/2 servings

ROAST THIS

▼ ▼ ▼

When fish is so fresh you can taste it, don't cover it up with fancy sauces or coatings. Instead, try the simplest and most satisfying way to prepare fish—roast it. Arrange fish fillets on a bed of fresh herbs, such as sprigs of rosemary, thyme, or sage in a baking dish and sprinkle more herbs on top. Fennel seeds are a nice addition, too. Brush the fish with some sea salt and cracked pepper, olive oil, season and scatter thin slices of lemon over and around the fish. Bake the fish at 450°F until it is cooked through.

Another lovely way to roast fish is on a bed of vegetables. Toss slices or chunks of carrot, turnip, rutabaga, butternut squash, potatoes (white or sweet), and/or fennel with a little olive oil, fresh thyme leaves, and a little salt and pepper. Spread the vegetables out in a baking dish and roast them in a 450°F oven until tender, about 20 minutes. Spoon the roast vegetables into the center of the baking dish so they can act as a bed for the fish. Place fillets on top, sprinkle them with herbs and lemon as above, and bake until fish is done, for a delicious rustic fish dinner.

Salmon with Basil and Tomatoes

Tomatoes and basil, a classic combo, make these salmon fillets moist, fragrant, and flavorful. How can so little effort result in something so tasty? Take three or four minutes to get these packets ready for the oven, and you'll find out.

Olive oil cooking spray
2 skinless salmon fillets
   (each about 6 ounces)
12 cherry tomatoes, halved
12 fresh basil leaves
1 tablespoon olive oil
Salt and black pepper

1. Preheat the oven to 450°F.

2. Tear off 2 pieces of heavy-duty aluminum foil each 12 inches long. Place the pieces of foil on a work surface and coat them with olive oil spray.

3. Place a salmon fillet in the center of each piece of foil. Top each fillet with 12 cherry tomato halves and 6 basil leaves. Drizzle 1 teaspoon of olive oil over each fillet, then season with salt and pepper.

4. Seal a packet by bringing together the two longest edges of foil and double folding them, leaving room for heat circulation inside. Crimp the edges to make a tight seal. Double fold and crimp the remaining 2 edges to finish sealing the

packet (there should be no gaps where juices can leak out). Repeat with the remaining piece of aluminum foil.

5. Transfer the foil packets to a rimmed baking sheet and bake them until the salmon is cooked through, 15 to 20 minutes, depending upon the thickness of the fillets. To test for doneness, carefully open a packet; when the salmon is cooked through, it will flake easily when pierced with a fork and will have turned light pink inside.

6. To serve, place the packets on serving plates and open them at the table, taking care to avoid the escaping hot steam.

SERVES 2

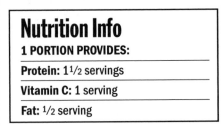

Nutrition Info
1 PORTION PROVIDES:

Protein: 1 1/2 servings

Vitamin C: 1 serving

Fat: 1/2 serving

Salmon Poached in Thai Carrot Broth

Intensely and intriguingly flavored with sweet carrots, pungent ginger, and cilantro, and tangy lime, this light-as-air salmon dish gives spa food a good name.

2 cups carrot juice

1 cup diced carrots

1 tablespoon minced peeled fresh ginger

2 teaspoons grated lemon zest

1 teaspoon grated lime zest

2 tablespoons fresh lime juice, or
**   more to taste**

3 scallions, both white and light
**   green parts, trimmed and sliced**

2 skinless salmon fillets
**   (each about 6 ounces)**

2 tablespoons chopped fresh cilantro,
**   plus more for garnish**

Salt and black pepper

1. Place the carrot juice, carrots, and ginger in a medium-size saucepan that is large enough to hold the salmon fillets without crowding and bring to a boil over medium-high heat. Reduce the heat and let simmer until the carrots are tender, about 5 minutes. Add the lemon and lime zests, lime juice, and scallions and let simmer until heated through, about 1 minute.

2. Add the salmon fillets to the pan, let it return to a simmer, cover, and cook until the salmon is just cooked through, about 10 minutes. Spoon the carrot broth over the fillets periodically.

3. Place the salmon fillets in shallow bowls. Add the 2 tablespoons of cilantro to the carrot broth, then season it with salt and pepper to taste, adding more lime juice, if desired. Pour the carrot broth over the salmon fillets, garnish with cilantro, and serve.

SERVES 2

FROM THE TEST KITCHEN **THE CARROT BROTH** is too good to save for just salmon. Try poaching halibut, sea bass, shrimp, scallops, or skinless, boneless chicken breasts in it, too.

Nutrition Info

1 PORTION PROVIDES:

Protein: 1½ servings

Green leafy and yellow vegetables and fruits: 2 servings; plus 2 more if you sip the carrot broth

Salmon Cakes with Tropical Salsa

Don't have the time (or the stomach) to stop by the fish market for fresh fillets? No harm in fishing some salmon out of a can. In fact, the soft bones in canned salmon provide a calcium bonus (you'll never notice them once they're mashed up). If there are any salmon cakes left over, you can have them cold for lunch.

1 can (14¾ ounces) pink salmon, drained and mashed with a fork
1 medium-size red bell pepper, cut into small dice
½ cup grated carrot
1 tablespoon drained capers
1 large egg
Zest of ½ lemon
4 tablespoons whole wheat bread crumbs
2 tablespoons wheat germ or ground flaxseed
Black pepper
2 teaspoons olive oil
1 cup pineapple chunks, fresh or canned
1 cup ripe mango chunks (from 1 large mango)
2 tablespoons balsamic vinegar
Pinch of crushed red pepper flakes

1. Place the salmon, half of the bell pepper, and the carrot, capers, egg, and lemon zest in a bowl and stir to mix.

2. Place the bread crumbs and wheat germ in a small bowl and whisk to mix. Add half of the bread crumb mixture to the salmon mixture and mix well. Season with black pepper to taste, then stir well to combine.

3. Divide the salmon mixture into 6 equal portions and pat into cakes, about ½ inch thick. Dredge both sides of the salmon cakes in the remaining bread crumb mixture.

Nutrition Info

1 PORTION (2 CAKES) PROVIDES:

Protein: 1 serving

Vitamin C: 2 servings plus

Calcium: 1 serving if made with bones

Green leafy and yellow vegetables and fruits: 1 serving

Whole grains and legumes: ½ serving

4. Heat the oil in a large skillet over medium-high heat. Add the salmon cakes and cook until golden brown and heated through, about 4 minutes per side. To check for doneness, insert a knife into the center of a salmon cake; if the knife feels hot when removed, the cake is done.

5. Meanwhile, place the remaining bell pepper and the pineapple, mango, balsamic vinegar, and red pepper flakes in a bowl and stir to mix.

6. Spoon the pineapple salsa onto serving plates and top with the salmon cakes.

MAKES 6 CAKES; SERVES 3

Pan-fried Trout with Tomatoes and Spinach

Adelicious cornmeal crust adds crunch to trout, then it's topped with a warm salad of tomato and spinach. This is what happens when fish leaves the campfire and goes uptown on the stove.

½ cup whole grain cornmeal
   (see Note)
2 tablespoons grated Parmesan
   cheese (optional)
1 teaspoon grated lemon zest
Salt and black pepper
Garlic powder
1 large egg
¼ cup buttermilk
2 large boneless trout fillet halves
   (about 6 ounces each)
Olive oil cooking spray
1½ tablespoons olive oil
1 tablespoon fresh lemon juice
4 ripe plum tomatoes, seeded and
   chopped

2 teaspoons chopped fresh tarragon
1 package (5 to 6 ounces) baby spinach,
   thick stems removed
2 teaspoons minced fresh chives
Lemon wedges, for serving

1. Place the cornmeal, Parmesan cheese, if using, lemon zest, and a pinch each of salt, pepper, and garlic powder in a shallow dish and stir to mix. Place the egg and the buttermilk in another shallow dish and gently whisk to combine.

2. Dip each trout fillet in the egg mixture, then in the cornmeal mixture, turning it to coat evenly and thoroughly.

3. Coat a large skillet with olive oil cooking spray, then heat 1½ teaspoons of the olive oil in it over medium heat. Add the trout and cook until the coating is browned and the fish is cooked through, about 4 minutes per side. Transfer the trout to a platter and cover with aluminum foil to keep warm.

4. Add the remaining 1 tablespoon of olive oil and the lemon juice to the skillet and scrape up the browned bits. Add the tomatoes and tarragon, reduce the heat to low, and cook until the tomatoes soften slightly, about 2 minutes. Add the spinach and cook, stirring, until barely wilted, about 2 minutes. Season with salt and pepper to taste. Top the trout with the tomato and spinach mixture, sprinkle with chives, and serve with lemon wedges.

SERVES 2

NOTE: Whole-grain cornmeal is available at health food stores and in the health food section of most supermarkets.

FROM THE TEST KITCHEN

THE COMBINATION of trout and nuts goes way back. For a change of pace, replace the cornmeal breading for the pan-fried trout with a combination of ¼ cup of ground toasted pecans or hazelnuts (see page 272), ⅓ cup of dry whole wheat bread crumbs, 4 tablespoons of finely chopped fresh parsley, 1 teaspoon of grated lemon zest, and a pinch each of salt and black pepper. Skip the egg and buttermilk bath; just moisten the trout fillets with milk before dredging them in the nut mixture. Pan fry the fish in a combination of 1½ teaspoons of butter and 1½ teaspoons olive oil. Sprinkle the trout with minced chives and lemon juice, and serve it with lemon wedges and a pilaf instead of the tomato and spinach salad.

Nutrition Info

1 PORTION PROVIDES:

Protein: 1½ servings

Vitamin C: 2 servings

Green leafy and yellow vegetables and fruits: 3 servings

Whole grains and legumes: ½ serving

Iron from the spinach

Fat: ½ serving plus

Shrimp with Feta

Here's a traditional Greek dish that's bound to become a tradition in your home, too—especially when you see how easy it is to make. Serve the shrimp over the grain of your choice.

1 tablespoon olive oil
1 medium-size red bell pepper,
  chopped
1 small fennel bulb, trimmed, halved,
  and thinly sliced crosswise
3 cloves garlic, minced
4 ripe plum tomatoes, seeded and
  chopped
1 tablespoon minced fresh oregano,
  or 1 teaspoon dried oregano
¾ pound shelled and deveined
  large shrimp
Fresh lemon juice
Black pepper
Hot sauce (optional)
½ cup crumbled pasteurized feta cheese
¼ cup toasted pine nuts
  (optional; see page 272)
Salt (optional)
2 tablespoons chopped fresh flat-leaf
  parsley

1. Heat the olive oil in a large skillet over medium-high heat. Add the bell pepper, fennel, and garlic and cook, stirring frequently, until the vegetables are softened, about 5 minutes. Add the tomatoes and oregano and cook, stirring frequently, until slightly softened, about 2 minutes. Stir in the shrimp and cook until it is cooked through and turns opaque, about 4 minutes.

2. Season the shrimp and vegetables to taste with lemon juice, black pepper, and hot sauce, if using. Add the feta cheese, stir well, and let simmer until the cheese begins to melt, about 30 seconds. Stir in the pine nuts, if using, and season with salt to taste (you may not need any since the feta is salty). Sprinkle the parsley on top and serve.

SERVES 2

FROM THE TEST KITCHEN

DON'T FEEL LIKE splurging on shrimp? Try substituting an equal amount of cubed skinless, boneless chicken breast or turkey tenders—or cubed firm tofu, for a good vegetarian alternative. Just cook the chicken or turkey until it's cooked through before adding it to the sauce. Add the tofu after the tomatoes and oregano.

Nutrition Info

1 PORTION PROVIDES:

Protein: 1½ servings

Calcium: 1 serving

Vitamin C: 3 servings

Green leafy and yellow vegetables and fruits: 1 serving

Fat: ½ serving

Italian Shrimp and Broccoli

Okay, so maybe stir-fry isn't the first thing you think of when you think Italian—but maybe it should be. This super-simple, yet super-tasty, dish combines the best of two cuisines. And using a package of broccoli florets will make it superfast. Serve the shrimp over rice or pasta.

1⅓ cups low-sodium chicken broth or vegetable broth
1 teaspoon cornstarch
1 tablespoon olive oil
¾ pound shelled and deveined large shrimp
1 tablespoon minced garlic
2 cups broccoli florets
2 ripe plum tomatoes, seeded and chopped
3 tablespoons chopped fresh basil
3 tablespoons chopped fresh flat-leaf parsley
Juice of ½ lemon, plus lemon wedges for serving (optional)

Nutrition Info

1 PORTION PROVIDES:

Protein: 1½ servings

Vitamin C: 2½ servings

Green leafy and yellow vegetables and fruits: 2½ servings

Fat: ½ serving

1. Whisk ⅔ cup of the chicken broth with the cornstarch and set aside.

2. Heat 2 teaspoons of the olive oil in a large nonstick skillet over medium heat. Add the shrimp and 1½ teaspoons of the garlic and cook, stirring frequently, until the shrimp is cooked through and turns opaque, about 4 minutes. Transfer the shrimp to a large bowl and cover to keep warm.

3. Heat the remaining 1 teaspoon of olive oil in the skillet over medium heat. Add the remaining 1½ teaspoons of garlic and the broccoli and cook, stirring, until the broccoli is coated with the garlic, about 1 minute. Add the remaining ⅔ cup of chicken broth and let come to a boil, then cover the skillet, reduce the heat to low, and let simmer until the broccoli is crisp-tender, 3 to 4 minutes. Transfer the broccoli to the bowl with the shrimp.

4. Add the reserved broth and cornstarch mixture, the tomatoes, and 2 tablespoons each of the basil and parsley to the skillet. Increase the heat to medium-high and cook, stirring frequently, until the tomatoes soften, about 3 minutes. Add the cooked shrimp and broccoli and the lemon juice and cook, stirring, until heated through. Sprinkle the remaining 1 tablespoon each of the basil and parsley on top and serve immediately, with additional lemon wedges, if desired.

SERVES 2

FROM THE TEST KITCHEN

FOR AN EXTRA PUNCH of protein, serve the Italian Shrimp and Broccoli on a bed of Leek and Tomato Quinoa (see page 418).

Seared Sea Scallops on Succotash

Silken sea scallops love nothing more than a good bed, and crunchy succotash makes a beautiful bed.

½ pound sea scallops
2 teaspoons fresh lemon juice
2 teaspoons olive oil
¾ teaspoon minced fresh tarragon, or ¼ teaspoon dried tarragon
Edamame Succotash (page 412)
Zest of ½ lemon
½ teaspoon minced fresh dill
½ teaspoon minced fresh parsley
Salt and cracked black pepper

1. Place the scallops in a mixing bowl. Add the lemon juice, olive oil, and tarragon and stir to coat the scallops evenly. Let the scallops marinate in the refrigerator, covered, for up to 30 minutes.

2. Preheat the broiler or set up the grill and preheat it to high.

3. Broil or grill the scallops until they are just cooked through, springy to the touch, and have a golden brown edge, 2 to 3 minutes per side.

4. Toss the succotash with the lemon zest, dill, and parsley and divide it evenly between 2 serving plates. Season the cooked scallops lightly with salt and pepper. Divide the scallops between the plates and serve at once.

SERVES 2

Nutrition Info
1 PORTION (WITHOUT THE SUCCOTASH) PROVIDES:

Protein: 1 serving

Seared Scallops on White Beans and Kale

This Spanish-influenced dish marries delicate scallops with a robust ragout of beans, tomatoes, and greens. The result is hearty, satisfying, and speedy to prepare, thanks to the canned beans and tomatoes.

2 teaspoons olive oil
1 small onion, chopped
2 cloves garlic, minced
1 bay leaf
1 can (14½ ounces) of diced tomatoes, drained
2 cups chopped kale
1 cup drained navy or cannellini beans, rinsed

1 tablespoon chopped fresh flat-leaf parsley, plus more for garnish (optional)
Salt and black pepper
1 teaspoon butter
2 teaspoons fresh lemon juice, plus more for seasoning the beans (optional)
½ pound sea scallops

SPEEDY SALSA

▼ ▼ ▼

Looking for a way to dress up protein? Try any of these salsas on grilled fish, meat, or poultry:

■ Chopped seeded ripe tomato, kalamata olives, red onion, garlic, and lemon juice

■ Chopped tomatoes, fresh yellow peaches, fresh mint, balsamic vinegar, and olive oil

■ Chopped pineapple, red bell pepper, jalapeño pepper, and fresh cilantro

■ Chopped seeded ripe tomato, roasted corn, chopped roasted red bell pepper, red onion, fresh cilantro, and lime juice

■ Diced mango, yellow bell pepper, jalapeño pepper, cumin, lime juice, and olive oil

■ Black beans (rinsed and drained), chopped tomato, yellow bell pepper, cilantro, scallions, lime juice, and olive oil

1. Heat the olive oil in a large nonstick skillet over medium-low heat. Add the onion, garlic, and bay leaf and cook, stirring frequently, until the onion is softened and golden brown, about 10 minutes. Add the tomatoes and kale and cook, stirring frequently, until the vegetables soften, about 10 minutes. Add the beans and parsley, stir to mix, and season to taste with salt, pepper, and if desired, fresh lemon juice. Set the bean mixture aside, covered, to keep warm.

2. Preheat the broiler.

3. Melt the butter in a small saucepan over low heat. Stir in the 2 teaspoons of lemon juice. Place the scallops in a broiling pan and brush the tops with half of the lemon butter. Broil the scallops close to the heat until browned, 2 to 3 minutes. Turn the scallops and brush them with the remaining lemon butter. Broil the second side until the scallops are just cooked through and springy to the touch, 2 to 3 minutes.

4. Divide the bean mixture between 2 serving plates. Lightly season the scallops with salt and pepper then arrange them on top of the beans. Sprinkle additional chopped parsley on top, if desired.

SERVES 2

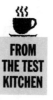

FROM THE TEST KITCHEN **MAKE THE WHITE BEANS** again (or cook extra), and just about any roast or grilled fish (halibut, salmon, sea bass), seafood (shrimp, calamari), poultry (chicken, turkey), or meat (pork, beef, lamb) will be tasty served on top.

Nutrition Info
1 PORTION PROVIDES:

Protein: 1½ servings

Vitamin C: 1½ servings

Green leafy and yellow vegetables and fruits: 1 serving

Other fruits and vegetables: ½ serving

Whole grains and legumes: 1 serving

Iron: from the beans

Fat: ½ serving

Vegetables and Other Sides

Have side dishes become . . . well, beside the point? Wondering how you can keep things interesting when it comes to vegetables and other sides? Luckily, these recipes are here to rescue you from the side dish doldrums. Using a variety of fresh vegetables, tangy herbs, pungent spices, chewy grains, and savory beans, these unusually tempting dishes will fill your veggie and grain requirements while adding terrific taste and texture to your meals. Since the idea is to use these side dishes to your dietary advantage, nutritional superstars (those vibrant yellows, greens, and whole grains) lead the pack, while veggies and grains that pale (literally) by comparison take a back seat. With recipes like Lemon Carrots with Rosemary, Balsamic Braised Red Cabbage, Green Mashers, Barley Risotto with Wild Mushrooms, Leek and Tomato Quinoa, and Edamame Succotash, you'll discover plenty of ways to make side dishes stellar, or even the main attraction.

Asparagus and Parmesan Curls

Serve this asparagus alongside a fish, chicken, or meat dish or as an elegant start to any meal.

½ pound asparagus stalks
2 teaspoons olive oil
Juice and zest of ½ lemon
Salt and black pepper
¼ cup Parmesan or
    provolone cheese shavings
    (about 1 ounce, see page 317)

1. Trim off and discard the tough stem ends of the asparagus stalks.

2. Steam the asparagus following the instructions below until just tender, 4 to 8 minutes, depending on the thickness of the asparagus.

3. Pat the asparagus dry and divide it evenly between 2 serving plates. Drizzle the olive oil and lemon juice over the asparagus and top it with the lemon zest. Season the asparagus with salt and pepper to taste, then top it with the cheese shavings.

SERVES 2

STEAMING SAVVY

▼ ▼ ▼

When it comes to vegetables, steaming beats boiling hands down. First, it retains far more nutrients. When you boil vegetables, the nutrients end up in the cooking water; that's fine if you're going to drink the cooking water—as in a soup—but not so fine if you'll be pouring the water down the drain. Second, steaming eliminates two steps: there's no waiting for a big pot of water to boil; no draining afterwards. Third, and possibly most important, steaming preserves flavor and texture.

If those aren't enough reasons to switch to steaming, here's one more: It couldn't be easier. Just pour water to a depth of 1 inch into a large pot with a tight-fitting cover and bring it to a boil. Add the steamer basket and the veggies (season them now if you won't later). Cover the pot and steam the vegetables over boiling water until they are just tender. Serve them as is with just a squeeze of lemon or toss them into any recipe that calls for cooked veggies. (Steaming is also an easy way to cook shrimp.)

STEAM TWICE AS MUCH asparagus as you want to serve, then chill the leftovers for the next day's salad. It's delicious tossed with a little lemon vinaigrette, as in Broccoli Vinaigrette, below. Like a green leafy option? Substitute broccoli or broccoli rabe for the asparagus.

Nutrition Info
1 PORTION PROVIDES:

Calcium: 1/2 serving

Vitamin C: 1 serving

Broccoli Vinaigrette

As much a salad as a veggie side, this delicious hybrid tops steamed broccoli with a vinaigrette made aromatic with herbs and shallots. Coarsely chopped nuts add a crunchy crowning touch. The broccoli is delicious the next day, too.

3 cups broccoli florets

2 shallots, minced

2 tablespoons fresh lemon juice, or more to taste

2 tablespoons extra-virgin olive oil

2 teaspoons chopped fresh tarragon

2 teaspoons chopped fresh chives

Salt and black pepper

1/4 cup coarsely chopped toasted pistachios or walnuts (see page 272)

1. Steam the broccoli following the instructions on page 391 until crisp-tender, 4 to 5 minutes. Place the broccoli in a large bowl.

2. Place the shallots, lemon juice, olive oil, tarragon, and chives in a small bowl and whisk to mix, then season with salt and pepper to taste. Pour the herb mixture over the broccoli and toss well to coat. Sprinkle the pistachios over the broccoli just before serving.

SERVES 4

Nutrition Info
1 PORTION PROVIDES:

Vitamin C: 1 serving

Green leafy and yellow vegetables and fruits: 1 1/2 servings

Fat: 1/2 serving

Broccoli and Tofu Stir-Fry

Y ou don't have to be a vegetarian to enjoy this nutritious Chinese favorite. It makes a tasty meatless meal, particularly when it's teamed with brown rice or *soba* noodles.

¾ cup plus 2 tablespoons vegetable
   broth
2 tablespoons low-sodium soy sauce
2½ teaspoons cornstarch
2 teaspoons unseasoned rice vinegar
2 teaspoons sesame oil
1 tablespoon canola oil
8 ounces extra-firm tofu, drained well
   on paper towels and cut into
   ½-inch cubes
Pinch of salt
2 cups broccoli florets
2 teaspoons minced garlic
1 tablespoon grated fresh ginger
   (optional)
1 cup sliced shiitake mushrooms
Crushed red pepper flakes (optional)

1. Place 2 tablespoons of the vegetable broth and the soy sauce, cornstarch, rice vinegar, and sesame oil in a small bowl and whisk to mix. Set the soy sauce mixture aside.

2. Heat the canola oil in a large nonstick skillet over medium heat. Add the tofu and salt. Cook, stirring frequently, until the tofu is golden brown all over, about 8 minutes. Remove the tofu from the skillet.

3. Add the broccoli, the remaining ¾ cup of broth, the garlic, and the ginger, if using, to the skillet. Cover and cook, stirring occasionally, until the broccoli is crisp-tender, about 4 minutes. Uncover the skillet, add the mushrooms and cook until softened, about 2 minutes. Add the soy sauce mixture and browned tofu to the broccoli and stir gently to coat. Season with red pepper flakes to taste, if desired. Cook, stirring occasionally, until the sauce thickens, about 2 minutes.

SERVES 2

Nutrition Info
1 PORTION PROVIDES:

Protein: ½ serving

Vitamin C: 2 servings

Green leafy and yellow vegetables and fruits: 2 servings

Other fruits and vegetables: 1 serving

Fat: 1 serving

Curried Broccoli and Tofu

From grains to green vegetables to vitamin C, this is actually a tasty one-dish meal that covers almost all of your Daily Dozen bases. Although it has a long ingredients list, it's easy to prepare and you can make it as mild or as spicy as you like.

1 package (14 ounces) extra-firm tofu
1 tablespoon sesame oil
1 medium-size red bell pepper, sliced
1 small red onion, halved and thinly
    sliced
2 teaspoons grated peeled fresh
    ginger
1 teaspoon curry powder
1 teaspoon ground coriander
1 teaspoon ground turmeric
1½ cups steamed small broccoli florets
    (see page 391)
1 can (14½ ounces) diced tomatoes
    (with their juices)
2 tablespoons vegetable broth,
    or more as needed
1 tablespoon low-sodium soy sauce
1 tablespoon white grape juice
    concentrate, Splenda, brown sugar,
    or honey
1 teaspoon chile-garlic sauce,
    or more to taste (optional; see Note)
Salt and black pepper
3 tablespoons chopped fresh cilantro
2 tablespoons chopped toasted
    cashews (see page 272)
1 cup cooked brown rice

1. Cut the tofu into roughly ½-inch cubes and place them in a single layer between paper towels to drain.

2. Heat the sesame oil in a large nonstick skillet over medium heat. Add the bell pepper and onion and cook until softened, about 5 minutes.

3. Reduce the heat to low, add the ginger, curry powder, coriander, and turmeric and cook, stirring frequently, until fragrant, about 2 minutes.

Nutrition Info

1 PORTION PROVIDES:

Protein: 1 serving

Calcium: ½ serving

Vitamin C: 4½ servings

Green leafy and yellow vegetables and
    fruits: 2½ servings

Other fruits and vegetables: 1 serving

Whole grains and legumes: 1 serving

Iron from the tofu

Fat: ½ serving

4. Add the drained tofu and the broccoli, tomatoes, vegetable broth, soy sauce, grape juice concentrate, and chile-garlic sauce. Increase the heat and let come to a boil. Reduce the heat and let simmer, covered, stirring occasionally, until the flavors blend, about 10 minutes. Add more vegetable broth if the mixture becomes too dry.

5. Taste for seasoning, adding more chile-garlic sauce as necessary, and salt and pepper to taste. Sprinkle the cilantro and cashews on top, and serve with hot brown rice.

SERVES 2

NOTE: Chile-garlic sauce is available in the Asian food section of the supermarket.

Roast Butternut Squash

Because squash is starchy, it can soothe an upset tummy. Packed with vitamin A, it will help fill your requirement for yellow vegetables. Enjoy leftovers the following day.

Olive oil cooking spray
1 medium-size butternut squash,
   peeled and cubed
1 tablespoon olive oil
1 tablespoon fresh thyme leaves,
   or 1 teaspoon dried thyme
1/2 cup grated Parmesan cheese

1. Preheat the oven to 400°F.

2. Coat a 9-by-13-inch baking dish with olive oil cooking spray, then add the squash. Drizzle the olive oil over the squash, sprinkle the thyme on top, and toss gently to coat evenly.

3. Bake the squash until tender and golden brown, about 25 minutes. Sprinkle the Parmesan cheese over the squash before serving.

SERVES 4

Nutrition Info

1 PORTION PROVIDES:

Calcium: 1/2 serving

Green leafy and yellow vegetables and
   fruits: 2 servings

Fat: 1/2 serving

Brussels Sprouts and Figs

No bitter brussels sprouts these. Figs lend a sweet taste, intriguing texture, and additional minerals to this much maligned vegetable. The result is an unlikely combination that you're likely to love.

1 teaspoon butter
2 small shallots, minced
1 cup apple cider
1 cup low-sodium chicken broth or
    vegetable broth
1½ cups small brussels sprouts
    (choose small ones), trimmed and
    tough outside leaves removed
    (you can also use frozen)
6 dried figs, cut in half
Salt and freshly ground black pepper

1. Melt the butter in a medium-size non-stick saucepan over low heat. Add the shallots and cook, stirring frequently, until softened and golden, about 2 minutes.

2. Add the cider and chicken broth to the pan, increase the heat slightly, and let come to a simmer. Add the brussels sprouts and figs, cover the pan, and let simmer, stirring occasionally, until just tender, 7 to 10 minutes (the larger the brussels sprouts, the longer this will take).

3. Using a slotted spoon, remove the brussels sprouts and figs from the cider mixture and set aside. Increase the heat to medium-high and cook until the liquid is reduced to about ¼ cup, 3 to 5 minutes.

4. Toss the figs and brussels sprouts with the reduced cider mixture, season them with salt and pepper to taste, and serve warm.

SERVES 2

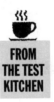

FROM THE TEST KITCHEN

DON'T LIKE your brussels sprouts quite so sweet? Add a squeeze or two of lemon juice before serving.

Nutrition Info
1 PORTION PROVIDES:

Vitamin C: 1½ servings

Other fruits and vegetables: 2 servings

Balsamic Braised Red Cabbage

Braising red cabbage in balsamic vinegar helps preserve its color and infuses it with a delectably sweet and complex flavor. Fresh and dried cranberries contribute to the color scheme, as well as to the nutritional content and tangy taste. Team this traditional holiday favorite with the Christmas goose, the Thanksgiving turkey—or Tuesday night's pork chop.

4 cups sliced red cabbage
2 cups vegetable broth or low-sodium
　　chicken broth
¼ cup balsamic vinegar
¼ cup white grape juice concentrate,
　　Splenda, honey, or brown sugar
1 cup fresh cranberries
⅓ cup dried cranberries

1. Preheat the oven to 400°F.

2. Place the cabbage, vegetable broth, balsamic vinegar, grape juice concentrate, and fresh and dried cranberries in a large mixing bowl and stir to mix. Transfer the cabbage mixture to a flameproof baking dish. Let the mixture come to a boil over medium heat, then cover the baking dish with aluminum foil.

3. Bake the cabbage mixture until tender, about 45 minutes. Serve the cabbage warm or at room temperature. The cabbage can be refrigerated, covered, for 2 days.

SERVES 4

FROM THE TEST KITCHEN

DON'T HAVE AN HOUR to spare? Simply place all of the ingredients for Balsamic Braised Red Cabbage in a large saucepan over medium heat and bring them to a simmer. Cover the pan and let the cabbage cook until it is tender, about 10 minutes. Another tip: Make this dish up to two days in advance—the flavors will deepen. Warm the braised cabbage before serving, or just let it return to room temperature.

Nutrition Info
1 PORTION PROVIDES:

Vitamin C: 1 serving

Other fruits and vegetables: 1 serving

Lemon Carrots with Rosemary

Baby carrots with a twist of lemon and a sprinkling of aromatic rosemary make a classic companion to roast chicken or store-bought rotisserie. They're also delish with fish.

2 teaspoons olive oil
1½ cups baby carrots
¼ cup low-sodium chicken broth
   or vegetable broth
1 clove garlic, minced
2 teaspoons fresh chopped rosemary,
   or ½ teaspoon dried rosemary
1 teaspoon grated lemon zest
Salt and black pepper
Fresh lemon juice

1. Heat 1 teaspoon of the olive oil in a large nonstick skillet over medium heat. Add the carrots and cook until beginning to soften, about 2 minutes. Stir in the broth and let come to a boil. Reduce the heat, cover the skillet, and let the carrots simmer until they are tender, about 10 minutes. Transfer the carrots to a bowl and set aside, covered, to keep warm.

2. Heat the remaining 1 teaspoon of olive oil in the same skillet over medium heat. Add the garlic and cook until beginning

to soften, about 1 minute. Add the rosemary and lemon zest and the cooked carrots and stir to coat.

3. Remove the carrots from the heat. Season them with salt, pepper, and lemon juice to taste and serve.

SERVES 2

FROM THE TEST KITCHEN

USING THYME LEAVES in the Lemon Carrots in place of the rosemary make them a perfect partner for poultry. Feeling fishy? Substitute 2 teaspoons of chopped fresh dill or ½ teaspoon of dried dill.

Nutrition Info

1 PORTION PROVIDES:

Green leafy and yellow vegetables and fruits: 3 servings

Glazed Carrots and Pineapple

Baby carrots are giants among vegetables when it comes to vitamin A. In this recipe, pineapple and ginger enhance the carrots' natural sweetness. Use the packaged peeled baby carrots found in the produce section, and they'll be ready in less than ten minutes. The recipe is easy to cut in half, if you prefer.

1 package (16 ounces) peeled baby carrots (about 2½ cups)
1 cup vegetable broth
3 to 4 tablespoons pineapple juice concentrate (use the larger amount for very sweet carrots)
1 tablespoon minced peeled fresh ginger
½ teaspoon ground cinnamon
½ teaspoon ground cumin
½ teaspoon cumin seeds
4 scallions, both white and light green parts, trimmed and thinly sliced

Place the carrots, vegetable broth, pineapple juice concentrate, ginger, cinnamon, ground cumin, and cumin seeds in a saucepan over medium-low heat, and let come to a simmer. Cook the carrots until just tender, 8 to 10 minutes. Toss the carrots with the scallions and serve warm or at room temperature. Leftover carrots can be refrigerated, covered, for up to 2 days.

SERVES 4

FROM THE TEST KITCHEN

CARROTS AND PINEAPPLE are pals from way back. Reunite them by tossing ¾ cup of drained crushed pineapple into the pot before cooking.

Nutrition Info

1 PORTION PROVIDES:

Vitamin C: ½ serving

Green leafy and yellow vegetables and fruits: 2½ servings

Minty Medley

The unexpected addition of mint and shiitake mushrooms to peas and carrots gives you a deliciously sophisticated take on the standard school cafeteria variety. You'll eat every carrot and pea on your plate when they're cooked this way. (Make it faster still by using frozen peas and carrots.)

¾ cup shelled fresh green peas,
   or ¾ cup frozen peas
½ cup thinly sliced carrots
1 tablespoon olive oil or butter
1 cup sliced shiitake mushrooms
1 shallot, minced
1 tablespoon chopped fresh mint
Salt and black pepper

1. Cook the peas and carrots separately until crisp-tender, following the steaming instructions on page 391 or the microwave oven instructions on the facing page, about 2 minutes for steamed peas or 1½ minutes in the microwave and 3 minutes for steamed carrots or 2½ minutes in the microwave.

2. Heat the olive oil in a saucepan over medium heat. Add the mushrooms and shallot and cook until beginning to soften, about 2 minutes. Add the cooked peas and carrots and the mint and stir gently until heated through. Remove the vegetable mixture from the heat and season with salt and pepper to taste.

SERVES 2

Nutrition Info

1 PORTION PROVIDES:

Vitamin C: ½ serving

Green leafy and yellow vegetables and
   fruits: 1 serving

Other fruits and vegetables: 1 serving

Fat: ½ serving

VEGETABLES IN A FLASH

▼ ▼ ▼

You can't beat steaming when it comes to retaining the nutrients found in vegetables, but you can beat the clock by using a microwave and bringing freshly cooked vegetables to the table in four minutes or less. When you need to save even more time, choose packaged vegetables that have already been rinsed, peeled and sliced, diced, or chopped. (You won't net as many nutrients as you would with freshly prepared produce, but you'll still get plenty.) Be sure to check the use-by dates carefully so you don't end up with expired carrots by the time you get around to zapping them. And keep in mind that not all vegetables microwave well (green beans, asparagus, and artichokes don't) but most do.

When you're ready to make microwave magic, arrange the vegetables in a single layer in a microwave-safe dish. Make sure the pieces are uniform in size. Add two tablespoons of vegetable or chicken broth (more for larger amounts of vegetables, but in general, keep the liquid to a minimum—that's where all the nutrients will end up). Season the vegetables with herbs (fresh or dried), a little salt and pepper, and a splash of lemon juice, if you like. Certain vegetables (think cauliflower or broccoli) can benefit from a handful or two of diced fresh or canned tomatoes. Tent the dish with microwave-safe plastic wrap leaving a small portion uncovered to vent the steam. Don't let the plastic wrap touch the vegetables. Microwave the vegetables on high until just tender, $1\frac{1}{2}$ to 4 minutes, depending on the thickness and how crisp you like them (larger amounts of vegetables may need longer cooking times). Let the vegetables stand for 3 to 5 minutes before serving.

Cauliflower and Cheese

Even the most resolute vegetable shunner will fancy this homey dish of cauliflower topped with a creamy cheese sauce that's packed with calcium and flavor.

1 head cauliflower, rinsed,
    patted dry, and cut into florets
    (about 2 cups)
1 cup milk
2 teaspoons cornstarch
1 cup grated cheddar cheese or
    Gruyère cheese, grated
Salt and white pepper

1. Steam the cauliflower following the instructions on page 391 until fork tender, 5 to 6 minutes. Set aside, covered, to keep warm.

2. Place the milk and cornstarch in a small saucepan and stir until the cornstarch dissolves. Bring the milk mixture to a boil over medium-high heat, then reduce the heat and let simmer until the mixture thickens, about 4 minutes.

3. Remove the saucepan from the heat; add the cheddar cheese and stir until it melts. Season the cheese sauce with salt and pepper to taste, then pour the sauce over the steamed cauliflower.

SERVES 4

FROM THE TEST KITCHEN

SAY CHEESE TWO WAYS: You can use a combination of Parmesan and cheddar in the sauce for the cauliflower. And because broccoli loves cheese, too, try this cheese sauce on steamed broccoli. Or make a combo of broccoli and cauliflower.

Nutrition Info
1 PORTION PROVIDES:
Calcium: 1 serving
Vitamin C: 1 serving

That's Italian Green Beans

Any green vegetables take a turn for the Tuscan when prepared with tomatoes, Italian herbs, and Parmesan cheese. Steamed broccoli is also good prepared this way. Add extra cheese on top for a calcium fix.

½ pound green beans, trimmed
½ cup canned Italian seasoned
    diced tomatoes
1½ teaspoons minced fresh oregano or
    basil, or ½ teaspoon dried oregano
    or basil
2 tablespoons grated Parmesan
    cheese
Pinch of crushed red pepper flakes
    (optional)

1. Steam the green beans following the instructions on page 391 until just tender but still crisp, 4 to 5 minutes.

2. Transfer the green beans to a saucepan, add the tomatoes, oregano, Parmesan cheese, and red pepper flakes, if using, and stir to mix. Cook over medium heat until heated through, about 1 minute.

SERVES 2

Nutrition Info

1 PORTION PROVIDES:

Vitamin C: ½ serving

Other fruits and vegetables: 1 serving

Spicy Greens with Ginger Dressing

The greens will be wilted, but the flavor will be lively. Add a dash of crushed red pepper flakes if you'd like it livelier still.

3 tablespoons seasoned rice
 vinegar
1 tablespoon light soy sauce
1 tablespoon sesame oil
2 teaspoons minced peeled fresh
 ginger
2 tablespoons chopped fresh cilantro
 (optional)
3 scallions, both white and
 light green parts, trimmed
 and sliced
1 package (5 ounces) Asian salad mix
 (see Note) or baby spinach
1 tablespoon toasted sesame seeds
 (see page 272)

1. Place the rice vinegar, soy sauce, sesame oil, and ginger in a small saucepan over low heat and cook, stirring, until hot, but not boiling, about 3 minutes. Stir in the cilantro, if using.

2. Place the scallions and the salad mix in a bowl and toss to mix. Pour the hot dressing over the greens, sprinkle the sesame seeds on top, and toss well. Serve immediately.

SERVES 2

NOTE: Asian salad mix is a spicy combination of such greens as spinach, mizuna, chard, and red mustard. Packages are available in supermarket produce sections.

Nutrition Info

1 PORTION PROVIDES:

Vitamin C: 1 serving

Green leafy and yellow vegetables and
 fruits: 3 servings

Iron: from the spinach

Fat: 1/2 serving

Kale and Shiitake Mushroom Salad

I s it a salad, or is it a stir-fry? Don't label it—just enjoy it, along with a day's worth of green and yellow vegetables and a bonus of soy protein.

1 small bunch kale, stems and tough
   center veins removed, rinsed well
2 tablespoons vegetable broth
1 tablespoon low-sodium
   soy sauce
1 tablespoon sesame oil
1 cup frozen shelled edamame
   (soybeans)
1¾ cups sliced shiitake mushrooms
¼ cup shredded carrots
2 tablespoons seasoned rice vinegar
2 teaspoons olive oil or canola oil
1 tablespoon toasted sesame seeds
   (see page 272)

1. Cut the kale into ½-inch strips.

2. Place the vegetable broth, soy sauce, and sesame oil in a large skillet over medium-low heat and let come to a simmer. Add the kale and edamame and toss to coat. Cover the skillet and cook just until the kale begins to wilt, 2 to 3 minutes. Transfer the vegetables to a salad bowl.

3. Add the shiitake mushrooms and carrots to the skillet and cook until just tender, 2 to 3 minutes. Add the mushroom mixture to the kale mixture and let come to room temperature.

4. Place the rice vinegar and olive oil in a small bowl and whisk to mix. Just before serving, toss the kale mixture with the dressing and sprinkle the sesame seeds on top.

SERVES 2

Nutrition Info

1 PORTION PROVIDES:

Protein: ½ serving

Calcium: 1 serving

Vitamin C: 1 serving

Green leafy and yellow vegetables and fruits: 3 servings

Other fruits and vegetables: 1½ servings

Whole grains and legumes: 1 serving

Fat: 1 serving

Oven-Roasted Cottage Potatoes

You don't need a trip through the golden arches when these golden but nearly greaseless potatoes are just twenty-five minutes from your plate.

Olive oil cooking spray

2 medium-size Yukon Gold red potatoes
   (about ¾ pound)

1 tablespoon olive oil

Salt and cracked black pepper

1. Preheat the oven to 425°F. Coat a large rimmed baking sheet with olive oil cooking spray.

2. Cut the potatoes into ¼-inch-thick slices, then pat them dry with paper towels. Place the potatoes in a bowl, drizzle the olive oil over them, then toss to coat evenly.

3. Arrange the potatoes on the baking sheet in a single layer and lightly season them with salt and cracked pepper.

4. Bake the potatoes until golden brown on top, about 15 minutes. Turn the potatoes over and continue baking until the second side is golden brown and the potatoes are tender, 10 to 15 minutes longer. If you like crisper potatoes, let them bake a little longer but watch them carefully so they don't burn.

SERVES 2

FROM THE TEST KITCHEN

FRIES WITH THAT? Cut the potatoes into thick french fry–shaped slivers. Toss them with olive oil, then place them in a single layer on a rimmed baking sheet that has been coated with cooking oil spray. Roast the potatoes in an oven preheated to 400°F for 15 minutes. Stir the potatoes to turn and continue roasting for another 10 minutes. For extra-crisp potatoes, stir them every 5 minutes. You can shake things up a bit by sprinkling some grated Parmesan cheese, garlic powder, or chili powder over them—or whatever flavor you fancy.

Nutrition Info

1 PORTION PROVIDES:

Vitamin C: 1 serving

Fat: ¹⁄₂ serving

Green Mashers

Festive on St. Patrick's Day, but so delicious you'll want to serve them all year round, the green—and a healthy dose, of protein—comes from the edamame the potatoes are mashed with.

1 cup frozen shelled edamame (soybeans)
2 small Yukon Gold potatoes,
    cut into 1-inch chunks
About 1 can (14½ ounces) low-sodium
    chicken broth or vegetable broth
⅓ cup milk or buttermilk,
    or more as needed
2 teaspoons olive oil (optional)
¼ cup grated Parmesan cheese
    (optional), or more to taste
Salt and black pepper

1. Let a saucepan of water come to a boil over high heat, add the edamame, and let return to a boil. Reduce the heat to medium and cook the edamame until very soft, about 12 minutes. Drain and set aside.

2. Place the potatoes and enough broth to cover them in a small saucepan. Let come to a boil over high heat, then reduce the heat and let simmer until the potatoes are tender, 10 to 15 minutes. Drain, reserving the cooking liquid.

3. Place the milk in a small microwave-safe bowl and microwave at medium-high-power until heated through, about 45 seconds.

MICROBAKED POTATOES

▼ ▼ ▼

Craving the creamy comfort of a baked potato without the wait? Skip the baking and head for the microwave instead. To microbake a potato, poke several small slits into the skin, then wrap the potato in a microwave-safe paper towel. Microwave on high power 7 minutes for one large baking potato or sweet potato, or 12 minutes for two (wrap each individually). One small potato will be ready in 5 minutes; two will be done in 7 minutes. To check for doneness, if a fork can pierce the flesh easily, it's ready. If it's not done, microwave it for another minute and try again.

4. Place the cooked edamame and a few tablespoons of the reserved potato cooking liquid in a food processor and process until smooth, then transfer to a bowl. Add the cooked potatoes, warm milk, and olive oil and Parmesan cheese, if using. Using a potato masher, mash to the desired consistency, adding more cooking liquid or milk as needed. Season with salt and pepper to taste and serve immediately.

SERVES 2

Nutrition Info
1 PORTION PROVIDES:

Protein: 1/2 serving

Calcium: 1/2 serving if made with Parmesan cheese

Vitamin C: 11/2 servings

Whole grains and legumes: 1 serving

Roasted Herbed Sweet Potatoes

Pop sweet potatoes in the oven when you're roasting poultry or meat, then pop the fragrant, golden brown wedges in your mouth anytime.

Olive oil cooking spray
1 medium-size sweet potato
 (about 1/2 pound), unpeeled
1 tablespoon olive oil
1 tablespoon chopped fresh rosemary,
 or 1 teaspoon dried rosemary
1 tablespoon chopped fresh oregano,
 or 1 teaspoon dried oregano
Dash of ground nutmeg
Dash of ground cumin
Salt and black pepper

1. Preheat the oven to 425°F. Coat a small baking dish with olive oil cooking spray.

2. Cut the sweet potatoes in half lengthwise. Cut each half into 6 wedges.

3. Place the sweet potatoes, olive oil, rosemary, oregano, nutmeg, cumin, and a sprinkle each of salt and pepper in a large bowl, and toss gently to coat evenly.

4. Place the sweet potato wedges in the baking dish and bake, uncovered, until tender and golden brown, about 45 minutes, gently stirring them halfway through.

SERVES 2

Nutrition Info
1 PORTION PROVIDES:

Vitamin C: 1/2 serving

Green leafy and yellow vegetables and fruits: 1 serving

Fat: 1/2 serving

Sweet Potato Chips

Bet you can't stop at just one Sweet Potato Chip—and there's no good reason why you should. You can get a chip fix and a hefty dose of vitamin A in the bargain.

Olive oil cooking spray
1 medium-size sweet potato
  (about 1/2 pound)
1 tablespoon olive oil
2 tablespoons grated Parmesan
  cheese
1 teaspoon chopped fresh rosemary
  or thyme
Salt and black pepper (optional)

1. Preheat the oven to 425°F. Coat a large rimmed baking sheet with olive oil cooking spray.

2. Peel the sweet potato, then cut into 1/4-inch-thick slices. Pat the slices dry with paper towels. Arrange the sweet potatoes on the baking sheet in a single layer and brush the tops with the olive oil.

3. Bake the sweet potatoes until the tops brown slightly, about 15 minutes. Turn the sweet potatoes over and continue baking until the second side is lightly browned and the potatoes are tender, 10 to 15 minutes longer. If you like crisper sweet potatoes, let them bake a little longer but watch them carefully so they don't burn.

4. Sprinkle the Parmesan cheese, chopped herbs, and salt and pepper, if desired, over the sweet potatoes before serving.

SERVES 2

Nutrition Info
1 PORTION PROVIDES:

Vitamin C: 1/2 serving

Green leafy and yellow vegetables and
  fruits: 1 serving

Fat: 1/2 serving

Italian Swiss Chard

This tasty sauté brings out the best in sturdy green leafy vegetables; try it with kale, too.

1 bunch Swiss chard, rinsed and
   patted dry
¾ cup chicken broth or vegetable
   broth
2 teaspoons olive oil
1 clove garlic, minced
1 shallot, minced
¼ cup grated Parmesan cheese
2 tablespoons toasted pine nuts
   (see page 272)
Salt and black pepper

1. Slice the leaves off the stems of the Swiss chard, then coarsely chop the leaves, and cut the stems crosswise into pieces that are about ½ inch wide and 2 inches long.

2. Place the chicken broth in a small saucepan and let come to a simmer over medium heat. Add the Swiss chard stems, reduce the heat to low, and cook until just tender, 8 to 10 minutes. Drain and set aside.

3. Heat the olive oil in a large nonstick skillet over medium-low heat. Add the garlic and shallot and cook, stirring occasionally, until softened, about 2 minutes. Add the Swiss chard leaves and the boiled stems and cook, stirring, until the leaves are just wilted, 1 to 2 minutes.

GREAT GREENS

▼ ▼ ▼

Many greens that you're used to eating raw in salads wilt well—tastily. And, since the greens cook down, you can pack far more vitamin power into an average portion. Try arugula or baby spinach wilted, following this recipe for Italian Swiss Chard, starting with Step 3, since these do not have tough stems. Tender greens like these wilt in no time. Serve wilted greens as a side dish or as a delicious bed for fish or chicken.

4. Add the Parmesan cheese and pine nuts to the Swiss chard and stir to mix. Season with salt and pepper to taste.

SERVES 2

Nutrition Info
1 PORTION PROVIDES:

Calcium: ½ serving

Vitamin C: ½ serving

Green leafy and yellow vegetables and
   fruits: 2 servings

Pan-Roasted Vegetables

The taste of autumn can come to your table any time of year. You'll love the way roasting brings out the best in vegetables, especially roots.

Olive oil cooking spray
4 medium-size red potatoes, halved,
    or 1 medium-size sweet potatoes,
    quartered
4 medium-size parsnips, peeled
4 medium-size carrots, peeled
1 small rutabaga (about 1/2 pound),
    peeled and cut into 1-inch chunks
1 large fennel bulb, trimmed and quartered
2 tablespoons olive oil
1 tablespoon fresh thyme leaves,
    or 1 teaspoon dried thyme
Salt and freshly ground black pepper
Zest of 1 lemon (optional)

1. Preheat the oven to 425°F. Coat a roasting pan with olive oil cooking spray.

2. Arrange the potatoes, parsnips, carrots, rutabaga, and fennel in a single layer in the roasting pan. Brush the vegetables with the olive oil and sprinkle the thyme over them. Season the vegetables with salt and pepper. Cover the roasting pan with aluminum foil.

3. Bake the vegetables until beginning to soften, about 25 minutes. Uncover the pan, stir the vegetables, and bake them, uncovered, until tender and golden brown, about 20 minutes longer.

4. Place the vegetables on a platter and sprinkle the lemon zest, if using, over

them. The vegetables can be refrigerated, covered, for up to 2 days. Reheat at 350°F until hot, about 10 minutes.

SERVES 4

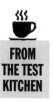

FROM THE TEST KITCHEN ROASTING BRINGS OUT the best flavor in just about every vegetable. You can use any of the following in place of, or in addition to, those in Pan-Roasted Vegetables: chunks of red onion, turnips, celery root, whole pearl onions, whole garlic cloves, whole baby beets, acorn squash, and/or butternut squash. Just be sure that they are roughly the same size or cut to comparable-size pieces.

And don't stop there. Roast cauliflower with cumin seeds, green beans with oregano, tomatoes with basil, and just about any vegetable with rosemary or sage.

Nutrition Info
1 PORTION PROVIDES:

Vitamin C: 1/2 serving

Green leafy and yellow vegetables and fruits: 2 servings if made with red potatoes; 21/2 if made with sweet potatoes

Other fruits and vegetables: 2 servings

Fat: 1/2 serving

Edamame Succotash

A far cry from the mushy, mostly nutritionless cafeteria variety, this succotash, made with crisp asparagus, bright red bell pepper, sweet corn, and chewy edamame is fresh tasting and packed with protein. Terrific, too, as a bed for fish fillets or chicken breasts.

1 tablespoon olive oil
1/2 cup chopped red bell pepper
1 cup vegetable broth
12 asparagus stalks, trimmed and
   cut into 1/2-inch chunks
1 cup shelled frozen edamame (soybeans)
1 cup yellow corn kernels
   (fresh or frozen)
2 tablespoons chopped fresh flat-leaf
   parsley
Salt and cracked black pepper

Heat the olive oil in a medium-size nonstick skillet over low heat. Add the bell pepper and cook until it begins to soften, about 3 minutes. Add the vegetable broth, raise the heat to medium, and let come to a simmer. Add the asparagus, edamame, corn, and parsley, cover the skillet, reduce the heat to low, and let simmer until just tender, about 4 minutes. Season the succotash with salt and cracked pepper to taste before serving.

SERVES 4

Nutrition Info

1 PORTION PROVIDES:

Protein: 1/2 serving

Vitamin C: 1 serving

Green leafy and yellow vegetables and fruits: 1 serving

Whole grains and legumes: 1/2 serving

Other vegetables and fruits: 1/2 serving

Fat: 1/2 serving

Grilled Tofu

Extra-firm tofu takes on an almost meaty texture when it's grilled, making this dish a great vegetarian alternative when you feel like passing on the sirloin. It's more like a meal than a side dish, especially when served over Spicy Greens with Ginger Dressing (see page 404) or in a sandwich.

1 package (14 ounces) extra-firm tofu, drained well on paper towels
¼ cup low-sodium soy sauce or tamari sauce
2 teaspoons sesame oil
1 teaspoon canola oil
1 tablespoon white grape juice concentrate, Splenda, honey, or brown sugar
2 teaspoons minced garlic (optional)
1 teaspoon chile-garlic sauce (see Note), or more to taste (optional)

1. Cut the tofu crosswise into 8 even slices. Place the tofu slices in a baking dish large enough to hold all of them in a single layer.

2. Place the soy sauce, sesame oil, canola oil, grape juice concentrate, and the garlic, and chile-garlic sauce, if using, in a small bowl and stir to mix. Taste for seasoning, adding more chile-garlic sauce if necessary. Pour the marinade over the tofu slices and let marinate in the refrigerator, covered, for 10 minutes, turning the tofu several times.

3. Meanwhile, set up the grill and preheat it to medium-high.

4. When ready to cook, oil the grill grate. Remove the tofu from the marinade and set the marinade aside. Grill the tofu until it's heated through and starts to brown, 3 to 4 minutes per side. As the tofu grills, brush it with the reserved marinade.

SERVES 2

NOTE: Chile-garlic sauce is available in the Asian food section of the supermarket.

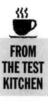

FROM THE TEST KITCHEN

FOR A DELICIOUS nutty taste and crunch, try sprinkling the marinated tofu with sesame seeds before grilling it.

Nutrition Info

1 PORTION PROVIDES:

Protein: 1 serving

Calcium: ½ serving

Vitamin C: 1 serving

Iron from the tofu

Fat: ½ serving

Stove-Top Brown Rice Pilaf

A sweet twist on traditional pilaf, this one, made with brown rice, may be particularly comforting when your morning sickness lasts through the dinner hour.

1 cup brown rice
3 cups vegetable broth, or more as needed
1/2 cup white grape juice concentrate
    or apple juice concentrate
1/2 teaspoon ground cinnamon
1/2 teaspoon ground cumin
1/2 cup raisins or chopped dried apricots
1/4 cup chopped toasted walnuts
    (see page 272)

1. Place the brown rice, vegetable broth, grape juice concentrate, cinnamon, cumin, and raisins in a medium-size saucepan and stir to mix. Let come to a boil over high heat, then reduce the heat, cover the saucepan, and let simmer until the rice is tender but not mushy, about 45 minutes. Stir the rice occasionally to be sure it's not sticking to the bottom of the saucepan, adding more vegetable broth if necessary.

2. Remove the saucepan from the heat and let sit, covered, for 10 minutes. Sprinkle the walnuts on top just before serving. The rice pilaf can be refrigerated, covered, for up to 4 days.

SERVES 4

Nutrition Info
1 PORTION PROVIDES:

Vitamin C: 1 serving

Green leafy and yellow vegetables and fruits: 1/2 serving if made with apricots

Other fruits and vegetables: 1/2 serving if made with raisins

Whole grains and legumes: 1 serving

Iron: from the dried fruit

Barley Risotto with Wild Mushrooms

Creamy and cheesy, this dish has all the best elements of a traditional risotto, making it a wonderful accompaniment to a hearty chicken or fish dish. The nutritious twist? Barley stands in for Arborio rice, lending more fiber and protein.

1 tablespoon olive oil
2 large shallots, chopped
2 cups coarsely chopped mushrooms,
    such as portobello, cremini, oyster,
    chanterelle, or button mushrooms
1½ tablespoons chopped fresh parsley
2 teaspoons fresh thyme leaves
2 cloves garlic, minced
½ cup barley
2½ cups vegetable broth or low-sodium
    chicken broth, or more as needed
1 tablespoon tomato paste
¾ cup grated Parmesan cheese
Salt and black pepper

1. Heat the olive oil in a medium-size nonstick saucepan over medium heat. Add the shallots and cook until softened, about 4 minutes.

2. Add the mushrooms to the saucepan and cook until browned, about 10 minutes.

3. Add the parsley, thyme, garlic, and barley, and cook, stirring, until heated slightly, about 1 minute.

4. Add 2 cups of the vegetable broth and let come to a boil. Reduce the heat, cover the pan, and let simmer until the liquid is almost absorbed and the barley is almost tender, 25 to 30 minutes.

5. Add the remaining ½ cup of vegetable broth and the tomato paste. Cook uncovered, stirring occasionally, until the barley is tender and creamy, about 10 minutes. If the barley becomes too dry, add a little more vegetable broth.

6. Stir in the Parmesan cheese and season with salt and pepper to taste.

SERVES 2

Nutrition Info

1 PORTION PROVIDES:

Protein: ½ serving

Calcium: 1½ servings

Other fruits and vegetables: 2 servings

Whole grains and legumes: 1 serving

Fat: ½ serving

Pomegranate Pilaf

Crunchy pomegranate seeds and chewy apricots add unexpected—and delightful—texture to this flavorful side dish of wild rice and barley.

1 tablespoon olive oil
1 shallot, finely chopped
¼ cup wild rice, rinsed and drained
¼ cup barley
1½ to 2 cups low-sodium chicken
   broth or vegetable broth,
   or more if necessary
½ cup pomegranate seeds
   (from about ½ pomegranate)
¼ cup chopped dried apricots
1 teaspoon grated lemon zest
1 tablespoon chopped fresh flat-leaf
   parsley
2 tablespoons chopped toasted pecans
   (see page 272)

1. Heat the olive oil in a medium-size nonstick saucepan over medium heat. Add the shallot and cook until softened, about 2 minutes.

2. Add the wild rice and barley and stir to coat with the oil. Add the chicken broth and let come to a simmer. Reduce the heat to low, cover the pan, and let simmer until the wild rice and barley are tender and most of the liquid has been absorbed, 45 to 50 minutes. Add more broth, if necessary.

THE GRAIN GAME

▼ ▼ ▼

There's a whole world of whole grains waiting at the natural foods store. Sure, right now you may not know how to pronounce some of them, never mind cook them, but there's no need to be intimidated. Actually, preparing whole grains isn't any trickier than preparing pasta, though in some cases the cooking time is a lot longer—from 30 minutes to as much as an hour. To save yourself time, consider cooking large batches, then refrigerating leftovers to be reheated in the microwave for hot cereal, pilaf, or stuffing or served cold in salads. They'll keep for up to one week. So experiment! Have fun! And remember, no matter how you serve whole grains, you'll be serving yourself a healthy dose of fiber, protein, B vitamins, and trace minerals.

3. Add the pomegranate seeds, apricots, lemon zest, parsley, and pecans to the pilaf. Fluff with a fork before serving.

SERVES 2

Nutrition Info

1 PORTION PROVIDES:

Green leafy and yellow vegetables and fruits: 1/2 serving

Whole grains and legumes: 1 serving

Fat: 1/2 serving

Quinoa Pearls with Wild Mushrooms

No need to fear this possibly unfamiliar pearl-like grain. It's easier to cook than to figure out how to pronounce (it's KEEN-wah). And you'll pronounce it delicious alongside poultry or beef.

1 cup vegetable broth or low-sodium
   chicken stock
1/2 cup quinoa, rinsed and drained
1 teaspoon fresh thyme leaves
1/8 teaspoon salt
1 tablespoon olive oil
2 cups sliced shiitake mushrooms
1 shallot, minced
1 tablespoon chopped fresh flat-leaf
   parsley
2 teaspoons balsamic vinegar

1. Place the vegetable broth in a medium-size saucepan and let come to a boil over high heat. Add the quinoa, thyme, and salt, then let the broth return to a boil. Reduce the heat to low, cover the pan, and cook until the quinoa is tender, about 15 minutes.

2. Meanwhile, heat the olive oil in a non-stick skillet over medium heat. Add the mushrooms, shallot, and parsley and cook until softened, about 5 minutes. Add the balsamic vinegar, cook just until heated through, about 30 seconds. Remove from the heat and toss the cooked quinoa with the mushrooms.

SERVES 2

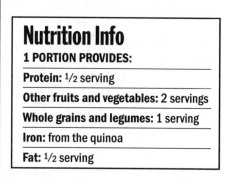

Nutrition Info

1 PORTION PROVIDES:

Protein: 1/2 serving

Other fruits and vegetables: 2 servings

Whole grains and legumes: 1 serving

Iron: from the quinoa

Fat: 1/2 serving

Leek and Tomato Quinoa

Never made quinoa before? Here's an easy and cheesy way to explore this intriguing grain.

½ cup quinoa, rinsed and drained
1 cup plus 2 tablespoons vegetable
    broth
1 tablespoon olive oil
1 large leek, both white and pale green
    parts trimmed, rinsed well, and
    finely chopped
1 medium-size tomato, seeded and
    chopped
2 tablespoons chopped fresh basil
    or flat-leaf parsley
½ tablespoon fresh lemon juice,
    or more to taste
Salt and black pepper
¼ cup grated Parmesan cheese,
    or more to taste

1. Place the quinoa and 1 cup of vegetable broth in a medium-size saucepan and let come to a boil over high heat. Reduce the heat to low, cover the pan, and let simmer until the quinoa is tender, about 15 minutes. Drain and set aside.

2. Meanwhile, heat the olive oil in a large nonstick skillet over medium heat. Add the leek and cook until it begins to soften, about 5 minutes.

3. Add the remaining 2 tablespoons of vegetable broth, cover the skillet, and let simmer until the leek is tender, about 5 minutes.

4. Add the cooked quinoa to the skillet and cook, stirring, until heated through, about 3 minutes.

5. Add the tomato, basil, and lemon juice and gently stir to mix. Taste for seasoning, adding more lemon juice as necessary and salt and pepper to taste. Sprinkle the Parmesan cheese on top and serve.

SERVES 2

Nutrition Info
1 PORTION PROVIDES:

Protein: ½ serving

Calcium: ½ serving

Vitamin C: ½ serving

Whole grains and legumes: 1 serving

Iron: from the quinoa

Fat: ½ serving

Three-in-One Pilaf

Bulgur, quinoa, and roasted buckwheat groats team up here for a deliciously different—and nutritious—pilaf. Peas or edamame add even more nutrients and a touch of color.

1 tablespoon canola oil
2 large shallots, chopped
1/2 cup coarse bulgur
1/4 cup quinoa, rinsed and drained
1/4 cup roasted whole buckwheat
   groats
2 3/4 cups vegetable broth
Pinch each of salt and black pepper
1/2 cup frozen peas or shelled edamame
   (soybeans)

1. Heat the oil in a medium-size non-stick skillet over medium heat. Add the shallots and cook until beginning to soften, about 2 minutes.

2. Add the bulgur, quinoa, and buckwheat groats to the skillet and cook, stirring, until coated, about 2 minutes, stirring.

3. Add in the vegetable broth, salt, and pepper and let come to a boil. Cover the skillet, reduce the heat and let simmer until almost all of the liquid is absorbed and the grains are tender, about 20 minutes.

4. Add the peas and let simmer until the peas are heated through, about 5 minutes. Season with more salt and pepper to taste before serving. Leftovers can be stored, covered, in the refrigerator for up to 3 days.

SERVES 4

Nutrition Info
1 PORTION PROVIDES:

Whole grains and legumes: 1 serving

Red Peppers Stuffed with Millet Pilaf

A festive addition to any fiesta, if you stuff a few extra peppers you can dress up tomorrow night's dinner, too. Pan roasting millet, a staple grain throughout Africa and Asia, brings out its nutty flavor.

¼ cup hulled millet seeds,
  rinsed and drained
1 cup vegetable broth
Pinch of salt
1 cup fresh or frozen corn kernels
  (from about 2 ears)
2 tablespoons chopped fresh cilantro
1 tablespoon fresh lime juice,
  or more to taste
1 teaspoon chopped peeled
  fresh ginger
2 scallions, both white and
  light green parts, chopped
½ cup chopped tomato
½ cup chopped yellow bell pepper
1 tablespoon olive oil
Salt and black pepper
2 large red bell peppers, cut in half
  and seeded

1. Preheat the oven to 375°F.

2. Place the millet in a large saucepan over medium heat and cook, stirring frequently, until the seeds are golden brown and fragrant, 2 to 3 minutes.

3. Add the vegetable broth and salt and let come to a boil. Cover the pan, reduce the heat to medium-low, and let simmer until the liquid is almost absorbed, about 20 minutes.

4. Add the corn to the millet and cook until heated through, about 5 minutes. Remove the saucepan from the heat. Add the cilantro, lime juice, ginger, scallions, tomato, yellow bell pepper, and olive oil to the millet and corn mixture and stir gently to mix. Season to taste with salt and pepper, and more lime juice if desired. Mound the pilaf in the red bell pepper halves, dividing it evenly among them.

5. Place the stuffed pepper halves on a baking sheet and bake until golden brown, 20 to 25 minutes.

SERVES 4

Nutrition Info
1 PORTION PROVIDES:

Vitamin C: 3 servings

Green leafy and yellow vegetables and fruits: 1 serving

Other vegetables and fruits: ½ serving

Whole grains and legumes: ½ serving

Wheat Berry Salad with Red Pepper, Carrots, and Red Onions

What do you get when you combine chewy wheat berries, crunchy vegetables, and a light dressing? A satisfying side dish that's perfect for a summer barbecue.

2 cups vegetable broth
Salt
2 cups water
1/2 cup wheat berries
2 tablespoons olive oil
1/2 medium-size red onion, finely chopped
2 tablespoons balsamic vinegar
2 scallions, both white and light green parts, trimmed and chopped
1 medium-size carrot, peeled and chopped
1 medium-size red bell pepper, chopped
Black pepper

1. Place the vegetable broth, a pinch of salt, and the water in a large saucepan over medium-high heat and let come to a boil. Add the wheat berries, reduce the heat, and let simmer until the wheat berries are tender, 45 minutes to 1 hour.

2. Meanwhile, heat 1 tablespoon of the olive oil in a medium-size nonstick skillet over medium heat. Add the red onion and cook until softened, about 5 minutes. Remove from the heat.

3. Place the remaining 1 tablespoon of olive oil and the vinegar in a small bowl and whisk to mix. Add the vinegar mixture to the red onion and set aside.

4. Place the cooked wheat berries, scallions, carrot, and bell pepper in a large bowl and toss to mix. Add the red onion mixture and toss to combine. Season with salt and black pepper to taste. The wheat berry salad can be served warm or at room temperature. It can be refrigerated, covered, for up to 3 days.

SERVES 2

Nutrition Info
1 PORTION PROVIDES:

Vitamin C: 2 servings

Green leafy and yellow vegetables and fruits: 2 servings

Whole grains and legumes: 1 serving

Fat: 1/2 serving

"Mocktails" and Smoothies

Think the party's over just because you're pregnant? Not so. Whether you're stocking your bar for a weekend brunch, a July Fourth barbecue, or a New Year's open house, don't forget to fill a pitcher or a blender with your favorite "mocktail" or smoothie so you can toast the occasion, too. But don't wait for a toast to enjoy these drinks. Sip them anytime you're thirsting (or in the case of smoothies, hungry) for a tasty treat. Some make satisfying before-dinner drinks—others can stand in for (or supplement) breakfast when you're in a hurry or too queasy to face solids.

First Blush

So sweet and satisfying, your First Blush may lead to a second. Substitute thawed frozen or fresh strawberries and add a little sparkling water if you'd like a more sippable drink.

1 cup diced seedless watermelon
1/2 cup frozen strawberries
1 cup calcium-fortified orange juice
2 tablespoons white grape, apple,
    or pineapple juice concentrate
8 fresh mint leaves (optional)
1/2 cup sparkling water (optional)

Place the watermelon, strawberries, orange juice, white grape juice concentrate, and mint leaves, if using, in a blender or food processor and process until the fruit is puréed and the mixture is well blended. Divide the drinks evenly between 2 tall glasses, stir 1/4 cup sparkling water, if desired, into each, and serve.

SERVES 2

FROM THE TEST KITCHEN

TURN YOUR FIRST BLUSH into a first-class smoothie by adding 1 cup of vanilla yogurt. You'll also turn a half-calcium serving into a whole one.

Nutrition Info
1 PORTION PROVIDES:

Calcium: 1/2 serving

Vitamin C: 2 servings plus

GET JUICED WITHOUT THE ACID

▼ ▼ ▼

The high acid levels in regular orange juice can definitely trigger tummy troubles in some expectant moms, particularly during the queasy early months. If that's true for you, shake up your shake without shaking up your stomach by using low-acid OJ or substituting another kinder, gentler juice, such as white grape. Many low-acid juices also come fortified with calcium.

Citrus Blueberry Blast

Very berry, very nutritious, very delicious—blissful blueberries, packed with antioxidants, combine with white grape and orange juice to make this "mocktail" a blast to drink.

1 cup frozen blueberries
¹/₂ cup unsweetened vitamin C–fortified
   white grape juice
1 cup calcium-fortified orange juice
1 cup sparkling water

Place the blueberries, grape juice, and orange juice in a blender or food processor and process until the fruit is puréed and the mixture is well blended. Divide the drinks evenly between 2 tall glasses, stir ½ cup sparkling water into each, and serve.

SERVES 2

Nutrition Info

1 PORTION PROVIDES:

Calcium: ¹/₂ serving

Vitamin C: 1¹/₂ servings

Other vegetables and fruits: 1 serving

Iced Watermelon Water

Refreshingly different—and just plain refreshing. It may not fill any Daily Dozen requirements, but it will be especially soothing to sip when you're queasy.

1 cup fresh mint leaves
3 tablespoons orange or white grape
   juice concentrate
4 cups diced watermelon
2 cups ice cubes
6 cups water

Place the mint and orange juice concentrate in a 4-quart pitcher and mash them with a wooden spoon. Add the watermelon, ice cubes, and water. Stir to mix. To serve, pour into glasses. Nibble on the fruit while you sip.

MAKES ABOUT 3 QUARTS

Tropical Temptation

Drink your vitamins. With a unique combo of flavors—orange, carrot, and peach or mango—this "mocktail" provides a taste of the tropics and a whole lot of nutrition.

$^1/_2$ cup calcium-fortified orange juice
$^1/_2$ cup carrot juice
1 cup sliced fresh ripe (or frozen) yellow
   peach or mango
1 tablespoon white grape juice
   concentrate, pineapple juice
   concentrate, Splenda, or honey

Place the orange juice, carrot juice, peach, and apple juice concentrate in a blender or food processor and process until the fruit is puréed and the mixture is well blended. Pour into a tall glass and serve.

SERVES 1

Nutrition Info

1 PORTION PROVIDES:

Calcium: $^1/_2$ serving

Vitamin C: 1 serving if made with peaches; 3 servings if made with mango

Green leafy and yellow vegetables and fruits: 3 servings if made with peaches; 4 servings if made with mango

Other fruits and vegetables: 1 serving if made with peaches

Ocean Breeze

Here's another taste of the tropics, with more vitamins than you can shake one of those little paper umbrellas at. Substitute vanilla yogurt for the sparkling water and you have yourself a tropical smoothie, plus an extra calcium serving.

1 cup diced ripe cantaloupe or mango
1 cup canned pineapple chunks
   in their juice, drained

$^1/_2$ cup calcium-fortified orange juice
1 cup sparkling water
2 fresh mint sprigs

Place the cantaloupe, pineapple, and orange juice in a blender or food processor and process until the fruit is puréed and the mixture is well blended. Divide the drinks evenly between 2 tall glasses and stir ½ cup sparkling water into each. Garnish each glass with a sprig of mint and serve.

SERVES 2

> **Nutrition Info**
>
> **1 PORTION PROVIDES:**
>
> **Calcium:** ½ serving
>
> **Vitamin C:** 2 servings
>
> **Green leafy and yellow vegetables and fruits:** 1 serving

Apple and Spice

Spice up your morning while calming your morning sickness with this big mama smoothie. Add yogurt (and maybe some flaxseed or wheat germ) if you'd like to make it a meal. Using frozen banana slices will make the smoothie even thicker.

1 cup pineapple juice
1 cup canned pineapple chunks
   in their juice, drained
1 small apple, peeled, cored,
   and chopped
1 ripe banana, sliced
1 piece (1-inch) fresh ginger,
   peeled and thinly sliced

Place the pineapple juice, canned pineapple, apple, banana, and ginger in a blender or food processor and process until the fruit is puréed and the mixture is well blended. Pour into a tall glass and serve.

SERVES 1

> **Nutrition Info**
>
> **1 PORTION PROVIDES:**
>
> **Vitamin C:** 3 servings
>
> **Other fruits and vegetables:** 2 servings

Breakfast Booster Shake

N o time to eat breakfast? Drink it, instead. This breakfast in a blender may be just the ticket, too, when solids don't appeal—or just aren't staying down.

1 cup calcium-fortified orange juice
½ cup vanilla yogurt
½ cup sliced ripe mango
  (from about ½ medium-size mango)
½ cup frozen or fresh blueberries
  (see Note)
½ banana, sliced (see Note)
3 ice cubes (optional; see Note)

Place the orange juice, yogurt, mango, blueberries, banana, and ice, if using, in a blender or food processor and process until the fruit is puréed and the drink is thick and creamy. Pour the drink into a tall glass and serve.

SERVES 1 GENEROUSLY

NOTE: If you like a really thick shake, freeze the banana slices. If you are using fresh blueberries and an unfrozen banana, add 3 ice cubes to chill the shake.

FROM THE TEST KITCHEN

BOOST YOUR BREAKFAST
Make a booster shake by trying these tips:

■ Add 1 or 2 tablespoons of wheat germ or ground flaxseed.

■ Add ¼ cup soft tofu (you'll get an extra protein boost without any change in flavor).

■ Substitute ½ cup of melon, peach, or apricot slices for the mango.

■ Sweeten the pot (or the blender), if you like, with juice concentrate, Splenda, or honey to taste.

Nutrition Info
1 PORTION PROVIDES:

Calcium: 1½ servings

Vitamin C: 3 servings

Green leafy and yellow vegetables and fruits: 1 serving

Other fruits and vegetables: 1½ servings

Razzleberry

Serve this drink thick and creamy—or thin it and make it fizz by adding sparkling water. Either way, it's yummy.

1¹⁄₃ cups frozen raspberries

1 cup calcium-fortified orange juice

12 fresh mint leaves (optional)

2 tablespoons low-fat vanilla yogurt or soft tofu

2 tablespoons white grape juice concentrate, Splenda, or honey, or to taste

1 cup sparkling water (optional)

Place the raspberries, orange juice, mint leaves, yogurt, and apple juice concentrate in a blender or food processor and process until the fruit is puréed and the drink is thick and creamy. Divide the drinks evenly between 2 tall glasses. If you want a thinner consistency, add ½ cup sparkling water to each before serving.

SERVES 2

Nutrition Info
1 PORTION PROVIDES:

Calcium: ¹⁄₂ serving

Vitamin C: 2 servings

Apricot Nectar

This rich-tasting smoothie is so thick, your straw may not be up to the job. Try a spoon for backup. For a less creamy drink, use fresh banana slices instead of the frozen.

1 cup canned apricot halves, fruit juice drained

1 frozen banana, sliced

1 cup vanilla soy milk or vanilla yogurt

Place the apricots, banana, and soy milk in a blender or food processor and process until the fruit is puréed and the mixture is thick and creamy. Divide the drink evenly between 2 tall glasses and serve.

SERVES 1

Nutrition Info

1 PORTION PROVIDES:

Calcium: 1 serving

Vitamin C: $1/2$ serving

Green leafy and yellow vegetables and fruits: 2 servings

Other fruits and vegetables: 1 serving

SOOTHING SMOOTHIES

▼ ▼ ▼

The name says it all—smoothies go down easily even when you're feeling a little rough. They can stand in for a meal when you don't feel like cooking or eating. Here are some general tips for making successful smoothies:

■ Start with a liquid: fruit juice, milk, or soy milk. For a smoothie that's more sippable, use at least a cup of liquid. For a thick smoothie worthy of a spoon—and an extra jolt of calcium—substitute yogurt for part of the liquid or use some in addition. Whenever possible, opt for juice that's been calcium fortified.

■ To make the smoothie creamy and custardy, use frozen fruits instead of fresh or freeze unsweetened, cut-up fresh fruit first.

■ Boost the smoothie's nutritional profile by adding a tablespoon or two of wheat germ, oat bran, ground flaxseed, nonfat milk powder, or soft tofu.

■ Turn any yogurt smoothie vegan by substituting soft tofu for yogurt. Just sweeten to taste with your sweetener of choice. Or use vanilla soy milk.

■ Ginger snaps the queasies for many women; try tossing a tablespoon of sliced peeled fresh ginger into any smoothie before blending.

■ Like your smoothies really sweet? Add some Splenda, honey, or a juice concentrate. Pick a flavor that will complement your choice of fruit—pineapple juice or mango concentrate in a tropical shake, for instance.

Mango Tango

This supernutritious drink will have your taste buds dancing all the way to the tropics. It's like paradise in a glass.

1 cup sliced chilled ripe mango
  (from 1 medium-size mango)
1 cup chilled pineapple juice
½ cup low-fat vanilla yogurt
½ teaspoon vanilla extract
2 to 3 ice cubes (optional)

Place the mango, pineapple juice, yogurt, vanilla extract, and ice cubes, if using, in a blender or food processor and process until the fruit is puréed and the ice is crushed. Pour into a tall glass and serve.

MAKES 1 TALL DRINK

FROM THE TEST KITCHEN

FOR A DAIRY-FREE smoothie, substitute ½ cup soft tofu for the yogurt. Sweeten to taste with juice concentrate, Splenda, or honey. Or use vanilla soy milk.

Nutrition Info

1 PORTION PROVIDES:

Calcium: ½ serving

Vitamin C: 4 servings

Green leafy and yellow vegetables and fruits: 2 servings

Desserts

Healthy isn't the first thing that usually comes to mind when you think dessert. Sweet, yes. Sinful, yes. But, healthy—not often . . . unless your idea of dessert is a ripe peach. Fortunately, with the recipes in this chapter, healthy desserts aren't just a pipe dream (or an oxymoron). On the pages that follow you'll find delicious cookies, cakes, pies, and cobblers designed to fill your nutritional requirements with whole grains and fruit, while filling your sweet tooth with joy. Does having such nutritious treats just a short recipe away (or stashed in the freezer) mean that you'll never want to reach for a truly decadent dessert (that molten chocolate cake, that glazed tart)? Maybe not. But it's nice to know you can have the option of reaching for a second slice of cake or a third cookie without a morsel of remorse. So dig in!

Fruity Oatmeal Cookies

These are way chewier than your average oatmeal cookie and a lot more nutritious, too. Handle them with care, or you'll find out just how this cookie crumbles (of course, the crumbs taste just as good as the cookie).

2 cups old-fashioned rolled oats
1/4 cup ground flaxseed
(see box on page 435)
1/4 cup wheat germ
2 teaspoons ground cinnamon
6 tablespoons (3/4 stick) butter, melted
1 large egg, lightly beaten
3/4 cup white grape juice concentrate
1/2 cup raisins, chopped
1/4 cup dried blueberries or cranberries,
or chopped dried apricots (optional)
1/3 cup chopped toasted pecans or
walnuts (see page 272)

1. Preheat the oven to 325°F. Set aside 2 nonstick cookie sheets.

2. Place the oats, flaxseed, wheat germ, and cinnamon in a mixing bowl and stir to mix well. Add the butter and stir to combine.

3. Place the egg and grape juice concentrate in another bowl, and whisk together. Pour the egg mixture over the oat mixture and stir well. Add the raisins, the blueberries, if using, and the nuts and stir to mix.

4. Drop the dough by tablespoonfuls onto the cookie sheets about 1 inch apart, then flatten slightly with the back of a fork (wet the fork slightly if the dough sticks to it) so they form irregular circles.

5. Bake the cookies until they are lightly browned and the edges are firm, about 15 minutes. Let the cookies cool completely before serving. The cookies can be stored in an airtight container for up to 5 days or frozen for up to 1 month.

MAKES ABOUT 30 COOKIES

Nutrition Info
1 PORTION (2 COOKIES) PROVIDES:

Vitamin C: 1/2 serving

Whole grains and legumes: 1/2 serving

Iron: from the dried fruit

Fat: 1/2 serving

Tropical Bar Nones

Chunky, chewy, a little gooey—and as nutritious as a bowl of granola. How's that for sweet revenge?

Vegetable oil cooking spray

1½ cups old-fashioned rolled oats

¾ cup chopped nuts, such as almonds, walnuts, Brazil nuts, pecans, or filberts

¼ cup wheat germ

2 teaspoons ground cinnamon

½ teaspoon ground ginger (optional)

½ cup plus 1 tablespoon flaked coconut, preferably unsweetened (see Note)

½ cup plus 2 tablespoons white grape juice concentrate

2 tablespoons Splenda or brown sugar

1 cup dried apricots

1 cup dried pineapple chunks, or
    ½ cup dried pineapple chunks
    and ½ cup dried mango chunks

3 tablespoons all-fruit apricot preserves

2 tablespoons pineapple juice concentrate

1. Preheat the oven to 350°F. Lightly coat a nonstick 9-inch-square cake pan with vegetable oil cooking spray.

2. Place the oats, nuts, wheat germ, cinnamon, ginger, if using, and ½ cup of the coconut in a food processor and process until the mixture resembles coarse meal. Add ½ cup of the grape juice concentrate and the Splenda or brown sugar and process until the mixture is crumbly and holds together when pressed.

3. Remove the oat batter from the processor and divide it in half. Lightly wet your fingers, then press half of the batter evenly over the bottom of the prepared cake pan.

4. Place the apricots, dried pineapple, apricot preserves, pineapple juice concentrate, and the remaining 2 tablespoons of grape juice concentrate in the food processor and process until the fruit is finely chopped. Spread the fruit mixture evenly over the batter in the cake pan.

NOT NUTS FOR NUTS?

▼ ▼ ▼

Nuts provide a healthy host of vitamins, minerals, and vital fatty acids. But if you'd like to leave them out of these recipes because you're not nuts for the taste, you have a nut allergy, or your doctor has advised you to avoid nuts during pregnancy, go right ahead. Omitting chopped nuts from a recipe won't affect the outcome significantly (toss in extra dried fruit if you like). If a recipe calls for ground nuts, substitute an equal amount of ground flaxseed, wheat germ, oats, or flour.

5. Spoon the remaining batter into the cake pan, then pat it down with your fingers so that it covers the fruit mixture evenly. Sprinkle the remaining 1 tablespoon of coconut over the top and press it into the batter.

6. Bake until lightly browned and firm, 25 to 30 minutes.

7. Let cool completely before cutting into 16 pieces, approximately 2¼ inches square. The bars can be stored in an airtight container for up to 4 days, or frozen for up to a mouth.

MAKES 16 BARS

NOTE: Unsweetened flaked coconut is available at health food stores.

FROM THE TEST KITCHEN

DON'T HAVE A TASTE for the tropics? Substitute any combination of dried fruit that strikes your fancy—dried blueberries, peaches, cherries, cranberries, apples, or pears—for the dried pineapple. Use orange, cherry, blueberry, peach, mango, or apple juice concentrate instead of the pineapple juice concentrate and match the flavor of the preserves.

Nutrition Info

1 PORTION (2 BARS) PROVIDES:

Vitamin C: ¹/₂ serving

Green leafy and yellow vegetables and fruits: ¹/₂ serving

Whole grains and legumes: ¹/₂ serving

Fat: ¹/₂ serving

Heavenly Chocolate Cake

Deep, dark, and delectable enough to satisfy any chocoholic. And who would have thought you could get a serving of vitamin C from a slab of chocolate cake?

Vegetable oil cooking spray
1 cup toasted almonds
¹/₂ cup all-purpose white flour
¹/₂ cup whole wheat flour
¹/₄ cup flaxseed (see box on the facing page) or wheat germ
2 teaspoons baking powder

1 teaspoon baking soda
³/₄ cup unsweetened cocoa (see Note)
2 cups white grape juice concentrate
4 tablespoons (¹/₂ stick) butter, melted
3 large eggs
1 tablespoon vanilla extract

1. Preheat the oven to 325°F. Lightly coat a nonstick 9-by-13-inch cake pan with vegetable oil cooking spray.

2. Place the toasted almonds in a food processor and pulse briefly to chop, then run the machine until the nuts are just ground, about 30 seconds. Do not over-process the almonds or you will end up with a paste. You should have about ½ cup of ground almonds.

3. Place the white and whole wheat flour, flaxseed, baking powder, baking soda, cocoa, and ground almonds in a mixing bowl and stir to mix well.

4. Place the grape juice concentrate, butter, eggs, and vanilla in another mixing bowl. Beat with an electric mixer at low speed or with a whisk until well mixed.

5. Slowly add the flour mixture to the grape juice mixture, continuing to beat at low speed just until thoroughly blended; be careful not to overmix. Pour the batter into the prepared cake pan.

6. Bake the cake until the top springs back when lightly pressed, about 30 minutes.

7. Let the cake cool slightly in the pan before turning it out onto a wire rack to cool completely or let it cool and serve it straight from the pan. For instructions on storing the cake see page 438.

MAKES ONE 9-BY-13-INCH CAKE (APPROXIMATELY 18 PIECES, EACH 2 X 3 INCHES)

NOTE: You can use less cocoa—as little as ½ cup—if you prefer a cake that has a less intense chocolate flavor.

FROM THE TEST KITCHEN

WHAT GOES BETTER with chocolate cake than whipped cream? If you like, top the Heavenly Chocolate Cake with freshly whipped cream that has been sweetened to taste. Vanilla frozen yogurt tops it well, too.

Nutrition Info

1 PORTION (1 PIECE) PROVIDES:

Vitamin C: 1 serving

I Can't See the Black Forest for the Cherries Cake

Chocolate, coconut, pecans, and lots of cherries combine to create a cake that's a rich, supermoist treat. A scoop of frozen yogurt or ice cream would put the cake over the top.

Vegetable oil cooking spray

1 cup pecans

½ cup all-purpose white flour

½ cup whole wheat flour

¼ cup ground flaxseed
   (see box on page 435)

½ cup unsweetened cocoa

2 teaspoons baking powder

1 teaspoon baking soda

1 cup black cherry juice concentrate
   (see Note)

1 cup white grape juice concentrate

4 tablespoons (½ stick) butter, melted

3 large eggs

½ cup all-fruit cherry preserves

1 tablespoon vanilla extract

½ cup coarsely chopped pitted fresh
   or frozen cherries

⅔ cup flaked coconut, preferably
   unsweetened

½ cup dried cherries

½ cup toasted pecan pieces
   (see page 272)

Whipped cream (optional), for serving

1. Preheat the oven to 325°F. Lightly coat a nonstick 9-by-13-inch cake pan with vegetable oil cooking spray.

2. Place the pecans in a food processor and pulse briefly to chop, then run the machine until the nuts are just ground, about 30 seconds. Do not overprocess the pecans or you will end up with a paste. You should have about ½ cup of ground pecans.

3. Place the white and whole wheat flour, flaxseed, cocoa, baking powder, baking soda, and ground pecans in a mixing bowl and stir to mix well.

4. Place the cherry juice concentrate, grape juice concentrate, butter, eggs, cherry preserves, and vanilla in another mixing bowl. Beat with an electric mixer at low speed or with a whisk until well mixed.

5. Slowly add the flour mixture to the juice mixture, continuing to beat at low speed just until thoroughly blended; be careful not to overmix. Pour the batter into the prepared cake pan.

6. Bake the cake until the top springs back when lightly pressed, about 35 minutes.

7. Let the cake cool slightly in the pan before turning it out onto a wire rack to cool completely or let it cool and serve it straight from the pan. Serve the cake with whipped cream, if desired. For instructions on storing the cake, see page 438.

MAKES ONE 9-BY-13-INCH CAKE
(APPROXIMATELY 18 PIECES,
EACH 2 X 3 INCHES)

NOTE: Black cherry juice concentrate is available in many health food stores and some supermarkets. If you can't find it, increase the amount of white grape juice concentrate to 2 cups.

Carrot Pineapple Cake

Slightly spicy, this luscious cake, chock-full of walnuts, raisins, carrots, coconut, and pineapple makes a nutritious snack or a satisfying dessert. There's no sweeter way to serve up your yellow vegetables.

Vegetable oil cooking spray
2 cups shredded carrots
²/₃ cup pineapple juice concentrate
1 tablespoon grated peeled fresh ginger
  (optional)
1 cup golden raisins
¹/₂ cup walnuts
1³/₄ cups whole wheat flour
¹/₂ cup ground flaxseed
  (see box on page 435), oat bran,
  or wheat germ, or a combination
2 teaspoons baking powder
1 teaspoon baking soda
1 tablespoon ground cinnamon
1 teaspoon ground ginger (optional)
2 cups white grape juice concentrate
¹/₄ cup canola oil
4 large eggs
1 tablespoon vanilla extract

¹/₂ cup chopped toasted walnuts
  (see page 272)
¹/₂ cup very well drained
  unsweetened crushed pineapple
¹/₂ cup diced dried pineapple
  chunks
Cream Cheese Frosting
  (recipe follows; see Note)

1. Preheat the oven to 350°F. Lightly coat 2 nonstick 9-inch round cake pans with vegetable oil cooking spray.

2. Place the carrots, pineapple juice concentrate, fresh ginger, if using, and water in a saucepan over medium heat. Cover the pan, let come to a simmer, and cook until the carrots are tender, about 10 minutes.

POP THEM INTO YOUR FREEZER

▼ ▼ ▼

No one expects you to eat an entire cake at one sitting (though you might be tempted to do so every now and then). Instead, bake the cake, cut it into individual servings, wrap the pieces in aluminum foil, and store them in the freezer for an easy dessert or anytime snack. (Don't forget to eat one slice first!) The cake slices will keep for up to a month in the freezer. To serve, simply let cake slices thaw at room temperature or in the fridge.

3. Transfer the cooked carrot mixture to a food processor, add the raisins and process until both are finely chopped. Remove from the processor and set aside.

4. Place the walnuts in the food processor and pulse briefly to chop, then run the machine until the nuts are just ground, about 30 seconds. Do not overprocess the walnuts or you will end up with a paste. You should have about ¼ cup of ground walnuts.

5. Place the whole wheat flour, flaxseed, baking powder, baking soda, cinnamon, ground ginger, if using, and ground walnuts in a large mixing bowl and stir to mix well.

6. Add the grape juice concentrate, oil, eggs, and vanilla to the flour mixture and beat with an electric mixer at low speed until well mixed. Fold the carrot and raisin mixture, the ground walnuts, and the crushed and dried pineapple into the batter. Pour the batter into the prepared cake pans, dividing it evenly between them.

7. Bake the cakes until a toothpick inserted into the center of each comes out clean, about 35 minutes.

8. Let the cakes cool completely on wire racks, then turn them out of the pans. Frost the top of one cake with the Cream Cheese Frosting. Place the second on top of the first, then frost the top of that cake. Refrigerate the cake after frosting. It may be refrigerated, covered, for up to 1 week.

MAKES ONE 9-INCH ROUND LAYER CAKE (8 TO 12 SERVINGS)

NOTE: If you don't want to bother with frosting, the cakes will still be tasty without it.

Nutrition Info

1 PORTION (⅛ OF A CAKE) PROVIDES:

Vitamin C: 2 servings

Green leafy and yellow vegetables and fruits: 1 serving

Other fruits and vegetables: 2 servings

Whole grains and legumes: 1 serving

Iron: from the raisins

Fat: ½ serving

Cream Cheese Frosting

Nothing tops a moist carrot cake better than cream cheese frosting. But this is not your run-of-the-mill frosting, full of fat and sugar. Dried pineapple and vanilla make it sweet and fragrant. It's light but bowl-licking good. Try it on the Banana Nut Cake, too (page 440).

½ cup dried pineapple chunks
1 package (8 ounces) light
  (not fat-free) cream cheese,
  at room temperature
2 teaspoons vanilla extract
3 tablespoons white grape juice
  concentrate or honey
Splenda, brown sugar, or another
  dry sweetener (optional)

Place the pineapple in a food processor and process until finely chopped. Add the cream cheese, vanilla, and grape juice concentrate and process until smooth. Taste for sweetness, adding Splenda 1 teaspoon at a time as necessary, if desired. The frosting is now ready to use.

MAKES ENOUGH TO FROST ONE 9-INCH LAYER CAKE

Gingerbread Mom

Ginger makes this cake especially soothing for a queasy tummy—and especially hard to resist.

Vegetable oil cooking spray
1 cup whole wheat flour
¼ cup ground flaxseed
  (see box on page 435)
¼ cup old-fashioned rolled oats
  or wheat germ
2 teaspoons ground ginger

1 teaspoon ground cinnamon
2 teaspoons baking soda
1 cup white grape juice concentrate
2 large eggs, lightly beaten
¼ cup canola oil
2 teaspoons minced peeled
  fresh ginger

1. Preheat the oven to 350°F. Lightly coat a nonstick 9-inch-square cake pan with vegetable oil cooking spray.

2. Place the whole wheat flour, flaxseed, oats, ground ginger, cinnamon, and baking soda in a mixing bowl and stir to mix well.

3. Place the grape juice concentrate, eggs, oil, and fresh ginger in another mixing bowl and beat with an electric mixer on low speed or with a whisk until well mixed.

4. Add the flour mixture to the grape juice mixture, continuing to beat at low speed just until thoroughly blended; be careful not to overmix. Pour the batter into the prepared cake pan.

5. Bake the cake until the top springs back when lightly pressed, about 30 minutes.

6. Let the cake cool slightly in the pan before turning it out onto a wire rack to cool completely or let it cool and serve it straight from the pan. For instructions on storing the cake see page 438.

**MAKES ONE 9-INCH CAKE
(8 TO 12 SERVINGS)**

Nutrition Info

1 PORTION (1/8 OF A CAKE) PROVIDES:

Vitamin C: 1 serving

Whole grains and legumes: almost 1 serving

Fat: 1/2 serving

Banana Nut Cake

B anana lovers will go ape for this extra moist cake. It's another good reason to break for coffee or, better still, milk.

Vegetable oil cooking spray

1 cup walnuts

2 medium-size bananas, cut into chunks

1/4 cup canola oil

3 large eggs

1 cup white grape juice concentrate

2 teaspoons vanilla extract

1 cup whole wheat flour

1/4 cup ground flaxseed
  (see box on page 435)

1/2 cup old-fashioned rolled oats

2 teaspoons baking soda

1 teaspoon baking powder

2 teaspoons cinnamon

1 teaspoon ground ginger
  (optional)

1/4 teaspoon ground nutmeg
  (optional)

1/2 cup coarsely chopped toasted
  walnuts (see page 272)

1. Preheat the oven to 325°F. Lightly coat a nonstick 9-by-13-inch cake pan with vegetable oil cooking spray.

2. Place the walnuts in a food processor and pulse briefly to chop, then run the machine until the nuts are just ground, about 30 seconds. Do not overprocess the walnuts or you will end up with a paste. You should have about ½ cup of ground walnuts. Remove from the processor and set aside.

3. Place the bananas in the food processor and process until puréed. Add the oil, eggs, grape juice concentrate, and vanilla and process until well blended.

4. Place the whole wheat flour, flaxseed, oats, baking soda, baking powder, cinnamon, ginger and nutmeg, if using, and ground walnuts in a mixing bowl and stir to mix.

5. Add the banana mixture to the flour mixture and beat with an electric mixer at low speed or with a whisk just until thoroughly blended; be careful not to overmix. Gently fold in the chopped walnuts. Pour the batter into the prepared cake pan.

6. Bake the cake until a toothpick inserted in the center comes out clean, 25 to 30 minutes.

7. Let the cake cool slightly in the pan before turning it out onto a wire rack to cool completely or let it cool and serve it straight from the pan. For instructions on storing the cake see page 438.

MAKES ONE 9-BY-13-INCH CAKE (APPROXIMATELY 18 PIECES, EACH 2 X 3 INCHES)

FROM THE TEST KITCHEN

WOULD YOUR WALNUTS like some sweet company in the banana cake? Fold in ½ to ⅔ cup of chopped dried fruit or raisins.

Nutrition Info

1 PORTION (2 PIECES) PROVIDES:

Vitamin C: ½ serving

Whole grains and legumes: ½ serving plus

Fat: ½ serving

Blueberry Oatmeal Cake

With a glass of milk or a smoothie, this crumbly, fruity cake could easily, and deliciously, pass for breakfast.

Vegetable oil cooking spray
¾ cup whole wheat flour
¼ cup ground flaxseed
   (see box on page 435)
¼ cup wheat germ, oat bran,
   or ground nuts
1 cup old-fashioned rolled oats
2 teaspoons baking powder
1 teaspoon baking soda
2 teaspoons ground cinnamon
1 teaspoon ground ginger
   (optional)
¼ teaspoon ground nutmeg
   (optional)
1½ cups white grape juice
   concentrate
4 tablespoons (½ stick) butter,
   melted
2 large eggs, lightly beaten
2 teaspoons vanilla extract
½ cup fresh or frozen blueberries
½ cup dried or dehydrated
   blueberries

1. Preheat the oven to 350°F. Lightly coat a nonstick 9-inch-square cake pan with vegetable oil cooking spray.

2. Place the whole wheat flour, flaxseed, wheat germ, oats, baking powder, baking soda, cinnamon, and ginger and nutmeg, if using, in a mixing bowl and stir to mix well.

3. Place the grape juice concentrate, butter, eggs, and vanilla extract in another mixing bowl. Beat with an electric mixer on low speed or with a whisk until well mixed.

4. Slowly add the flour mixture to the grape juice mixture, continuing to beat at low speed just until thoroughly blended; be careful not to overmix. Gently fold the fresh and dried blueberries into the batter. Pour the batter into the prepared cake pan.

5. Bake the cake until the top springs back when lightly pressed, about 40 minutes.

6. Let the cake cool slightly in the pan before turning it out onto a wire rack to cool completely or let it cool and serve it straight from the pan. For instructions on storing the cake, see page 438.

**MAKES ONE 9-INCH-SQUARE CAKE
(APPROXIMATELY 8 TO 12 SERVINGS)**

Nutrition Info

1 PORTION (⅛ OF A CAKE) PROVIDES:

Vitamin C: 1½ servings

Whole grains and legumes: 1 serving

Fat: ½ serving

Tropical Fruit Cake

Not your Aunt Ida's fruit cake, this is a tropical cousin of the pineapple upside-down cake. It has moist pineapple and peaches, chewy coconut, and crunchy nuts upside down, right side up, and inside out.

Vegetable oil cooking spray

1 cup flaked coconut, preferably
  unsweetened (see Note)

$^1/_2$ cup drained unsweetened
  pineapple chunks, diced

1 large ripe peach, pitted and
  chopped (about $^2/_3$ cup) or $^2/_3$ cup
  chopped thawed frozen peaches

$^1/_2$ cup chopped Brazil nuts

2 tablespoons Splenda or brown sugar
  (optional)

1 cup whole wheat flour

$^3/_4$ cup all-purpose white flour

$^1/_4$ cup ground flaxseed
  (see box on page 435)

1 tablespoon ground cinnamon

2 teaspoons baking powder

1 teaspoon baking soda

1 cup white grape juice concentrate

$^1/_2$ cup pineapple juice concentrate

3 large eggs

$^1/_4$ cup canola oil

1 tablespoon vanilla extract

$^1/_2$ cup chopped dried pineapple,
  peaches, or mangoes

1. Preheat the oven to 325°F. Lightly coat a nonstick 9-by-13-inch cake pan with vegetable oil cooking spray.

2. Combine the coconut, pineapple chunks, peach, and Brazil nuts in a mixing bowl. Taste for sweetness and add up to 2 tablespoons of Splenda, if desired.

3. Place the whole wheat and white flour, flaxseed, cinnamon, baking powder, and baking soda in another mixing bowl and stir to mix well.

4. Place the grape and pineapple juice concentrates, eggs, oil, and vanilla in a third mixing bowl and beat with an electric mixer on low speed or with a whisk until well mixed.

5. Slowly add the flour mixture to the juice mixture, continuing to beat at low speed just until thoroughly blended; be careful not to overmix. Gently fold the coconut mixture and the dried fruit into the batter. Pour the batter into the prepared cake pan.

6. Bake the cake until a toothpick inserted into the center comes out clean, 25 to 30 minutes.

7. Let the cake cool slightly in the pan before turning it out onto a wire rack to cool completely or let it cool and serve it straight from the pan. For instructions on storing the cake see page 438.

MAKES ONE 9-BY-13-INCH CAKE (APPROXIMATELY 18 PIECES, EACH 2 X 3 INCHES)

NOTE: Unsweetened flaked coconut is available at health food stores.

Nutrition Info

1 PORTION (2 PIECES) PROVIDES:

Vitamin C: 1½ servings

Whole grains and legumes: 1 serving

Fat: ½ serving

Apple Cranberry Crisp

Cozy up to this homey crisp any time of the day. It makes a satisfying dessert à la mode topped with whipped cream or a breakfast treat or snack topped with yogurt. Baking the apples and cranberries releases their natural sugars and results in a perfect balance of sweet and tart flavors.

FOR THE TOPPING:

½ cup old-fashioned rolled oats

½ cup toasted walnuts, pecans, or almonds (see page 272)

¼ cup whole wheat flour

3 tablespoons white grape juice concentrate

2 tablespoons Splenda or brown sugar

2 tablespoons (¼ stick) butter, at room temperature

2 teaspoons ground cinnamon

½ teaspoon ground nutmeg (optional)

¼ teaspoon salt (optional)

FOR THE FILLING:

6 medium-size baking apples, peeled, cored, and sliced, each slice cut in half

½ cup dried cranberries

¼ cup raisins

1 cup white grape juice concentrate or apple juice concentrate

2 tablespoons quick-cooking tapioca

1 tablespoon ground flaxseed (see box on page 435)

2 teaspoons ground cinnamon

Vegetable oil cooking spray

1. Preheat the oven to 375°F.

2. Prepare the topping: Place the oats, walnuts, whole wheat flour, grape juice concentrate, Splenda, butter, cinnamon, and nutmeg and salt, if using, in a food processor, and process until the mixture is crumbly.

3. Prepare the filling: Place the apples, cranberries, raisins, grape juice concentrate, tapioca, flaxseed, and cinnamon in a mixing bowl and stir to mix well.

4. Lightly coat a nonstick 8- or 9-inch square baking pan with vegetable oil cooking spray (an 8-inch pan will produce a chunkier crisp; in a 9-inch pan the apples will become more caramelized). Spoon the fruit filling into the prepared baking pan, spreading it out in an even layer. Spread the topping evenly over the fruit, patting it down with a spoon (the topping won't completely cover the filling).

5. Bake until the topping is golden brown, about 35 minutes. Let cool slightly and serve warm. Any leftovers can be refrigerated, covered, for up to 3 days. Let come to room temperature or rewarm in a 300°F oven before serving.

MAKES ONE 8- OR 9-INCH CRISP (APPROXIMATELY 8 SERVINGS)

FROM THE TEST KITCHEN

THERE'S MORE than one way to make a delicious crisp. Instead of apples, try using sliced pears (choose ones that are ripe but firm) or ripe yellow peaches (you'll get a serving of yellow fruit with this version).

Nutrition Info
1 PORTION (1/8 CRISP) PROVIDES:

Vitamin C: 1 serving

Other fruits and vegetables: 1 serving

SWEET DREAMS?

▼ ▼ ▼

Most of the baked goods in this book will come out sweet, but not too sweet. That's because they're sweetened with fruit, which is by nature (so to speak) a subtler sweet than sugar. If the baked goods of your dreams are sweeter, adding 2 to 4 tablespoons of Splenda, honey, or another sugar may help make your dreams come true.

Cherry Cobbler

Nothing says summer quite like a cherry cobbler. Of course, with the year-round availability of frozen cherries, there's no need to wait until Memorial Day to start serving this fruity favorite, topped with a crunchy oat topping.

FOR THE FILLING:
4 cups pitted, halved fresh sweet
    cherries
¼ cup all-fruit black cherry preserves
¼ cup white grape juice concentrate
¼ cup cherry juice concentrate,
    or ¼ cup more white grape juice
    concentrate
¼ cup quick-cooking tapioca
¼ cup Splenda or brown sugar
Vegetable oil cooking spray

FOR THE TOPPING:
¼ cup whole wheat flour
½ cup old-fashioned rolled oats
⅓ cup toasted slivered almonds
    (see page 272)
⅓ cup flaked coconut, preferably
    unsweetened (optional; see Note)
¼ cup white grape juice concentrate
2 tablespoons (¼ stick) unsalted
    butter, at room temperature
2 tablespoons Splenda or brown sugar,
    or more to taste
1 teaspoon ground cinnamon

1. Preheat the oven to 350°F.

2. Prepare the filling: Place the cherries, cherry preserves, grape and cherry juice concentrates, tapioca, and Splenda, in a mixing bowl and stir to mix well. Lightly coat a nonstick 9-inch square glass or ceramic square baking pan with vegetable oil cooking spray. Spoon the fruit mixture into the prepared baking pan, spreading it out in an even layer. Set the filling aside for 10 minutes to thicken.

3. Meanwhile, prepare the topping: Place the whole wheat flour, oats, almonds,

THE PIE THICKENS

▼ ▼ ▼

Sweetening fruit for a cobbler or pie filling with juice concentrate can mean a soggy, soupy (yet delicious) mess—unless you thicken things up before baking. That's why these fillings call for tapioca.

coconut, grape juice concentrate, butter, Splenda, and cinnamon in a food processor and process until the mixture is crumbly. Spread the topping evenly over the fruit patting it down with a spoon (the topping won't completely cover the filling).

4. Bake the cobbler until the topping is crisp and slightly golden, 35 to 40 minutes. Let cool slightly and serve warm or at room temperature. Any leftovers can be refrigerated, covered, for up to 3 days. Let come to room temperature or rewarm in a 300°F oven before serving.

MAKES ONE 9-INCH COBBLER (APPROXIMATELY 8 TO 10 SERVINGS)

NOTE: Unsweetened flaked coconut is available at health food stores.

Nutrition Info
1 PORTION (⅛ RECIPE) PROVIDES:

Vitamin C: 1 serving

Other fruits and vegetables: ½ serving

CAN YOU TOP THIS?

▼ ▼ ▼

Pies and crisps cry out for an à la mode topping (okay, maybe that was you crying out). Treat your next slab to a spoonful of whipped cream or a scoop of ice cream, frozen yogurt, or low-fat yogurt.

FROM THE TEST KITCHEN

FRESH OUT of fresh cherries? Or it's the season for frozen? Substitute 4 cups unsweetened frozen sweet cherries. Let the cherries thaw, then cut them in half and drain them thoroughly or your cobbler will be watery and not as sweet. Of course, any fresh or thawed frozen berry will also produce a delicious cobbler; just substitute the appropriate juice concentrate and preserves.

Berry Peachy Pie

Don't let the summer-fruit season pass you by without a pie baking session or two. Fresh peaches and blueberries make a delicious combination. Using a ready-made crust (you'll find whole wheat ones at health food stores) will save you time and energy.

FOR THE PIE AND FILLING:

1 frozen 9-inch pie crust
(preferably whole wheat), thawed
1 large egg, slightly beaten
4 cups sliced fresh ripe peaches
(from about 8 medium-size
yellow peaches)
1 cup fresh blueberries
⅔ cup white grape juice concentrate
⅓ cup all-fruit peach preserves
3 tablespoons quick-cooking tapioca
2 tablespoons Splenda or brown sugar,
or more to taste

FOR THE TOPPING:

½ cup dried peaches or apricots
⅔ cup old-fashioned rolled oats
⅔ cup almonds or walnuts
¼ cup whole wheat flour
5 tablespoons white grape juice
concentrate
2 tablespoons (¼ stick) butter,
at room temperature
2 tablespoons Splenda or brown sugar,
or more to taste
1 teaspoon ground cinnamon

1. Preheat the oven to 400°F.

2. Make the pie: Brush the pie crust lightly with the beaten egg and bake it in the aluminum foil pan until lightly browned, about 10 minutes.

3. Meanwhile, prepare the filling: Place the peach slices, blueberries, ⅔ cup grape juice concentrate, peach preserves, tapioca, and Splenda or brown sugar in a mixing bowl and stir to mix well.

4. Prepare the topping: Place the dried peaches, oats, almonds, whole wheat flour, 5 tablespoons of grape juice concentrate, butter, Splenda or brown sugar, and cinnamon in a food processor and process until the mixture is crumbly.

5. Spoon the filling into the baked pie crust, spreading it out in an even layer. Spoon the topping over the filling so that it covers the fruit completely, then pat it down with a spoon.

6. Place the pie on a baking sheet. Bake the pie for 10 minutes, then reduce the heat to 350°F and continue baking until the filling bubbles around the edges and the top is golden brown, about 20 minutes. If the crust begins to brown too quickly, cover it lightly with a piece of aluminum foil.

7. Let the pie cool slightly on a wire rack before serving. The pie can be refrigerated, covered, for up to 3 days. Let come to room temperature or rewarm in a 300°F oven before serving.

**MAKES ONE 9-INCH PIE
(APPROXIMATELY 8 TO 12 SERVINGS)**

FROM THE TEST KITCHEN

DON'T STOP with peaches and blueberries. Fill your pies with nectarines, strawberries, raspberries, blackberries, or a combination of summer fruits. You'll need a total of 5 cups of fruit. Summer's over? Cheer up—you can easily switch to frozen fruit, just thaw and drain it thoroughly before mixing the filling. Or use fall's harvest to bake up apple or pear pies.

Nutrition Info
1 PORTION (⅛ PIE, NOT INCLUDING CRUST) PROVIDES:

Vitamin C: 1 serving

Green leafy and yellow vegetables and fruits: 1 serving

ROLLING IN DOUGH

▼ ▼ ▼

Is pie just not pie unless you've made the crust from scratch? Knock yourself out if you want—but not before you've considered this. A crust made entirely with whole wheat will be tasty (and certainly nutritious) but a little on the heavy side. Make that a lot on the heavy side. You'll get a lighter texture without sacrificing any nutrition by combining all-purpose white flour with wheat germ. For a very wheaty crust, use ¼ cup wheat germ for every ¾ cup of white flour. For a less wheaty but still nutritious crust, bring the proportions of wheat germ down: ¾ cup plus 2 tablespoons of white flour to 2 tablespoons of wheat germ, for instance. Another option: Combine whole wheat flour with white flour, in any proportion that works for you. Experiment until you find the crust that suits your taste—and your favorite pie recipe.

Pumpkin Cream Pie

Here's a pie for those who enjoy the creamier things in life. The lighter, no-bake pumpkin filling packs in the yellow fruits.

1 frozen 9-inch pie crust
  (preferably whole wheat), thawed
2 envelopes unflavored gelatin
1¼ cups white grape juice concentrate
1 can (15 ounces) unsweetened solid
  pack pumpkin purée
2 teaspoons vanilla extract
2 teaspoons ground cinnamon
1 teaspoon ground ginger (optional)
½ teaspoon ground nutmeg
  (optional)
2 tablespoons Splenda or brown sugar
½ cup heavy (whipping) cream

1. Bake the pie crust in the aluminum foil pan according to the directions on the package. Set the crust aside on a rack to cool.

2. Place the gelatin and ½ cup of the grape juice concentrate in a small saucepan, stir to mix, and let stand until the gelatin softens, about 1 minute. Place the gelatin mixture over medium-high heat and let come to a boil, stirring constantly, then remove the saucepan from the heat. Continue stirring until the gelatin is completely dissolved.

3. Place the pumpkin, the remaining ¾ cup of grape juice concentrate, and the vanilla, cinnamon, ginger, nutmeg, and Splenda in a mixing bowl and stir to mix well. Add the gelatin mixture and beat with an electric mixer until well combined. Refrigerate the pumpkin mixture

just until it begins to thicken but don't let it set, about 20 minutes.

4. Meanwhile, place the heavy cream in another mixing bowl and beat with an electric mixer until soft peaks form. Fold the cream into the pumpkin mixture and whisk just until well blended; don't overmix.

5. Pour the pumpkin mixture into the cooled pie crust. Refrigerate the pie, covered loosely with plastic wrap, until set, about 2 hours. The pie may be refrigerated, covered, for up to 2 days.

**MAKES ONE 9-INCH PIE
(APPROXIMATELY 8 TO 12 SERVINGS)**

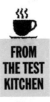

FROM THE TEST KITCHEN

THIS CREAMY PIE would be just as delish set in a graham cracker crust. If you make your own, look for whole-grain graham crackers.

Nutrition Info
1 PORTION (⅛ PIE, NOT INCLUDING CRUST) PROVIDES:

Vitamin C: 1 serving

Green leafy and yellow vegetables and fruits: 2 servings

Fat: ½ serving

Poached Pears with Ginger

Yes, these elegant pears are perfect for company. But why should company have all the fun? They're easy enough to make midweek, too. Have the leftovers for breakfast or as a snack.

4 Bosc pears
3 cups unsweetened vitamin C–fortified
   apple juice
1 cup white grape juice concentrate
1 teaspoon vanilla extract
1 piece (1 inch) fresh ginger,
   peeled and thinly sliced
4 small wedges aged cheddar cheese
   (1 to 1½ ounces each)

1. Peel the pears, then arrange them, stem end up, in a deep saucepan just big enough to hold them tightly in place. Add the apple juice, grape juice concentrate, vanilla, ginger, and just enough water to cover the pears.

2. Place the saucepan over medium-high heat and let the poaching liquid come to a boil. Reduce the heat, partially cover the pan, and let the pears simmer until soft but not mushy, about 20 minutes.

3. Let the pears come to room temperature in the poaching liquid, then remove them and set aside.

4. Place the saucepan over high heat, let the poaching liquid come to a boil and continue boiling until reduced by half, 10 minutes.

5. To serve, place the pears on serving plates and drizzle some of the poaching liquid over them. Serve a wedge of cheddar cheese alongside each pear.

SERVES 4

Nutrition Info

1 PORTION PROVIDES:

Calcium: 1 serving

Vitamin C: 2 servings

Other fruits and vegetables: 2 servings

Cool Fruit Gels

When you need something cool and a little sweet to settle a queasy tummy, eat a wiggly cube or two! Add pieces of the fruit of your choice for a chunky texture (and extra nutrients), or keep it smooth and soothing.

4 envelopes unflavored gelatin

2 cups unsweetened fruit juice (any juice or combo will work, as long as it doesn't include pineapple)

½ cup white grape juice concentrate

2 cups fresh fruit, such as blueberries, quartered strawberries, sliced bananas, cubed mango, and/or cubed peaches (optional)

1. Place the gelatin and 1 cup of the fruit juice in a bowl, stir to mix, and let stand until the gelatin softens, about 1 minute.

2. Place the remaining 1 cup of fruit juice and the grape juice concentrate in a small saucepan over medium heat and let come to a simmer.

3. Remove the heated juice mixture from the heat and pour it in the gelatin mixture. Stir until the gelatin is completely dissolved.

4. Pour the juice mixture into an 8-inch-square glass baking dish and add the fruit, if using. Refrigerate until set, about 2 hours.

5. Cut the fruit gels into roughly 2-inch squares. The fruit gels can be refrigerated, covered, for up to 3 days.

MAKES 16 FRUIT GELS

NOTE: Nutrition information depends on the juice and fruit used.

Conversion Table

Approximate Equivalents

1 stick butter = 8 tbs = 4 oz = 1/2 cup

1 cup all-purpose presifted flour or
dried bread crumbs = 5 oz

1 cup granulated sugar = 8 oz

1 cup (packed) brown sugar = 6 oz

1 cup confectioners' sugar = 41/2 oz

1 cup honey or syrup = 12 oz

1 cup grated cheese = 4 oz

1 cup dried beans = 6 oz

1 large egg = about 2 oz = about 3 tbs

1 egg yolk = about 1 tbs

1 egg white = about 2 tbs

Weight Conversions

U.S.	METRIC	U.S.	METRIC
1/2 oz	15 g	7 oz	200 g
1 oz	30 g	8 oz	250 g
11/2 oz	45 g	9 oz	275 g
2 oz	60 g	10 oz	300 g
21/2 oz	75 g	11 oz	325 g
3 oz	90 g	12 oz	350 g
31/2 oz	100 g	13 oz	375 g
4 oz	125 g	14 oz	400 g
5 oz	150 g	15 oz	450 g
6 oz	175 g	1 lb	500 g

NOTE: All conversions are approximate but close enough to be useful when converting from one system to another.

Liquid Conversions

U.S.	IMPERIAL	METRIC
2 tbs	1 fl oz	30 ml
3 tbs	11/2 fl oz	45 ml
1/4 cup	2 fl oz	60 ml
1/3 cup	21/2 fl oz	75 ml
1/3 cup + 1 tbs	3 fl oz	90 ml
1/3 cup + 2 tbs	31/2 fl oz	100 ml
1/2 cup	4 fl oz	125 ml
2/3 cup	5 fl oz	150 ml
3/4 cup	6 fl oz	175 ml
3/4 cup + 2 tbs	7 fl oz	200 ml
1 cup	8 fl oz	250 ml
1 cup + 2 tbs	9 fl oz	275 ml
11/4 cups	10 fl oz	300 ml
11/3 cups	11 fl oz	325 ml
11/2 cups	12 fl oz	350 ml
12/3 cups	13 fl oz	375 ml
13/4 cups	14 fl oz	400 ml
13/4 cups + 2 tbs	15 fl oz	450 ml
2 cups (1 pint)	16 fl oz	500 ml
21/2 cups	20 fl oz (1 pint)	600 ml
33/4 cups	11/2 pints	900 ml
4 cups	13/4 pints	1 liter

Oven Temperatures

°F	Gas	°C	°F	Gas	°C
250	1/2	120	400	6	200
275	1	140	425	7	220
300	2	150	450	8	230
325	3	160	475	9	240
350	4	180	500	10	260
375	5	190			

NOTE: Reduce the temperature by 20°C (68°F) for fan-assisted ovens.

Index

Hemorrhoids, 6, 29
Herbal teas, 174, 228
Herbs, 121, **138–42,** 233
  breastfeeding and, 228
  fresh vs. dried, 139
  medicinal (supplements),
    103, 124, 139
High blood pressure.
  See Hypertension;
  Preeclampsia
Holiday eating, 193–94
Honey, 32, 173
Hormones, 13, 14, 22, 24, 26,
  27, 37, 63, 73, 99
Hors d'oeuvres, at parties, 192
Hot weather, fluid needs in,
  101, 221
Hummus, 223
Hunger, 43
  between-meal, planning for,
    116
  food cravings and, 23
  food shopping and, 120
  nausea triggered by, 14
  see also Appetite
Hydrogenated fats, 145, 146
Hypertension, 5, 45, 99
  in pregnancy. *See*
    preeclampsia

I

Iceberg lettuce, 91, 93, 126,
  127
Ice chewing, craving for, 22
Immune system, 24, 60, 63,
  144, 163, 201, 202
Indian restaurants, 188
Indigestion. *See* Heartburn and
  indigestion
Ingredients lists on food labels,
  146, 147
Insomnia, 35
Insulin, 68, 69, 72, 211
Iodine, **68–69,** 220
  salt and, 69, 70, 99, 220
Iron, **69,** 71, 103, 176, 205
  anemia and, 6–7, 22, 36, 37,
    65, 69, 95, 220, 222
  animal vs. plant sources of,
    95–96
  planning for pregnancy and,
    233–34
  in postpartum period, 220
  -rich foods, in Daily Dozen,
    95–96, 105
  sources of, 69, 126, 129,
    131, 132, 134, 137, 138

supplements and, 18, 28–29,
  69, 96, 102, 103, 205
vegetarians and, 207
Vitamin C and absorption
  of, 66, 95, 205
Italian restaurants, 187

J, K, L

Japanese restaurants, 187
Job, eating well at, 179–81
Juices. *See* Fruit juices
Juicing citrus fruits, 130
Junk foods, 10, 77

Kasha (buckwheat), 85, 95, **132**
Kidney beans, **135**
Kitchen, evaluating food in,
  119
Kitchen equipment, 197
Kitchen safety, 152–53
Kiwis, 27
Knives, 153, 197

Labels on foods, 146–50
  definitions of terms on,
    148–49
  fats and, 145, 148, 149
  ingredients lists on, 146, 147
  misleading terms on, 147
  nutrition information on,
    146–49
  organic foods and, 124–25
  "sell by" and "use by" dates
    on, 154, 155
  whole grains and, 133, 146
Labor and delivery, 5, 7–8, 236
  excess weight gain and, 45
  preterm, 7, 44, 61, 65, 66,
    69, 72, 103, 121, 163
Lactase, 209
Lactose, 173
Lactose intolerance, 143,
  208–10
Laxatives, 29, 86
Lead in water, 174, 175
Leaf lettuces, 91, **127–28**
Leafy greens. *See* Green leafy
  vegetables
Leftovers:
  safety and, 155, 160
  time constraints and, 198–99
Leg cramps, 6, 36–37, 69
Legumes, 138, 217
  in Daily Dozen, 94–95, 105
  as protein servings, 84
  see also Beans
Lentils, 65, 69, 71, 84, 95, **135**

Lettuces, 91, **127–28**
  washing and drying,
    129–30, 157, 268
Lifestyle, tailoring healthy
  eating habits to, 115
Linoleic acid, 37, 137, 144
Listeria, 157, 161, 163, 171
Low-carb diets, 78, 232
Low-carb foods, 50
Lunch, 34, 117–18
  brown-bag, 179–80, 195
  at work, 179–81
Luncheon meats, 160–61
Lycopene, 97, 140

M

Macadamia nuts, **138**
Magnesium, 7, 29, 35, 36, 37,
  69, 103, 205
  sources of, 69, 90, 94, 131,
    132, 134, 136, 137, 138
Malnutrition, maternal, 4, 233
Manganese, **69–71,** 132, 134,
  136, 137
Mannitol, 173
Margarine, 97, 145
Marinating, 158, 168
Marjoram, **140**
Meals:
  lifestyle realities and, 115
  planning ahead, 115, 116–17
  skipping, 76–77, 116–18,
    212, 217
  small, frequent, 14, 16, 32,
    34, 76, 205, 222
Meats, 84, 96, 234
  defrosting, 153, 158
  doneness of, 160, 161
  lean forms of, 144
  nutrients in, 63, 64, 65, 67,
    68, 71, 72
  safety and, 153, 154,
    158–61, 171–73
  shopping for, 122
  smoked and cured, 171–73
  see also Beef
Mesclun greens, **128**
Metabolism, 34–35, 39, 51, 61,
  62, 63, 64, 65, 66, 69, 82
Metallic taste in mouth, 26
Mexican restaurants, 188
Microwave, 14, 130, 197
  cooking fish in, 372
  cooking potatoes in, 253, 407
  cooking vegetables in, 130,
    401
  defrosting in, 158

Recipe Index

A

B